AN ILLUSTRATED HISTORY

Western Medicine

EDITED BY

IRVINE LOUDON

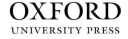

OXFORD
UNIVERSITY PRESS

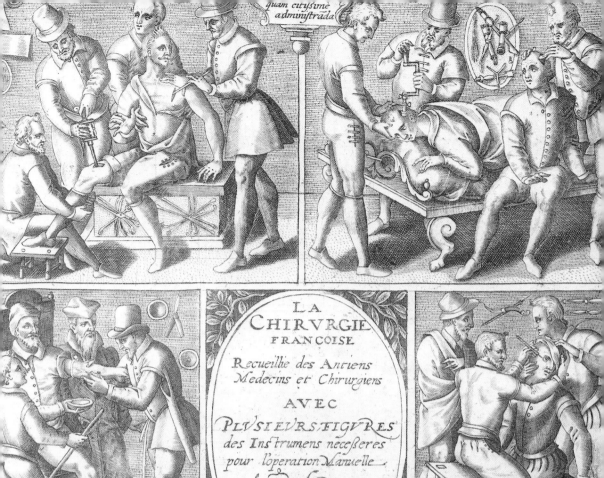

quam cityssimè
administrada

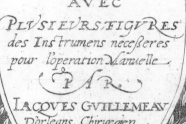

LA
CHIRVRGIE
FRANÇOISE
Recueillie des Antiens
Medecins et Chirurgiens
AVEC
PLVSIEVRS FIGVRES
des Instrumens neceseres
pour l'operation Manuelle
PAR
IACQVES GVILLEMEAV
D'Orleans, Chirurgien
du Roy et Iuré
A Paris.

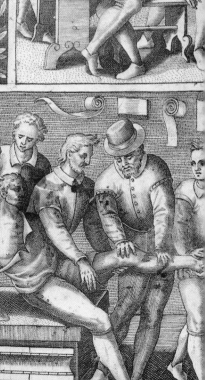

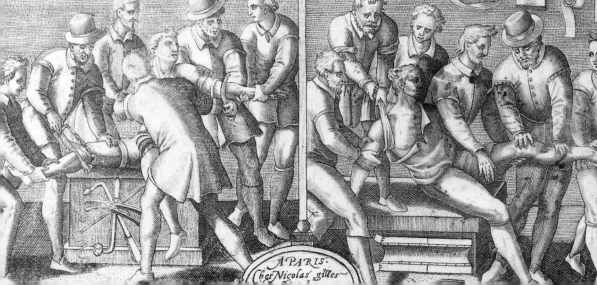

A PARIS.
Chez Nicolas gilles

AN ILLUSTRATED HISTORY

Western Medicine

EDITED BY

IRVINE LOUDON

Oxford   New York

OXFORD UNIVERSITY PRESS

1997

OXFORD

UNIVERSITY PRESS

Great Clarendon Street, Oxford OX2 6DP

Oxford University Press is a department of the University of Oxford.
It furthers the University's objective of excellence in research, scholarship,
and education by publishing worldwide in

Oxford New York

Athens Auckland Bangkok Bogotá Buenos Aires Cape Town
Chennai Dar es Salaam Delhi Florence Hong Kong Istanbul Karachi
Kolkata Kuala Lumpur Madrid Melbourne Mexico City Mumbai Nairobi
Paris São Paulo Shanghai Singapore Taipei Tokyo Toronto Warsaw
with associated companies in Berlin Ibadan

Oxford is a registered trade mark of Oxford University Press
in the UK and in certain other countries

Published in the United States
by Oxford University Press Inc., New York

British Library Cataloguing in Publication Data

Data available

Library of Congress Cataloging in Publication Data

Data available

ISBN 0–19–820509–0 (hbk.)
ISBN 0–19–924813–3 (pbk.)

10 9 8 7 6 5 4 3 2 1

Printed in Great Britain on acid-free paper by
Butler & Tanner Ltd., Frome

2270   P

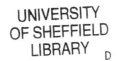

PREFACE

What is medical history, and who are medical historians? The reader may well ask, because many people, if they have heard of medical history at all, believe it is something to do with medical schools and doctors—a sideline in medicine. Even those who are familiar with such subdivisions of history as social, political, economic, and military may be unaware that medical history has expanded so rapidly that it has now become a new and firmly established branch of history, attracting researchers from a wide variety of backgrounds.

Before 1960 there were a few distinguished historians of medicine, such as Charles Singer, Fielding Garrison, Henry Sigerist, Erwin Acknernecht, and George Rosen—most, it should be noted, US scholars—but it is scarcely an exaggeration to say that the sum total of such medical historians could be counted on the fingers of both hands. All this has changed over the last thirty years. There has been a rapid expansion of medical history in North America and Europe. In the UK, where it is increasingly true that a new academic discipline can thrive only if it attracts funds, there can be no doubt that the expansion of medical history owes a great deal to Sir Henry Wellcome, the founder of the pharmaceutical firm first known as Burroughs-Wellcome, then as the Wellcome Foundation, and recently (as the result of a merger) as Glaxo-Wellcome.

In his will, Wellcome left instructions that the profits from his company should, through the creation of the Wellcome Trust, be used to support medical research. He also stipulated that a proportion of those funds should be used to support the history of medicine. The Trust has thrived and the annual expenditure of the Trust on the history of medicine has grown (in round figures) from £49,000 in 1976/7 to £233,000 in 1980/1, £1.8 million in 1989/90, and £3.7 million in 1993/4. A large part of these funds has been used to support and expand the Wellcome Institute for the History of Medicine in London, which began as a museum and a library with only a few staff and is now by far the largest institution of its kind in the world. The Trust has also created history of medicine departments (known as 'Wellcome Units') in a growing number of universities, and provided funds to establish lectureships, fellowships, and scholarships.

The character of medical history has changed as it has expanded. Before the 1960s it was largely concerned with the history of the 'great men' of medicine, medical discoveries, and famous medical institutions. Now the emphasis has shifted towards the social history of medicine, with emphasis on the sick as well as their doctors, and on the health of populations. Strong links have been established between medical history, on the one hand, and social and economic history, historical demography and geography, and epidemiology, on the other. Before the 1960s very little had been published, for example, on the politics and economics of medical care, on the influence of changes in social, economic, and medical factors on the health of the populations, or on the history of medical education, the medical profession, public health, psychiatry, nursing, and midwifery; and very little had been written on the statistics of mortality and morbidity. All have now become subjects of intense historical research. Furthermore, before the 1960s there was a general feeling that 'proper' medical history was concerned only with the distant past—for example, Galen and Hippocrates, William Harvey, the Black Death, and the perils and agonies of surgery before anaesthesia. The notion that twentieth-century medicine, up to and including the last few years, was a proper subject for historical research would have been suspect. Now, however, the field has broadened to include not only the traditional subjects, but also (and with a growing input from oral history) various aspects of twentieth-century medicine, such as the National Health Service, medical genetics and molecular medicine, and the history of current aspects of health such as contraception and 'the Pill', drug abuse, and AIDS.

Another significant change is that nowadays only a minority of fully committed historians of medicine are medically qualified. The list of the contributors to this book shows that historians of medicine come from a wide variety of backgrounds. There is little doubt that this is the factor which is largely responsible for the rapid and exciting development of the discipline over the last few decades.

A brief word about the structure of this book, and a disclaimer. It does not pretend to be encyclopaedic or comprehensive. That would be impossible in a book of this length, and unnecessary, because some excellent encyclopaedias of medical history have recently been published. Instead, it is a series of illustrated essays on a number of selected themes. The illustrations in this volume have been chosen carefully as an integral part of each chapter. The importance of the illustrations is emphasized by placing the chapter by Martin Kemp, which explores the nature, purpose, and impact of visual imagery on medicine, at the beginning of the book. The rest of the work is divided into two parts. In Part I, which is chronological, the authors provide an overview of the main features of the history of medicine in their respective periods stretching from medicine in the classical world to the present. Part II consists of essays on a number of selected themes. Although there are many other themes which might have been included if space had allowed, those which have been selected are broadly speaking representative of the subjects which have been central to the development of the history of medicine over the past few decades. A Glossary and a Chronology are included, and lists of Further Reading have been compiled by the authors of each chapter.

I.S.L.L.

ACKNOWLEDGEMENTS

Thanks are due to the Wellcome Institute for the History of Medicine, London, and particularly to William Schupbach, for assistance in the selection of illustrations, for which the Wellcome Iconographic Collections Videodisc has been an invaluable source. Dr Richard Smith played the major part in designing the contents of the book and inviting the appropriate authors. Both Richard Smith and the editor gratefully acknowledge the assistance provided in the early stages by Humaira Erfan-Ahmed, previously Secretary/Administrator to the Wellcome Unit for the History of Medicine in the University of Oxford. Dr James Longrigg is grateful to the President and Fellows of Wolfson College for the award of a Charter Fellowship in 1993–4 which enabled him to write his chapter 'under ideal circumstances' and to the Research Committee and Department of Classics in the University of Newcastle for their generous funding. Margaret Pelling is grateful to Professor Pietro Corsi for assistance in translating some difficult passages of Italian. The editor is very grateful to Anne Lyons, the picture researcher, and to Hilary Walford, copy-editor, for their meticulous and excellent work; it is no exaggeration to say that their contribution to the production of this book has been immense.

CONTENTS

Contents

LIST OF COLOUR PLATES

LIST OF CONTRIBUTORS

Harold J. Cook received his Ph.D. in History from the University of Michigan (1981). He is Professor of the History of Medicine, Wellcome Trust Centre, University College London. He has published on early modern English medicine, on Anglo-Dutch medical and scientific relationships, and on the centrality of medicine and natural history to the 'scientific revolution' in the Dutch Golden Age, which he is currently working on for a book.

Anne Digby, MA, Ph.D., FRHS, is Professor of Social History at Oxford Brookes University. Among her publications in the social history of medicine are *Madness, Morality and Medicine: A Study of the York Retreat, 1790-1914* (Cambridge, 1985), and *Making a Medical Living: Doctors and Patients in the English Market for Medicine, 1720-1911* (Cambridge, 1994). She is currently undertaking research in the history of general practice in Britain from 1850 to 1948.

Mary Dobson, BA (Oxon) 1st class hons. in Geography 1976, AM (Harvard) 1980, MA (Oxon) 1980, D.Phil. (Oxon) 1982. Harkness Fellowship at Harvard University 1978-80. E. P. Abraham Prize Research Fellow (Nuffield College, Oxford) 1981-2. Open Prize Research Fellow (Nuffield College, Oxford) 1982-4. Demonstrator/Lecturer, School of Geography, 1983-9. Research Fellow, Wolfson College, Oxford, 1987-94. Wellcome Fellow in the Department of Community Medicine and General Practice, Oxford, 1989-90. She is Director of the Wellcome Unit for the History of Medicine in the University of Oxford. Her publications include 'Malaria in England: A Geographical and Historical Perspective', in W. F. Bynum and B. Fantini (eds.), *Malaria and Ecosystems: Historical Aspects (Parasitologia,* 36 (1994)), and *Contours of Death and Disease in Early Modern England* (Cambridge University Press, 1997).

Martin Kemp is British Academy Wolfson Research Professor and Professor of the History of Art at the University of Oxford. He studied Natural Sciences and Art History at Cambridge and at the Courtauld Institute of Art, London. He is the author of *Dr William Hunter at the Royal Society of Arts* (1975), *Leonardo da Vinci: The Marvellous Works of Nature and Man* (1981, winner of the Mitchell Prize), *The Science of Art: Optical Themes in Western Art from Brunelleschi to Seurat* (1990), and numerous studies of the relationships between representation in art and science. He is currently researching issues in scientific representation and writing a book on anatomical, physiognomic, and natural themes in art from the Renaissance to the nineteenth century.

Jane Lewis, previously Professor of Social Policy at the London School of Economics, is Barnett Professor of Social Policy, St Cross College, University of Oxford. She is the author of a large number of books and articles on the history of social policy, including: *What Price Community Medicine? The History of Public Health since 1918* (1985); *Women and Social Action in Victorian and Edwardian Britain* (1991); and *The Voluntary Sector, the State and Social Work in Britain* (1995).

Stephen Lock qualified in medicine from Cambridge and St Bartholomew's Hospital Medical School in 1953 and worked as a clinical haematologist for ten years until he joined the staff of the *British Medical Journal*. He served as Editor from 1975 until 1991, taking a particular interest in peer review and research misconduct. Since retirement he has worked as Research Associate at the Wellcome Institute for the History of Medicine, London, where he has formed part of the Steering Group of the History of Twentieth-Century Medicine Group. His current research interests include the history of publication and of the treatment of breast cancer. He is an Associate Editor of the *New Dictionary of National Biography* and a co-editor of *The Oxford Medical Companion* (Oxford, 1994).

James Longrigg, BA (Dunelm), M.Litt. (Oxon), is Reader in Ancient Philosophy and Science, University of Newcastle upon Tyne. He has been Carl Newell Jackson Research Fellow in Classics, Harvard University; Senior Research Fellow, Warburg Institute, London; Visiting Professor, Institute for the Humanities, University of Wisconsin-Madison; Wellcome Fellow in the History of Medicine (twice), and Charter Fellow in the History of Science, Wolfson College, Oxford. His book *Greek Rational Medicine* was published by Routledge in 1993.

Irvine Loudon, DM (Oxford), FRCGP, DRCOG, ARE, qualified in medicine from Oxford University in 1951 and subsequently worked as a general practitioner in Wantage, Oxfordshire. He became interested in the history of medicine around 1970. When he was awarded a Wellcome Research Fellowship in the History of Medicine in 1981 he resigned from general practice and has worked full-time as a medical historian ever since. His main interests have been the history of the medical profession, medical education, medical institutions, diseases, and childbirth. His publications include: *Medical Care and the General Practitioner, 1750–1850* (Oxford, 1986); *Death in Childbirth: An International Study of Maternal Mortality, 1800–1950* (Oxford, 1992); *Childbed Fever: A Documentary History* (New York, 1995). He is currently writing a monograph on the history of puerperal fever and co-editing a book on the history of general practice under the National Health Service.

Michael McVaugh received his BA degree in History and Science from Harvard (1960) and his Ph.D. in History from Princeton (1965). He is Professor of History at the University of North Carolina (Chapel Hill), where he has taught since 1964. His most recent book is *Medicine before the Plague* (Cambridge, 1993). He has also been one of the general editors of the *Arnaldi de Villanova Opera Medica Omnia* since the inception of the series in 1975.

Michael Neve is Senior Lecturer in the History of Medicine at the Wellcome Trust Centre, University College London. He has an MA in History from Cambridge and a Ph.D. from the University of London. He teaches the history of life sciences and the history of psychiatry to both undergraduates and postgraduates. His recent work includes the conclusion to *The Western Medical Tradition* (1995), which was produced with his colleagues from the Institute, and he has co-edited with Janet Browne Darwin's *Voyage of the Beagle* for Penguin Classics.

Katharine Park studied History and History of Science at the Warburg Institute of the University of London and Harvard University, where she received her Ph.D. in 1981. She is Professor of History at Wellesley College, in Wellesley, Massachusetts, and has written two books: *Doctors and Medicine in Early Renaissance Florence* (Princeton University Press, 1985) and, with Lorraine Daston, *Wonders and the Order of Nature, 1150–1750* (Zone Books, 1996). She is currently finishing a series of articles on the history of human dissection in medieval and Renaissance Europe and is co-editing *The Cambridge History of Early Modern Science.*

Margaret Pelling, BA (Melb.), M.Litt. (Oxon), is Reader in the Social History of Medicine in the Modern History Faculty of the University of Oxford. Her main area of interest is medical practice and social conditions in early modern England. Recent research includes articles on gender and the iconography of healing in *The Task of Healing* (Erasmus, 1996), edited with Hilary Marland; a volume of her essays, *The Common Lot: Sickness, Medical Occupations and the Urban Poor in Early Modern England* (Longman, 1998); and a monograph on the College of Physicians and irregular practitioners in London, 1550–1640, to be published by Macmillan.

Cay-Rüdiger Prüll was born in Katzenelnbogen, Germany. He qualified in medicine (MD, Freie Universität Berlin, 1992) and in History and Philosophy (MA, University of Giessen, 1990). He worked as physician at the Schering AG, Berlin, from 1990 to 1991. He was then appointed assistant first at the Institute of the History of Medicine in Aachen (1991–2) and, since 1992, at the Institute of the History of Medicine in Freiburg. He is the author of *Der Heilkundige in seiner geographischen und sozialen Umwelt. Die Medizinische Fakultät der Universität Giessen auf dem Weg in die Neuzeit (1750–1918)* (1993) and he is currently working on the history of pathology in Berlin and London from 1900 to 1945.

Lisa Rosner was born in New York. She was awarded a BA from Princeton University and a Ph.D. in the History of Science from Johns Hopkins University. She is currently Associate Professor of History at Richard Stockton College in New Jersey. She is the author of *Medical Education in the Age of Improvement: Edinburgh Students and Apprentices 1760–1826* (Edinburgh, 1991).

Emilie Savage-Smith, BA in Classics, DePauw University, Ph.D. in the History of Science, University of Wisconsin-Madison, has, since 1991, been a member of the Faculty of Oriental Studies at the University of Oxford. For the previous fifteen years she was with the Center for Near Eastern Studies and the History of Medicine Division of the Department of Anatomy at the University of California, Los Angeles. Her most recent publications include a chapter on Islamic celestial mapping in J. B. Harley and D. Woodward (eds.), *The History of Cartography* (Chicago, 1992), *Islamic Culture and the Medical Arts* (Bethesda, Md., 1994), published to coincide with an exhibition for which she was guest curator at the National Library of Medicine, and a study of attitudes towards dissection in the medieval Islamic world (*Journal of the History of Medicine*, 1995).

Anne Summers, Ph.D., is a Curator in the Department of Western Manuscripts at the British Library, anbd a founding editor of *History Workshop Journal.* Her previous post was at the Wellcome Unit for the History of

Medicine, University of Oxford, where she was a Wellcome Research Fellow. She is the author of *Angels and Citizens: Women as Military Nurses, 1854–1914* (1988), and of numerous articles on the history of philanthropy, nursing, and military medicine.

Tilli Tansey studied neurotransmitter distribution in octopus brains for her Ph.D. and has worked on the pharmacology of Parkinson's disease at the MRC Brain Metabolism Unit in Edinburgh, and on the biochemistry of multiple sclerosis at St Thomas's Hospital, London. In 1986 she moved to the Wellcome Institute for the History of Medicine, and completed a second Ph.D. on the scientific career of Sir Henry Dale, FRS (1875–1968). She is currently Senior Lecturer in the History of Medicine at the Wellcome Trust Centre and Honorary Senior Lecturer in the Department of Anatomy, University College London. She has published on the history of modern physiology and pharmacology and is co-editor of *Women Physiologists* (Portland Press, 1993).

Ulrich Tröhler was born in Berne, Switzerland. He qualified in medicine (MD, University of Zurich, 1972) and engaged in a career in physiological research, which he interrupted from 1976 to 1978 to complete a Ph.D. in the history of medicine in London. He has been Professor and Chairman of the History of Medicine at the Universities of Göttingen (1983–94) and Freiburg, Germany (since 1994). His major publications concern the history of the quantification of clinical experience, the history of surgery, anti-vivisection, and eighteenth-century medical students. He is currently working on the origins and impact of ethical codes and guidelines in twentieth-century medicine.

John Walker-Smith, MD (Sydney), FRCP (Edin.), FRCP (London), FRACP. Senior Lecturer (1973), and then Professor (1985) of Paediatric Gastroenterology in the University of London, first at St Bartholomew's Hospital from 1985 and then at the Royal Free Hospital from 1995. He is a member of the History of Twentieth-Century Medicine Group at the Wellcome Institute, London, and has studied infantile diarrhoeal mortality in the Edwardian period.

Michael Worboys graduated in biology from the University of Sussex and completed his doctorate on colonial science and medicine at the same university. He has been in the Department of History at Sheffield Hallam University (formerly Sheffield City Polytechnic) since the mid-1970s. He retains research interests in the history of colonial science and medicine, though most of his recent work has been on the history of medical bacteriology and immunology, and the prevention and treatment of infectious diseases in the period 1860–1940.

1 | Medicine in View: Art and Visual Representation

MARTIN KEMP

THE visual legacy of Western medicine is richer than that for any other scientific or technical activity. A vast range of images has been generated both within the practice of medicine and by outside observers of medical practice. Every era and culture that has produced visual images concerned with the human condition in a social context has generated what may be called 'medical art'. If we attempt to define what we mean by medical art, it is difficult to know where to draw the boundaries. Any image which is made to perform some kind of role in how we perceive our bodies and alter our state of health can potentially be included. The broadest definition of medical art would include not only the obvious illustrative material in the Western tradition, such as the great picture books of anatomy and photographs of surgical procedures, but also talismanic objects which are meant to effect some change in our well-being through invisible agencies. I am thinking of such items as a witch doctor's magic charm or an altarpiece containing an image of one of the two major plague saints, St Roch and St Sebastian. The great folding altarpiece which Matthias Grünewald produced for the Anthonite monastery at Isenheim in the second decade of the sixteeth century is a spectacular case in point. The monks of the hospital were dedicated to the treatment of skin diseases and most especially 'St Anthony's fire' (ergot poisoning), which savagely disfigures the joints of the body. The inmates would pray before the altarpiece in its fully open form, saying their devotions before the scourged body of Christ, whose distorted limbs and disfigured skin spoke to the afflicted with special resonance. They would seek the intercessions of St Anthony, who exercised a special power over his 'fire', and of St Sebastian, whose miraculous resistance to the executioners' arrows provided a source of succour for those assailed by the darts of outrageous misfortune.

Medical histories have long drawn on the evidence of this great visual legacy. But in talking about the 'evidence' provided by visual representations we need to exercise two big cautions. The first concerns the need to understand each image in terms of the context of its own generation. A representation is made to serve one or more specific functions in particular circumstances and involves a series of choices that reflect the values and priorities of the makers of the image and its intended viewers. An artist, looking at medicine as an outsider, or even as the subject of its ministrations, will obviously be making a personal statement. To understand this statement as evidence—even as evidence of the artist's attitude—we need to be alert to the way that kinds of art actually operate in their own context. A seventeenth-century genre painting may look at first sight like a piece of documentary *reportage*, but such paintings worked very much within their own special set of communicative conventions. When we look at the more technical and apparently objective representations generated within medicine, we may think that the evidence can be read in a more straightforward manner. However, in producing even the most sober illustration, choices are always made—advertently and inadvertently. What we are presented with is a selective depiction of what is selectively perceived. Even the specialist medical artist of today, providing a functional illustration for, say, an anatomy book for trainee doctors, is indulging in a highly selective form of visual pointing, which involves a series of value judgements about what is important in relation to the perceived needs of the spectators. The value judgements will be locked into the system of beliefs which motivate the institutional practice of medicine at this particular time. All the illustrations in this volume declare in overt or covert ways where they stand in relation to accepted values of their own time.

The second big caution concerns how subsequent viewers, including ourselves, can see the images other than through later preconceptions. Different spectators, particularly those from different historical or ethnic cultures, will work with the visual images within different frameworks of expectation and knowledge, frameworks which may entirely transform the original function of the image. Each age expects visual images to work in certain ways and to perform certain functions, and will look at the past through anachronistic eyes. While the problems of historical and cultural remove cannot be wholly avoided, the historian can work towards a reconstruction of the original 'message' of the images in terms of functions, intention, and contemporary reception. This reconstruction will involve asking about the makers of the images, their motivations (overt and covert), their procedures, the media to which they had access, the particular types of books, paintings, prints, journals, broadcast media, and so on that were available, the particular role of visual imagery in any era (not least in relation to verbal records), and the parameters within which contemporary viewing took place.

The reader who begins by leafing through the pages of the present volume will immediately see that an extraordinary range of imagery is involved, from highly technical illustrations in sober black and white to magnificent paintings in full colour. The choices of illustrations for the other chapters are supplemented here by some examples of types of image which otherwise seem to have been under-represented. The overall intention of this chapter is less to provide a comprehensive discussion of the full array of illustrative material than to review the *types* of visual material that are available and how we might interpret them in a manner that is sensitive to the original purposes of the images. My strategy is to move from relatively technical questions of the how and what of representation to the human presence which must ultimately lie at the very core of art and medicine.

From the Scalpel to the Pen: Showing it for Real

Virtually all the items we regard as 'medical art' were concerned with what I am calling 'showing it for real'. I use the term 'the real', not simply in terms of the kind of accuracy of representation which has been one of the goals of medical illustrators since the Renaissance, but more widely in terms of what is perceived at any one time to be the reality of how the body functions, both in itself and in relation to external agencies. Thus, for someone who believes that the state of the body and the mind is under the avoidable dominance of the stars, the designation of astrological signs as governing different parts and functions of the body is as real as the signs of mental activity in a modern brain scan using positron emission tomography. How the signs embedded in the representations can be read is the subject of the next section. For the moment I want to look at the more obvious question of the means of representation within the more standard areas of medical illustration.

We should, before we embark on our quest, remind ourselves that there is in fact nothing 'obvious' about medical illustration. Visual representation has played a central, instructional role within the special tradition of Western medicine only since the Renaissance. There were strong proscriptions against illustration in classical medicine, above all in the succession of Galen, although, as we shall see, other forms of visual imagery did play a role in ancient practice. The prime justification for the proscription, which remained a persistent undercurrent in later centuries, was that the real body itself was the true illustration. The body was the book which was to be read. Even Vesalius, who in 1543 effectively established illustration at the heart of anatomical learning, reminded his readers that pictures were not a substitute for the real thing. Once representations assumed the magnificence and visual conviction of those in Vesalius' *Fabrica*, they were readily taken as 'showing it for real'. The potency a picture tends to assume over the real thing and indeed over the descriptive text is linked not least to systems of memory. Thus the traditional 'wound man' of the late Middle Ages and Renaissance, adorned with an apparently incongruous array of weapons adhering to various parts of his body, plays a powerful mnemonic function in the fixing of the typology of wounds in the minds of the field surgeon and those concerned with field surgery. Schematic diagrams in a modern textbook play similar roles with respect to the student's learning process.

Within the special tradition of Renaissance and post-Renaissance Western medicine, representations which claim to be carrying precise and memorable information range from highly detailed 'pictures' of what can be seen to overtly diagrammatic illustrations of particular aspects of the seen forms. At their most elaborate, naturalistic depictions aim to provide a surrogate for the experience of seeing what lay in front of the eyes of the draughtsman. The skills possessed by Renaissance draughtsmen, spectacularly exemplified by Leonardo da Vinci, meant that illustrations could convince the viewers that they were effectively seeing reality portrayed from life. The visual impact and

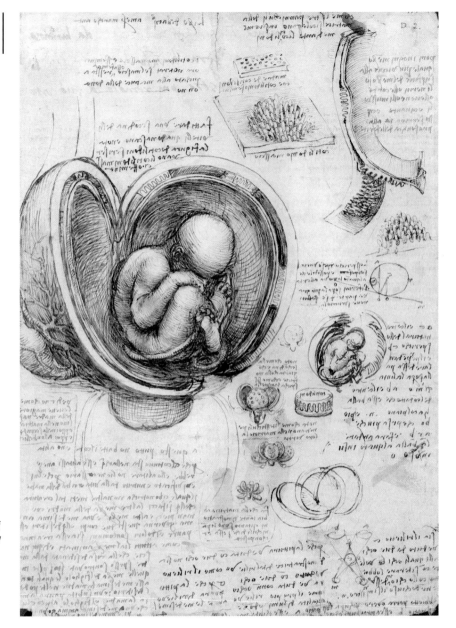

Foetus in the womb and other studies, by Leonardo da Vinci. The main image, drawn around 1513, shows a beautifully characterized foetus in a womb with a cotyledonous placenta, derived from Leonardo's dissection of the uterus of a cow. Other studies show some of the varied types of illustration devised by Leonardo, including that used to demonstrate the interdigitations of the placenta and uterus.

inventive illustrative techniques of the famous drawing by Leonardo which shows the foetus in the womb give it an air of total conviction, much as more recent observers have tended to trust a photograph as an accurate record of reality—though Leonardo himself acknowledges on the same page that a drawn image can never convey the full effect of an actual object viewed with two eyes. The great picture books of anatomy, from the time of Vesalius' *Fabrica* to modern photographic atlases, all share the aim of 'showing it for real' in various ways. In the eighteenth century the aspiration to present the unvarnished truth as visible in a single specimen—warts and all—became an absolute goal, especially in Britain with books like William Hunter's *Gravid Uterus*. It was this ambition to create an image of compelling realism, almost hyper-realism, which fuelled the enthusiasm for the three-dimensional casts and elaborately coloured wax models which became the speciality of a few highly skilled practitioners from the seventeenth century onwards and later of specialist firms. However, we need to be aware that high skill in fabricating apparently realistic images is a double-edged sword. The false can potentially be portrayed with the same conviction as the true. Thus Leonardo gives us a vivid picture of the interdigitations of a cotyledonous placenta, which was in fact derived from his dissections of a cow and differs radically from a human placenta.

With the advent of photography in 1839, it seemed that a new tool to achieve unmediated realism was at hand, but its use in medicine proved highly problematic, for a number of reasons. Most particularly, a photograph of the inner parts of a body, especially before colour photography became a practical proposition, not only posed all the difficulties of looking into a real body but also suffered from an absence of clear spatial and colouristic differentiation. Furthermore, the reproduction of photographs on a mass scale did not become practical until the 1870s with the invention of the collotype and related processes of printing. The area colonized most rapidly and successfully by photography was the illustration of some grosser abnormalities and pathologies, particularly those visible on the naked body. Some of the most successful of the early attempts to overcome the legibility of photographs involved stereoscopic images, in which two photographs were taken from positions equivalent to those of the left and right eyes and the resulting photographs viewed in a special apparatus. Stereo-photographs of pathological specimens could be very striking and not a little repellent in their three-dimensional realism. In 1905 the Scottish anatomist David Waterston produced a *Stereoscopic Atlas of Anatomy*, which gave a vivid impression of the inner spaces and plastic shapes of the organs of the body, in a way not dissimilar to some of the teaching aids that have become available on computer in the late twentieth century.

Alongside the techniques which claimed to show in a literal fashion what the eye sees, there were varieties of traditional diagrams which gave highly selective or schematic renderings of forms, often driven by a clear sense of the functional implications of the drawn structures. Vesalius referred to some of his line diagrams, like one to show the criss-cross arrangement of fibres in tissues, as both 'rudimentary' and 'true'. The use of diagrams and charts has characterized medical texts virtually from the beginning. Although some of the schematizations in early manuscripts, printed books, and individually printed sheets may seem crude to our eyes, they served clear educative and mnemonic functions in the contexts of contemporary medicine and the audience for medical texts. Diagrammatic charts and maps such as that in the fifteenth-century *Vademecum* in the Wellcome Institute in London could act as an effective *aide-mémoire* on such vital matters as bloodletting and diagnosis from the inspection of urine in special glass flasks. The principle of diagrammatic succinctness is not essentially different from that in a modern line diagram of a neural pathway in the most advanced textbook of neurophysiology. Even illustrations produced by the most technologically advanced means are frequently accompanied by simplified line drawings which act to guide our detection of the most salient features.

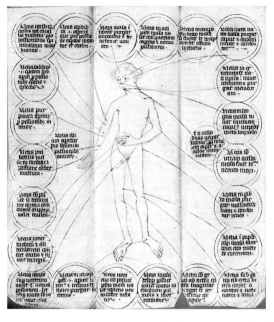
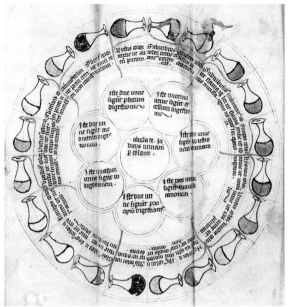

Fifteenth-century vade-mecum. Composed from a series of folding sheets, this manuscript was designed to provide the physician with a portable crib of philosophical and applied knowledge. The diagrammatic illustrations on these pages show crucial points for blood-letting and a guide for diagnosis from the examination of urine in glass flasks.

The poised beauty of the illustrations in Albinus' great picture-book of the human body (*facing*), produced in intimate collaboration with his draftsman, Jan van Wandelaar, was deemed appropriate for the divine 'architecture' of the body. The picturesque backgrounds were ostensibly intended to reduce the starkness of the paper.

Whether we are dealing with an artist making a detailed rendering, a draughtsman devising an effective diagram, or a photographer who judges lighting, exposures, and printing, complex series of choices are made which involve what we may call artistry, in the sense of using skill to give a selective, effective, and even appealing depiction. In the case of a traditional medical artist, using normal drawing media, the artistry is obvious. Artistry may be welcome or unwelcome to the anatomist or doctor who is in charge of the project. For Vesalius, and his successors in the seventeenth and eighteenth centuries, such as Bidloo and Albinus, the stylishness of their illustrators' products was an integral part of the enterprise, both to show the beauty of nature's supreme machine and to produce books which were themselves prestigious products. A book such as Albinus' *Tables of the Skeleton and Muscles* was as much at home in an aristocrat's library or in the life room of an academy of art as in the surgery of a doctor.

Increasingly, as the teaching of medicine became more institutionalized, so there was a demand for a manner of illustration which breathed an air of sober truth, without visual flourishes and without overt signs of the artist's transformative eye and hand. The first edition of Gray's *Anatomy* in 1858 is a monument to the ambition to operate with what may be called the 'non-style'—one drained of any apparently subjective appeal—but which is, of course, a style in its own right, expressive of what Gray and his contemporaries believed was the true nature of medical instruction. A precursor of the sober non-style is the one and only plate in William Harvey's seminal work of 1628. New media in the nineteenth century, such as lithography and photography, enabled huge numbers of identical images to be produced at a relatively modest cost to meet the growing demands of the expanding world of professional medicine. Yet the great atlases did not fade away entirely, and the large-scale lithographic plates produced in the nineteenth century by Bougery in France and Quain in Britain still traded on overtly stylish visual appeal. More recently, colour pho-

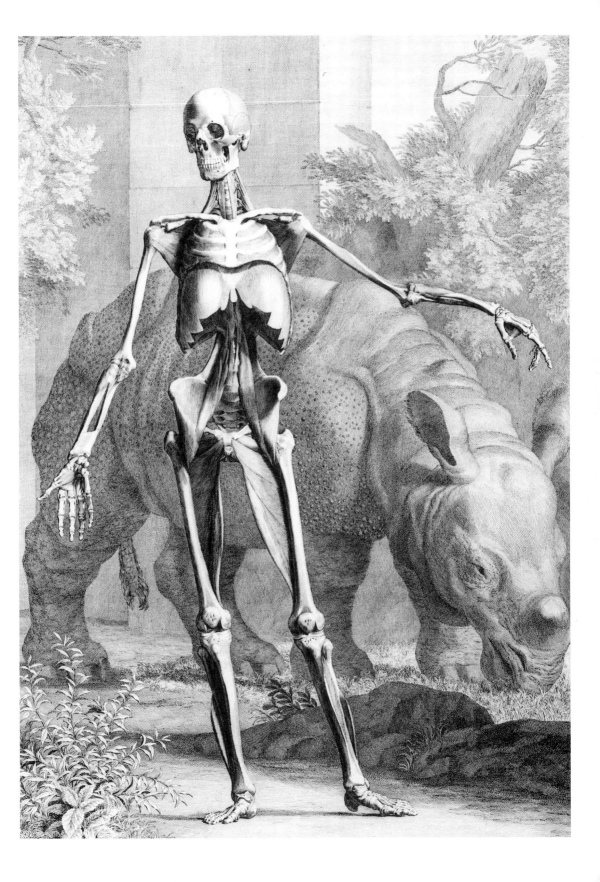

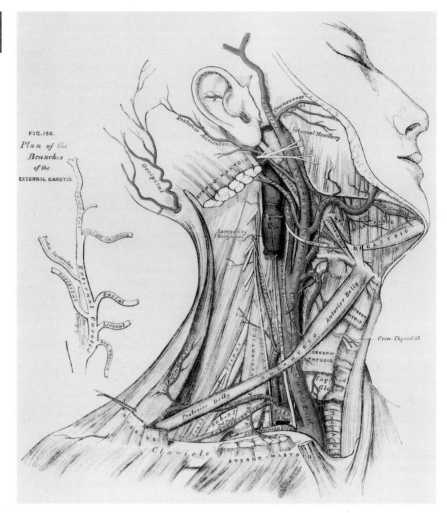

Gray's _Anatomy_. Henry Gray's utilitarian text for students of surgery is supported by Henry Vandyke Carter's clear and functional line drawings, reproduced in plain woodcuts, in conscious contrast to the visual magnificence of earlier picture-books of the human body.

tography and computer imagery have sustained the production of visually striking depictions of the body, and even the later editions of _Gray's Anatomy_ have become vehicles for some trendily flashy visuals.

For all these images, from the artistic pictures in Renaissance books to the polished graphics of the computer, each of the processes involved in making and viewing can be seen as purposeful and partial, according to overt and covert intentions and proclivities. This is not to say, however, that the results are arbitrary and contain nothing more than subjective views of multiple realities. Within the kind of shared context of communication which prevails in, say, the nineteenth-century teaching of anatomy, knowledge of a repeatedly verifiable and efficacious kind was being transmitted. It was an incomplete and selective knowledge, but it could justly claim to be knowledge. It gave those charged with intervening in the body a powerful though fallible guide in knowing what could be done and what might be encountered. Without visual tools for the transmission of cumulative knowledge, many of the techniques that we now take as routine are unlikely to have been developed.

Seeing the Unseen

In the modern era important instruments have increasingly been utilized to provide visual access to forms and phenomena which are invisible to the unaided eye. The earliest of those to be invented was the microscope, apparently developed in Holland around 1600 as a genuinely practical and potent device for the viewing of features as potentially small as the contents of a nucleus. Small instruments employing a single biconvex lens were used with particular acumen by the Dutch 'amateur' Anthony von Leeuwenhoek, to produce stunning revelations of a world of tiny mechanisms, automata, and animalcules, though the medical utility of many of the observations was not to be realized until the framework of medical assumptions had changed. Not the least of the difficulties with the microscope, as with the telescope, was interpreting what was seen in coherent terms and achieving accurate renderings, given the lack of established frames of visual reference for perception and representation at such unfamiliar scales. From the first, proponents of microscopy needed to combat the charge that what they saw was more a product of the instrument than a true picture of reality.

In the twentieth century, major discoveries have been made using instrumental systems of perception, in which invisible emissions, such as X-rays, are used in conjunction with a 'perceiving machine' to give a picture of something which lies outside the normal range of vision. X-ray photography, announced in 1895 by Wilhelm Röntgen, has transformed our ability to see inside the body without surgery, exercising a major impact upon the popular imagination no less than on professional medicine. A film like *The Man with X-Ray Eyes* relies in equal measure upon public information and misinformation about visual techniques which are both admired and feared. More recent methods of scanning, such as ultrasound, magnetic resonance imaging, and positron emission tomography, are set up to provide highly filtered and processed images of what we wish to render visible. Thus ultrasound is used to 'see' the unborn foetus in the womb; an endoscope provides astonishing pictures of what happens within tiny parts of a living body; and a PET scan supplies data for a computer to assemble sectional views of the brain in order to map levels of cerebral activity. Such methods of scrutiny provide potent tools with which the doctor can distinguish between what is defined as normal and abnormal in morphological and physiological terms. The highly selective rigging of these technological systems of artificial perception is not in principle different from the rigging of our own systems of perception and representation, though the human faculty of vision has a complexity and fluidity which gives it a quite different range of potential from any instrumental system, which is basically designed to do one kind of thing.

The fact that the data generated by new scanning techniques and recorded in digital form are so regularly translated into conventional 'pictures' confirms the continuing potency of the visual image as a means of comprehension and communication. The addition of colour in the so-called 'false-colour' images adds a further layer of pictorial convention. To some extent, the designation 'false-colour images'—which indicates that features in bodies of data are signalled by the arbitrary assigning of a different colour to each of

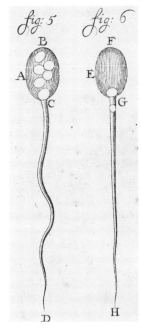

Spermatozoa. Using the simplest microscopes, remarkable observations of unseen forms revealed new miracles of design, though the full implications of many of the observations were only realized over the course of succeeding centuries. From Anthony von Leeuwenhoek's *Opera omnia* (1722).

9

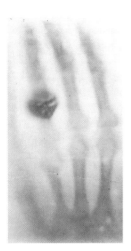

X-ray of the hand.
Discovered when Wilhelm
Röntgen was experi-
menting with cathode ray
tubes in 1895, X-rays
became an overnight
sensation in the popular
press. They assumed huge
importance as the first
visual tool to extend our
capacity for 'seeing' into
realms beyond the normal
range of visible light.

them—is a misnomer, since the principle is essentially no different from that of the human eye. Our eye and perceptual system take in stimuli of light at different wavelengths and differentiate them in terms of what we call colour, but the object we see as coloured is not literally of such-and-such a colour. Indeed, eyes of other organisms are adapted to encode stimuli in a different way and presumably do not see the same colours as we do. Thus the assigning of colours to such properties as zones of temperature or levels of neurological activity is not so much 'false' as relying on an encoding through colour, analogous to that accomplished by our eyes. Often the choice of colour is not actually arbitrary in terms of how we view colour in our normal visual world. Zones of 'hot' activity are characteristically designated as red or orange, while the darker and cooler hues are used to express lesser concentrations and energies.

The ability to convert the unseeable into visible images has been enormously extended in the twentieth century by such techniques as electron microscopy and X-ray diffraction crystallography, which have provided data about far smaller features than can be resolved with the use of visible light. Electron microscopy has revealed very important features of the tissues and cells of the body and of the agents of infection, while X-ray diffraction has provided data for the assembly of models of the complex organic molecules which provide the basic building blocks of the body. These models, increasingly familiar in the form of brilliantly coloured and animated computer graphics, do not show us literally what the viruses or molecules 'look' like, because the forms are not visible in any real sense. What they represent is the conversion of selected data into visual forms which work with our normal conventions of representation. The resulting images, such as those of the AIDS (acquired immune deficiency syndrome) virus, can provide potentially powerful tools when, say, researchers wish to construct a chemical which will lock onto part of the virus in a three-dimensional bond in order to neutralize the ability of the virus to colonize white blood cells.

In all these areas of seeing and depicting the unseen, medicine has increasingly constructed a visual world of invisible forms and phenomena which can only be verified with special equipment and interpreted with specialist knowledge. In such circumstances, the public is required to take even more on trust than has always been the case with visual representations of things which the spectator has not seen or could not see.

Seeing the Signs

If looking and representing, whether by human hand and eye or by machine, are necessarily highly selective and even partial, the partiality is heavily directed by interests which are concerned with meaning—the whole range of significances and associations which centre on the body. The significances and associations are often of a highly emotive or symbolic kind, relating to such issues as health and illness, beauty and deformity, sanity and madness, and the seats of reason, emotion, sexuality, and the soul. In the astrological figure the symbolic connotations are overt, but even in the modern era many artists and scientists have been drawn irresistibly to the key organs of the brain and the heart, the traditional centres of the intellect and emotions and indeed of life itself. A brain scan, revealing the localized charges of energy in response to a particular stimulus, and a heart transplant operation still carry *frissons* of interest beyond, say, an X-ray of the large intestine. There are many taboos, attractions, repulsions, and sexual connotations involved with the viewing of bodies, real or represented, and even the most ostensibly unemotive rendering cannot hope to control the associations brought to the image by the spectator—or even hide connotations which the author of the image might not wish to acknowledge.

No field is richer in metaphor than the body. I am less concerned here with the use of metaphors drawn *from* the body—such as 'the heart of the matter'—than with metaphors *for* the body. In the Renaissance the metaphors were predominantly cosmological and architectural. The body was a 'miniature world', a microcosm, embodying all the essential aspects of universal design. Thus Leonardo in 1513 displays the foetus in a womb which opens like a seed-case to reveal the secret of life within, while the tree-like configuration of the blood vessels on the outside of the womb makes overt visual reference to Leonardo's analogies between branching structures in plants, rivers, and veins. Not the

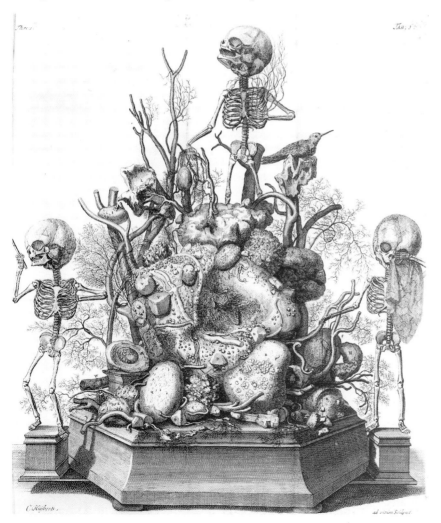

Montage of stones, cast vessels, skeletons, etc. Frederik Ruysch was a pioneer of casting vessels by injection. The resulting 'trees' were assembled into elaborate tableaux, with stones from bodily organs and other natural items, as philosophical curiosities in which the earthly and human bodies are paralleled.

least astonishing manifestations of the microcosmic urge are the *tableaux* of anatomical items assembled in the early eighteenth century by Frederik Ruysch, who made elaborate montages of stones taken from human organs, casts of blood vessels, infants' skeletons, and other curious forms. The essentially serious, philosophical nature of such apparently bizarre creations is confirmed by the publication of folding plates of his constructions, which appeared in his volumes of serious essays on medical topics. The microcosmic body was also viewed as a temple or a house, the functioning elements of which must be maintained in equilibrium. God was the supreme *artifex* of the temples of the body and the cosmos. Anatomists from Vesalius to Albinus were able to justify the publications by claiming to reveal the divine secrets of the architecture of the human body as a form of homage to the Almighty. The disclosing of the miracle of microcosmic design was undertaken in a theatre, like the fictional structure illustrated in the frontispiece to the *Fabrica*, which provided a suitable arena for the most dramatic performance of all. During the seventeenth century, the mechanical analogies became increasingly prominent, and by the nineteenth surgeons were seen as undertaking the necessary training to transform themselves into mechanics of the body. The new technologies of the twentieth century have produced their own metaphors and analogies, not least that of the brain as the greatest computer of all. In one sense or another no one involved in medical illustration can avoid our propensity to take the body as a field for metaphorical readings, whether by direct representation or by allusion to things and places associated with the bodily functions of health and illness.

The whole concept of health is and always has been deeply concerned with visible signs. The gross overall concept of health is intimately linked to how someone 'looks', in the sense of 'you look well today'. Each age develops its own image of the ideal and thus healthy body—or perhaps of various ideals, depending on context and spectator. Not for nothing was a magazine which provided a vehicle for photographs of delectable nudes ogled by generations of schoolboys called *Health and Efficiency*. There has been a perpetual strain between the visual rhetoric of the body beautiful perpetrated by makers of images and the reality of what most of us have been given. In the anatomy books, the male bodies which always provided the main focus for demonstration characteristically assumed heroic Apollonian or Herculean airs. The first book in Italy to carry the new style of illustration, Berengario da Carpi's *Commentaria* of 1521, showed nude male figures in heroic Roman poses or implicit dramas, while the muscle-men in Vesalius' *Fabrica* act out a monumental dance of death as they are stripped down to their very bones. Some of Vesalius' demonstrations of internal organs are set in part-figures that overtly recall famous fragments of ancient sculpture. Anatomies of women were largely reserved to showing how they differ from men, with displays of reproductive organs set in bodies that not infrequently make overt reference to the most admired prototype of the beloved and fecund body, that of Venus herself.

The diagnosis of illness—of what renders the body ugly and diseased—has, of course, always been linked with 'seeing the signs', but in a very different way from modern diagnostic observation. In the long period of medicine from classical antiquity to the eighteenth century which was dominated by the theory

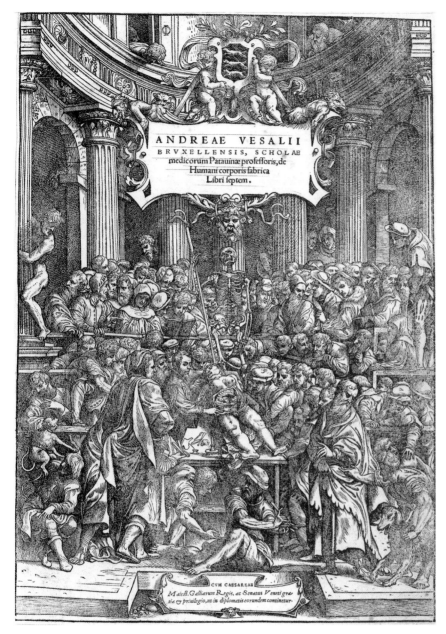

In the title-page of his great book of anatomy, Vesalius is shown as conducting the dissection himself, rather than leaving the practical procedures to an assistant. The grand theatre with supporting cast and symbolic allusions is an exercise in visual rhetoric rather than a portrayal of an actual situation.

of the four humours, complexions, and temperaments—the sanguine, choleric, phlegmatic, and melancholy—the physician's observations were primarily directed to the detection of gross imbalances, using such signs as the colour and smell of urine, but not to the systematic observation and recording of the detailed symptoms and physical changes which reveal to modern medicine which part of the machine is breaking down and why. A Renaissance physician's crib, like the *Vademecum*, is designed to operate in precisely this context. Albrecht Dürer's elaborately symbolic evocation of *Melencolia*, paralysed into introverted inaction by a superfluity of black gall, is locked into precisely the system of cosmological and astrological beliefs that characterized much

13

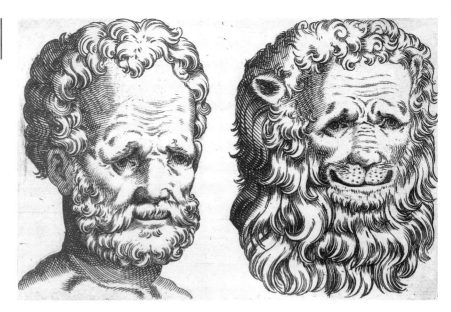

Since the time of Aristotle, the science of physiognomy had promised to ascertain the inner natures of people from the reading of facial 'signs'. Apparent parallels with animal types indicated a temperament like that of the corresponding beast. Comparison of a man and a lion from Giovanni Battista della Porta's *De Humana physiognomia* (1586).

medieval and Renaissance medical practice. Temperamental peculiarities could be read particularly clearly from facial signs according to the ancient science of physiognomy, later to be amplified by phrenological analyses of the cranium. The way in which Giovanni Battista della Porta's book on physiognomy in 1586 sought analogies with the wider world, in this case with animals, was typical of the philosophical framework for early medicine. If such physiognomic studies should seem merely to be curious instances of ancient superstitions, it is worth noting that the reading of facial expression was still the subject of serious investigation in the era of photography, when in 1862 Duchenne de Boulougne published his *Mécanisme de la physiognomie humaine*, which contained Tournechon's remarkable photographs of facial motions stimulated by electric charges. In earlier humoral medicine, smell, touch, sound, and even taste played large roles in the diagnosis of temperamental imbalances. It is this earlier concept of diagnosis which largely explains why systematic and detailed visual representations of pathology arrived so late on the scene, when the techniques for depiction were long since available. Only with the concepts of disease and pathology developed by physicians like Sir William Jenner (1815–98) did small visual discriminations of series of associated physical signs assume a crucial role in the education of the practitioner.

Illustrations of pathology, sometimes involving the visual recording of extremes of deformity and abnormality, became increasingly prominent during the nineteenth century, with photography assuming a major role. Alongside the obvious clinical role of such pictures, there has been a strange and persistent current of voyeurism, with spectacular photographs of gross abnormalities attracting a fascinated if repelled audience outside the strictly medical arena. Such a fascination is nothing new. The grotesque carvings of the Gothic cathedrals, the monstrous forms of Bosch and Bruegel, the bizarre heads drawn in such numbers by Leonardo, and the sometimes hideous drolleries of Dutch seventeenth-century genre paintings and prints all testify to widespread fascination with what may be termed 'pathological ugliness'. Related to this fascination is the way that books of anatomical dissections, especially the great picture books, were aimed at markets which extended beyond professional doctors. Indeed, some of the very expensive eighteenth-century atlases, like Hunter's *Gravid Uterus* in 1774, were sold by subscription to the great and the good. That the inner landscapes of the body and distortions from the perceived norm should find spectators beyond the world of medicine clearly testifies to a fundamental and enduring trait in how we handle and mediate a complex range of deep feelings about the body, including, not least, a sense of fear.

Amongst the representations of what is seen as the bizarre and abnormal, the portrayal of the clinically insane, or more generally of mad and deviant behaviour, has been a conspicuous genre in its own right. At least some of the manic activities in the paintings of Bosch and Bruegel portray the insanity to which the human race is regarded as prone, in a way that is analogous to the literary tradition of the 'ship of fools'. Stock representations of the fool or idiot persist from the Middle Ages to (at least) the nineteenth century. Specific depictions of the denizens of madhouses occur in increasing numbers in the eighteenth and nineteenth centuries, either as freaks evoking horrified fascination or in the context of a wider allegorical meaning or social and moral narrative. Hogarth, for instance, notably characterized various kinds of madness (as then defined) in the asylum scene in the last of the paintings and engravings in his 1735 series devoted to the *Rake's Progress*, in which the intemperate rake ends his days in Bedlam. Searching and potentially sympathetic explorations of insanity are rarer than those of a derisory nature. The earliest example of what may be described as an analytical image is Dürer's engraving of *Melancolia* (1514), in which the deep speculations characteristic of those with a melancholic temperament have reached such a pathological extreme that all practical action—symbolized by the discarded tools—is obstructed. Only with more sustained exploration of the symptoms of insanity in the eighteenth and nineteenth centuries were portrayals of the insane used as front-line tools of medical analysis and pedagogy. The most notable examples, at least in terms of artistic quality, are the series of portraits produced by Théodore Géricault in 1822–3 for Dr Étienne-Jean Georget, medical officer at the Salpêtrière Hospital, where people afflicted with various kinds of insanity were housed. It is clear, looking at the five surviving examples, such as the *Woman Exhibiting the Monomania of Envy*, that the crude prescriptions of the physiognomists and phrenologists have been transcended in favour of a far subtler and elusive response to the relationship between inner thoughts and outward appearance. It was at the Salpêtrière after 1862 that Dr Jean-Martin Charcot undertook the most ambitious of all the attempts to create what may be called 'visual psychology', in which a heightened awareness of the visual played a central role in diagnosis, recording, clinical suggestion, treatment, and the design of the patients' surroundings. With his assistant, Paul Richer, who had previously trained as an artist, he embarked in 1888 on a richly illustrated series of annual publications devoted to the *New Iconography of the Salpêtrière*, in which he demonstrated a 'method of analysis that completes written observations with images'. Richer also illustrated Charcot's *Demoniacs in Art* in 1887, which surveyed what he identified as artists' representations of devilish convulsions, spiritual possession, and hysteria from the fifth century onwards.

In the case of the representation of insanity by artists it might be argued that the more artistically subtle the image, as is the case with Géricault's portraits, the less direct utility it possesses as an illustrative tool. However, I think it would be truer to say that the most sensitive of the depictions serve to illustrate that neither the technical matter of diagnosis nor a humane personal response can be reduced to a series of crude signs and stereotyped characterizations. In such a field, medical art can both convey a human truth and at the same time be of limited technical utility.

Spaces and Things

Medical interventions have tended over the years not to take place just anywhere and under any circumstances. The designation of special spaces for the doctor's activities has served both functional and symbolic purposes. There have been obvious reasons for the bringing-together of sick people in specially dedicated buildings. Treatment is rendered more efficiently if the patients are in close proximity and readily available to the physician or surgeon. There have also been good reasons for removing the sick from their normal habitations and from the general community. Isolating the sick and the insane, and the rapid disposal of the dead, were established practices long before modern notions of disease and contagion were developed. Dedicated spaces may range from the custom-built hospital or madhouse to the 'sickroom' in the patient's own house, generally a bedroom which is temporarily equipped with various permutations of herbs, potions, pills, basins, medical paraphernalia, and talismanic objects. The symbolic role of the spaces is no less integral to their functions. The visual rhetoric of the places of healing is integral to establishing a relationship between treater and treated. Since the Middle Ages, the specialized hospital—typically with neat beds in neat rows with neat sheets and neatly minimal arrays of furniture—and the doctor's surgery as a privileged territory have come to acquire particular kinds of 'look' which write indelible messages in the minds of the patients. We all know the clinical look of a modern hospital. Indeed 'clinical' has become a metaphorical adjective for a practical kind of visual style—one that is stripped to essentials, undecorative, austere even, breathing an air of cleanliness and efficiency, with no dark corners for germs or the wandering mind. The style has a rationale in function. Even the light surfaces have a role, since they show up contaminating grime. But the style has gone beyond function and has become a metaphorical system of communication in which many of the institutional stratifications and subjugations of modern medicine are embodied.

Pictorial representations of spaces within which medicine has been practised—or was ideally seen as being practised—featured quite regularly in medieval manuscripts, above all in those produced for wealthy patrons in which the illuminations were less concerned with communicating medical knowledge to fellow practitioners than directed towards establishing the physician's status and the gentlemanly nature of his calling, or towards the religious incentives of those charged with caring for the sick. Representations

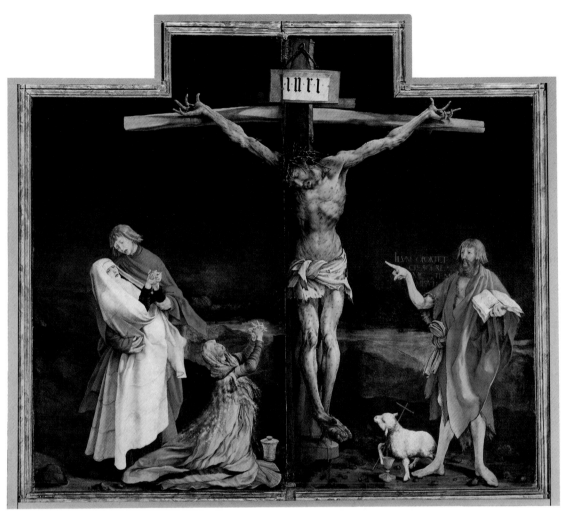

Matthias Grünewald, *Crucifixion with Saints Anthony and Sebastian, and the Lamentation over the Dead Christ.* This large folding altarpiece was painted around 1513 for the Anthonite Monastery at Isenheim, where the monks in the hospital specialized in treating 'St Anthony's Fire' (ergot poisoning), which causes grossly disfigured joints. The images in the open and folded altarpiece feature sufferings with which the afflicted could empathize, messages of redemption, and images of intercessory saints.

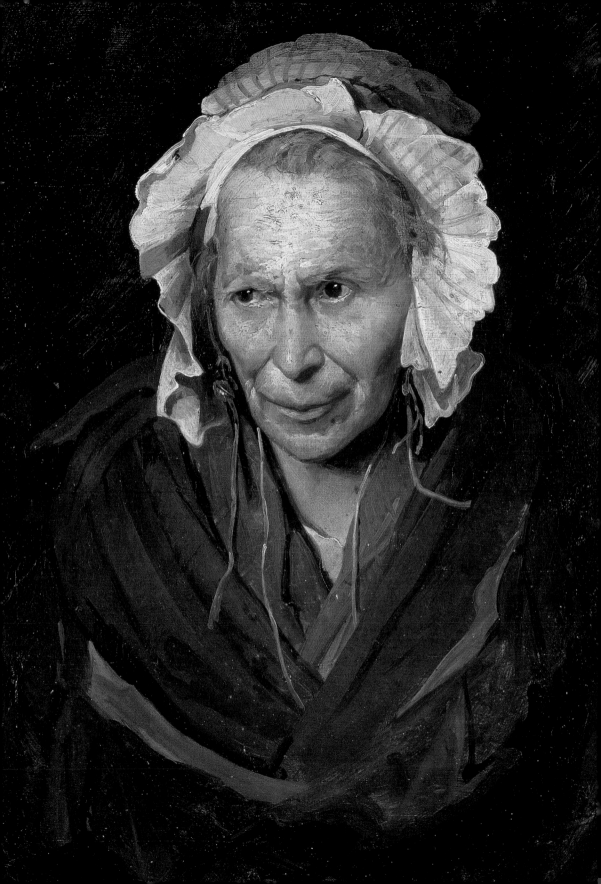

of the interiors of hospitals became increasingly common from the seventeenth century onwards in the context of the extension of art into many more areas of the everyday life of the community. In particular, the much-vaunted madhouses of the eighteenth century were recorded in their full architectural glories, since the spaces for treatment, scrutiny, and supervision were seen as essential levers on the architecture of the human mind. Illustrations of tidy wards with caring, clean-robed nurses, attentive doctors, compliantly cheerful patients, healing equipment, and the inevitable flowers and grapes have become stock images—part of the propaganda surrounding the experience of hospitalization which is designed to allay fears and instil confidence. Such images have proliferated in the medium of photography, serving propagandistic functions in various overt and covert ways, as is apparent in a number of the illustrations of essentially cheerful institutions in this volume. The reality of the patient's perceptions may be very different. Featureless corridors, the visual sterility of the wards, the brisk professional courtesies of the doctors on their rounds, the imposed routines of meals and bedpans, can all too easily jar with the ragged perceptions of those who are seriously ill. Such jarring seems to be of concern to a small minority of medical professionals and a few architects of hospital buildings. Often it is the artist, the insider–outsider, who can bring the sharpest visual perspectives on the loss of those human values that enter through the eye.

No less integral to the visual rhetoric of medicine is the presence and design of the paraphernalia of treatment. Some of the earliest medical illustrations in the Middle Ages involved arrays of equipment, knives, hooks, saws, and various alarming devices for insertion into the orifices of the body. In the sixteenth century some books of surgery illustrated elaborate mechanical devices, much in the style that was already common in books of engineering marvels. Edited books by classical and Arabic surgeons, and treatises by modern authors such as Girolamo Fabrici, openly paraded the machinery of medicine in technical illustrations of the highest skill and visual impact. The representations served an obviously descriptive function, but they also came to act as certifiers of a kind of activity and competence on the behalf of surgeons, and to underscore the view of the body itself as a piece of engineering. The apparent lack of discomfort which characterizes many of those shown as the beneficiaries of the machinery also serves a reassuring function. Books of anatomy, inspired not least by Vesalius' *Fabrica*, often contain prominent illustrations of tools, dissecting boards, pins, and clamps as a way of declaring to the viewer that what is seen in the illustrations is literally the result of first-hand experience. In the era of high-tech medicine, in which the patient is encouraged to feel better in direct ratio to the expense of the equipment used, illustrations of the latest devices, such as X-ray machines for the treatment of cancers and ultrasound scanners in maternity hospitals, are important parts of the visual marketing of medical services—now in the context of the false market being established within the British National Health Service (NHS) no less than in the financially rapacious world of US medicine. For these purposes the equipment has to breathe the visual air of high tech, whether of a white box with dials or the more visceral structures of devices which display their working parts.

No less significant in the treatment of routine illnesses is the kind of para-

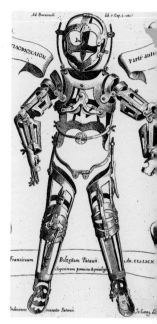

Prosthetic apparatuses. The book of surgery by Girolamo Fabrici, appointed as professor at Padua in 1565, provides a superb example of the use of technological illustrations in emulation of Renaissance engineering books as a way of certifying the surgeon's mastery of advanced techniques.

Théodore Géricault, *Woman Exhibiting the Monomania of Envy* (*facing*). One of the five known examples of ten portraits produced by Théodore Géricault in 1822–3 for Dr Etienne-Jean Georget, medical officer for the insane at the Salpêtrière Hospital, presumably as clinical records of facial signs, though their precise function is not documented.

phernalia which is provided for the patient in a domestic setting. I suppose the common thermometer is the most familiar and widely used of the home devices. The traditional mercury thermometer, emerging from its velvet-lined metal sheath, shining and clinically scaled, carries associations for generations of sufferers from high temperatures. Now the computerized, instant thermometer is taking over, speaking the visual language of electronic technology. One of the most important but neglected aspects of such medical design has involved the containers for medicaments. The orientalizing *albarello* (the handle-less, decorated ceramic jar of the Renaissance and later centuries) and the great vessels of the apothecary's shop represent species of specialized design which speak their own languages. The labelled bottles, ointment jars, pill boxes, and squeezy tubes of more modern medicine have all acquired their own distinct and evolving looks over the years. Even a tube of toothpaste, invariably white, with secondary adornments of bright primary colours (especially blues) and typically incisive typefaces, is a piece of visual rhetoric. The visually distinct types of medical container are linked to function, not least that of declaring that they contain medicine which might be dangerous if misused, but the function and the style are inseparable if we wish to understand why a container looks as it does.

Such objects are often stored together in particular ways. Few modern homes in Westernized societies do not have a medical cabinet in which medicines, bandages, thermometers, and related items are collected together. Indeed the cabinet has been a constant feature of medicine since the sixteenth century. The earliest cabinets, the kinds of *wunderkammer* or 'cabinet of curiosities' assembled by physicians, contained a wider range of strange and magic objects of artificial and natural origins than we would expect in a modern medical cabinet, but the principle is not so very different. The early cabinets of 'collectibles', such as that constructed by Ferrante Imperato at Naples, served to display the owner's high understanding of the world and evidence of his command over items that might be efficacious in a variety of often incomprehensible ways. Ruysch's extraordinary *tableaux* spoke of the kind of philosophical grasp of the nature of things which was seen as underpinning the physician's ability to retune discordant components in the ailing body. When an apothecary hung the corpse of an alligator from the ceiling of his shop, he was setting his practice in a nexus of secret knowledge of the exotic mysteries of how nature really worked in all its manifest variety and how it could be brought to bear on the human constitution. It is one of the ironies that the functioning objects collected in cabinets themselves become collectible in different ways as they assume functional obsolescence, entering collections as eloquent visual reminders of other medical cultures. The visual paraphernalia of past ages speak, as they say, volumes. We are less good at noticing the significance of the signs of our own age.

Heroes and Victims (and Heroines?)

Underpinning all the elaborate apparatus of pedagogic representations, systems of signification, operational spaces, and eloquent paraphernalia lies the human presence. In the final analysis, medicine is exercised by people on people within social structures. The relative status of those performing the actions and those being acted on is articulated in complexly different ways in different societies, and the internal statuses of both categories are subject to important and changing differentiations.

The most obvious depiction of the humans at the centre of the endeavour is through portraiture. Being deemed to be a subject worthy of a portrait or being able to afford a portrait (at least before the era of mass photography) was itself a significant measure of status. For a physician or even more notably for a hands-on surgeon to acquire the status of a 'gentleman' was an important sign, both for the recognition of the individual and for the profession as a whole. The whole point of the great majority of medical portraits before the nineteenth century was to imply or overtly to display the elevated status of the sitter rather than to display him in the baser business of practical procedures. The tradition was begun in classical antiquity, with such images as marble busts of Hippocrates, and was sustained by the author 'portraits' included in some medieval and Renaissance manuscripts. It continued unabated into the era of the great printed picture books. Thus Bidloo, in his splendid book of dissections in 1685, is displayed by Gerard de Lairesse, the 'Dutch Poussin', as a gentleman and scholar, elegantly dressed and addressing us through Latin humanist inscriptions. At most, a few attributes—a scalpel, an anatomical model, or suitably titled books—might be included in a conventional portrait to allude to the sitter's profession. The Athenian tombstone of Jason portrays the young patient as an 'attribute' of the caring physician rather than illustrating treatment in realistic action. Six hundred years later, the posthumous portrait of William Hunter, first Professor of Anatomy at the Royal Academy of Arts in London, painted in 1788–9 by the Academy's President, Joshua Reynolds, conforms to the accepted norm. The genre of scientists with attributes has persisted with undiminished vigour into the era of photography, as is shown nicely by the famous photograph of Watson and Crick with their model of the double helix of DNA, the model which has become such an icon of modern biomedical research.

The relatively scarce 'action portraits' commissioned by or for medical men before the nineteenth century were occasioned by special motives, like Vesalius' wish to show himself in the frontispiece of the *Fabrica* reading the physical book of an actual body on his own account, or in Nicholas Tulp's desire to show himself demonstrating the wonders of the bodily machine in the elaborate allegory of human knowledge painted by Rembrandt. The increasing likelihood of a doctor being shown 'on the job' in the nineteenth and twentieth centuries, most commonly in the kind of contrivedly informal photographs with which we are familiar in a variety of publications, is linked to a complex series of changed perceptions about medicine and the system of values into which it has become locked in our scientific and technological society. A particularly nice fusion of new imagery and an old medium is the image of Sir Alexander Fleming, saint of the discovery of penicillin, in a stained-glass window in St James's Church in Paddington, near St Mary's Hospital. The laboratory, like the operating theatre, has become an admired site for the exercise of minds and hands, and is therefore a fit subject for representation in the most prestigious contexts. The genres of medical portraiture have been overwhelmingly male

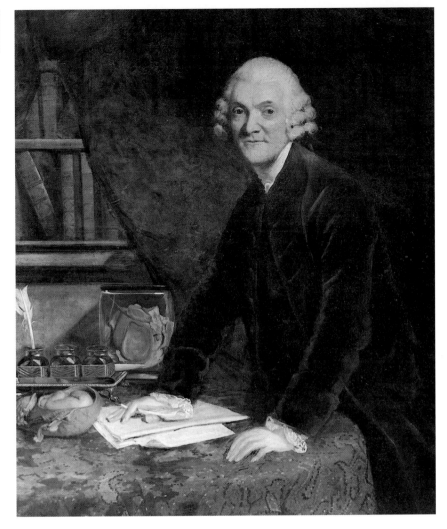

William Hunter, Scottish obstetrician to Queen Charlotte, and collector of works of art, books, manuscripts and scientific objects, was the first Professor of Anatomy at the Royal Academy of Arts. He is shown with books, anatomical models, and writing implements in a memorial portrait by Sir Joshua Reynolds, the Academy's first president.

in character, largely until the rise of the professional nurse under the inspiration of Florence Nightingale. The great majority of medical portraits of women, either individually or more typically in the act of caring, still occur in the field of nursing—mirroring the professional differentiations which have far from dissolved with the advent of feminism.

More general depictions of medical practice have featured throughout the course of Western medicine, but in their earlier guises are far removed in function from illustrations of procedures in modern textbooks. Ancient and medieval images portray the kind of thing that is happening—serving as general illustrations—rather than offering instruction in how to undertake specific interventions. When medicine was more frequently shown in action in the seventeenth and eighteenth centuries, it was predominately in the fields of genre painting and social satires. Many of these representations concerned vernacular, popular, even vulgar medicine—the practice of itinerant dentists, barber-surgeons, quack sellers of incredible potions, and suchlike. A genre of medical imagery developed, most especially in English satirical art in the eighteenth century, in which a medical narrative was used to allude to some other topic, such as the state of the nation or the foibles of the monarchy. Doctors, official professionals no less than the quacks, became prominent butts of visual satire—not altogether unwillingly in some instances, since there is evidence of practitioners seeking to gain notice by commissioning satirical images of themselves. Looking at the range of narratives, we need to be continually alert to the dangers of too literal a reading of the images as if they are documentaries. All the representations exist within defined fields of types of image, each of which has its own rules, compositional types, inclusions, and exclusions. Each image was designed selectively to make a point, not necessarily in all cases about medicine itself. The inclusion of symbolic references, such as a skull on the ground, should alert us to the way that images are artificially constructed within a context of shared expectations about how meaning is conveyed.

With modern photography of medicine in action we seem at first sight to be moving into a more objective, 'documentary' mode of imagery, and the way we react to the image as a record of something real has been significantly conditioned by our knowledge of how a photograph is made. Yet it is doubtful if any of the photographs in this volume arose in contexts in which implicit or explicit values did not motivate the staging of the situation and the taking of the 'snapshot'. The most obvious staging is when a politician is shown taking pointed interest in a laboratory or a hospital ward, but more covert strategies are apparent in every image of an admired professor in action, a doctor on the job, a patient calling for our sympathy, and a heart-rending child requiring treatment. The modern photograph, unless it has been manipulated by computer or other form of 'fakery', is not a fiction in the same sense as a genre painting or a Hogarth print, but neither is it a disinterested presentation of neutral facts—least of all when portraying subjects in which so much human emotion is invested.

Genre paintings and prints are perhaps most revealing of how the victims of the medical professions saw the business of medicine. The majority of the makers of the narratives possessed limited medical knowledge, and few of the images were made under the supervision of doctors. The narratives are thus valuable witnesses for the social history of medicine, most particularly with respect to the perceptions of the recipients of treatment, either on an individual or on a more collective basis. Early images of diabolic activity and brutish death give a particularly vivid impression of concepts of human strife and life in relation to divine purposes, for which images of intercessory saints promise to provide the other side of the picture. In later ages the genre of science fiction, in books like Mary Shelley's *Frankenstein* or the horror films which centre on medical themes, tells us much in particular periods about popular perceptions and fears of what science might achieve when unleashed into realms of the inhuman, devilish, and irrational.

When artists are portraying their own direct experiences, either through the depiction of things they have witnessed in hospitals and other medical establishments or by the most direct act of all—self-portraiture while ill or under treatment—the potential for the most direct and compelling communication of the mental states induced by medicine is vividly apparent. Such medical self-images range from Dürer in the Renaissance, pointing in a nude drawing of himself to the spot which hurt, to Edvard Munch's moving painting of himself standing forlornly beside a bed and clock shortly before his death, and Vincent van Gogh's self-portraits when he was deemed to be insane. Equally telling in their own way are the artefacts produced by deeply disturbed or mentally disadvantaged individuals, whether they are seen as having diagnostic or therapeutic value. Some of the images generated by artists, sane and insane, may not be comfortable for the medical professions, but the perceptions they embody are ignored at the peril of ignoring the personal dimension of healing in favour of the technological.

The Eloquence of the Visual

The great territory of medical art, of which we have explored only a fraction, is densely signposted, but the directions on the signs can be adequately interpreted only if we learn to decipher each kind of image in terms of what kind of signpost it is—who made it and for what purpose—and whether we can now tell if it is still pointing in the right direction. Messages in visual images are never rigidly stabilized, even within quite technical fields of illustration. The present book, as an 'illustrated history', bears sustained witness to the eloquence of the visual within the history of medicine. The depictions provide notable bodies of evidence about medical practices and attitudes in past and foreign cultures, but it is vital to understand that this 'evidence' needs to be teased out with the greatest discretion in relation to historical contexts and modern viewings. Interpreted with such discretion, the visual legacy of medicine provides a uniquely valuable testimony not only to the technical history of practice but also to the kind of human values without which medicine loses its heart.

From the Hippocratic *Corpus* to Twentieth-Century Medicine

2 | Medicine in the Classical World

JAMES LONGRIGG

ONE of the most impressive contributions of the ancient Greeks to Western culture was their invention of rational medicine. It was the Greeks who first evolved rational systems of medicine free from magical and religious elements and based upon natural causes. Here for the first time in the history of medicine were displayed strikingly rational attitudes that resulted in a radically new conception of disease, whose causes and symptoms were now accounted for in terms of purely physical causation.

Medicine in the Heroic Age

It is clear from our earliest literary sources, however, that attitudes towards sickness and disease in the heroic age of Greece were not essentially different from those of the ancient Egyptians and Babylonians, who invoked supernatural agencies to explain the causes of disease. In Egypt and Babylon diseases were held to be caused by malignant demons. Similarly, in ancient Greece sickness and disease were linked with the supernatural. As the Roman encyclopaedist Cornelius Celsus has written, 'morbos . . . ad iram deorum immortalium relatos esse' (diseases were attributed to the wrath of the gods). In ancient Greece, however, it was generally believed that the gods, for the most part, acted directly and not through the intermediary of demons or evil spirits. In the opening book of the *Iliad*, for example, the plague that decimates the Greek army besieging Troy is represented as supernatural in origin, sent by Apollo in punishment for Agamemnon's arrogant treatment of his priest, Chryses, who had come to the Greek camp to ransom his captured daughter. In Hesiod's *Works and Days* it is Zeus this time who sends famine and plague, which kill men and render women barren. On a more individual level, the arrows of Apollo and those of his sister Artemis are held to be the causes of the sudden onslaught of disease. Among their victims are numbered the six sons and the six daughters of the unfortunate Niobe, who had boasted that she was superior to their mother, Leto, who had produced only two children.

It has been claimed that Hesiod earlier in the *Works and Days* puts forward a different conception of disease from that found elsewhere in Greek epic and believes that diseases come upon mankind in the natural order of things and are not dispatched in accordance with divine whim. Here Hesiod describes how Zeus, angered by Prometheus' theft of fire on behalf of mortals, sought vengeance by creating the woman Pandora, so called because all the Olympians gave her a gift as a 'bane to men who eat bread'. When he had created this 'insurmountable snare', he sent her with Hermes as a gift to Epimetheus and the latter, unmindful of his brother's forewarning, accepted her. Previously the 'tribes of men' had lived on earth free from ills and grievous diseases. But Pandora took the lid from the jar that contained the gifts and scattered these evils abroad. (Only Hope remained within the jar.) Consequently 'Countless plagues wander among men; for the earth is full of evils and the sea is full. Diseases spontaneously [*automatai*] come upon men continually by day and by night silently bringing mischief to mortals; for wise Zeus took away speech from them.'

Upon the basis of the above it has been claimed that these diseases came upon men, not as the result of divine agency, but entirely of their own accord. It should not be overlooked, however, that, even though the diseases are described as having the power to act spontaneously, they were initially the (deadly) gifts of the gods. It should also be borne in mind that the object of the Olympians' collective wrath is mankind as a whole and not any particular group or individual. The form of the myth explains its lack of specificity here. Hesiod's conception of disease, then, is not essentially different from that found elsewhere in Greek epic. Like Homer, he remains committed to an ontological conception of disease, regarding it as an entity possessing a separate existence of its own. Even though the diseases here have the capacity to act spontaneously, Hesiod, like Homer, believes that their origin is ultimately divine.

Epimetheus opening Pandora's Box. In this seventeenth-century engraving by Sébastien Le Clerc, it is not Pandora herself but Epimetheus, 'one of her lovers', who is depicted in her boudoir opening the deadly jar and releasing ills for mankind.

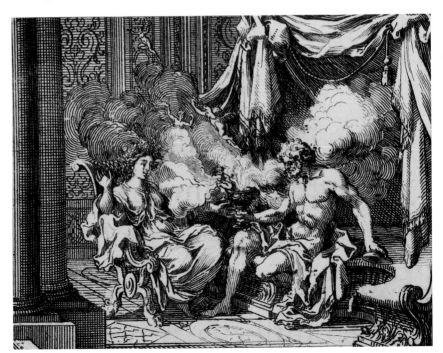

Religious Medicine in Ancient Greece

In addition to causing disease and death, the gods also cured diseases and healed wounds. In ancient Greece, as in Egypt, religious medicine became firmly established. Priests in their temples and sanctuaries catered to an eternal human need. The sick in ancient Greece were able to turn to a wide range of gods and demigods who practised the art of healing. Initially Apollo was the most important; but he was subsequently eclipsed by his son, Asclepius, who was transformed in the last third of the fifth century from a minor cult-hero into a major god.

The tiny figure of Telesphorus, the child-god of convalescence, stands by the right foot of Asclepius, reading from a scroll. Detail from a ceremonial ivory diptych carved in late Roman style.

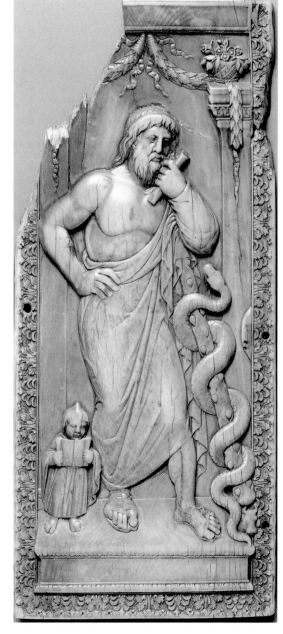

Until not so very long ago, it was widely assumed that Asclepius' temple at Cos was the cradle of Greek medicine. By the early Roman imperial period the story had become widespread that Hippocrates, the 'Father of Medicine', had learned medicine from studying the *iamata* (descriptions of the cures effected by the god) on display in the temple. According to Pliny, Hippocrates is said to have copied out these cures and employed the knowledge derived from them to invent rational medicine. This story was given added credence by the arguments that, just as Egypt and Mesopotamia had priest-physicians, so, in similar fashion, the priests of Asclepius were physicians; that his temples were centres of research and training, where medical experience was accumulated and transmitted to subsequent generations; that Hippocrates was himself an Asclepiad, a member of the hereditary priesthood, and, finally, that Hippocrates was said to have been 'the first to separate medicine from philosophy', thereby creating rational medicine at Cos. But the general attitude of contemporary Greek authors, who regarded medicine as an established art progressively developed by a protracted process of trial and error, is strongly against such a standpoint, as, indeed, is so paradoxical an origin for rational medicine. Moreover, the Asclepieion at Cos was not, in fact, built until the late fourth century BC and archaeological investigation has revealed no trace of an earlier temple on the site. By the fourth century, of course, the island was already famous for its secular medicine. It is true that there exist striking affinities between Hippocratic medicine and the healing practices employed within the temples of Asclepius, but these similarities are better explained as the result of the influence exercised upon religious medicine by its secular counterpart

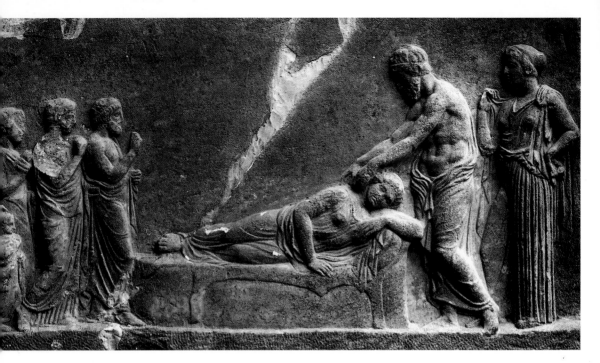

rather than vice versa. The healing dispensed within the precincts of the temple seems to have been conceived with the Hippocratic doctors' practice as its model. Accordingly, the origin of Greek rational medicine must be sought elsewhere.

The Invention of Rational Medicine

Our earliest evidence of Greek medicine reveals, then, that, as in Egypt and Mesopotamia, the causation of disease and the operation of remedies administered to the sick were so linked with superstitious beliefs in magic and supernatural agencies that a rational understanding of disease, its effect upon the body, or of the operation of the remedies administered was impossible. The sixty or more treatises of the Hippocratic *Corpus*, however, provide a striking contrast and are virtually free from magic and supernatural intervention. In this collection, for the first time in the history of medicine, complete treatises have survived which display an entirely rational outlook towards disease, whose causes and symptoms are now accounted for in purely natural terms. The importance of this revolutionary innovation for the subsequent development of medicine can hardly be overstressed.

This emancipation of (some) medicine from magic and superstition did not originate from temple practice, but was rather the outcome of precisely the same attitude of mind which natural philosophers from the Ionian city of Miletus were the first to apply to the world about them. Attempts made by these thinkers in the sixth century BC to explain their environment in terms of its physical constituents without recourse to supernatural explanation brought about a transition from mythological conjecture to rational explanation. Just as these first philosophers had sought to account in purely natural terms for frightening phenomena such as earthquakes, thunder and lightning, and eclipses, which had previously been regarded as manifestations of supernatural powers, so the same outlook was later applied by medical authors to explain frightening diseases such as epilepsy and apoplexy. The clearest evidence of this relationship between Ionian philosophy and Hippocratic medicine may be seen in the fact that the medical literature of the fifth and early fourth centuries BC is written in the Ionic dialect. Although Cos and Cnidus, whence the bulk of the treatises in the Hippocratic *Corpus* seems to have emanated, were both Dorian settlements, the *Corpus* itself is written throughout in Ionic.

Without this background of Ionian rationalism, Hippocratic medicine could not have been conceived. Virtually all that differentiates it from earlier and contemporary medicine has been derived from its philosophical background—that is, its conviction that man should be regarded as a product of his environment, made of the same substances and subject to the same physical laws as the world at large; its belief that diseases possessed their own individual natures and ran their courses within set periods of time, totally independent of supernatural interference.

A striking illustration of this new rational attitude can be seen in the treatise *Sacred Disease*, whose author seeks to demonstrate that epilepsy, a disease that even now is regarded with superstitious dread because of its dramatic and frightening symptoms, has a natural cause like any other disease. A similar attitude is displayed in *Airs, Waters, and Places*—a work possibly by the same author—which attempts to account for diseases generally as due to the effect of climatic and environmental factors. This rejection of belief in supernatural causation and the efficacy of spells and incantations represents medicine's greatest and most enduring debt to philosophy. Although particular explanations of disease were often highly speculative and naïve—epilepsy, for example, was held to be caused by an accumulation of phlegm blocking the passages from the brain—this innovation, whereby doctors now sought to account for sickness, both physical and mental, upon a rational, natural basis, paved the way for medicine's future development as a science. It should be noted, however, that irrational elements were not completely eradicated from Greek medicine. Then, as now, superstitious beliefs and irrational practices continued to be rife. It was, for example, actually during the Fifth Century Enlightenment, under the impact of plague, that the healing cult of Asclepius experienced a dramatic acceleration in its expansion throughout Greece.

Medicine and Philosophy in the Fifth Century BC

As Pliny has complained, the history of Greek medicine is shrouded in darkness down to the Peloponnesian War. A few fragments surviving from the work of Alcmaeon of Croton (fl. second quarter of the fifth century BC), however, flicker in the darkness and, sparse though they are, throw a fitful light to guide our steps. Alcmaeon is the only pre-Hippocratic medical author whose theories have survived in any form. He has been variously described as 'the Father of Anatomy', 'the Father of Physiology', 'the Father of Embryology', 'the Father of Psychology', 'the Creator of Psychiatry', 'the Founder of Gynaecology', and even, comprehensively, as 'the Father of Medicine' itself. Given the scanty nature of our evidence, it would be prudent to avoid such extravagant assessments; but it is, nevertheless, apparent that Alcmaeon is a figure of great importance in the interrelationship between medicine and philosophy. Whether or not he himself actually originated the theories attributed to him is of subsidiary importance. What is important is that his medical views reveal precisely the same rational outlook characteristic of the Ionian philosophers before him and other pre-Socratic thinkers after him.

Alcmaeon's theory of health, preserved by a later writer, reveals a totally different conception of disease from that encountered previously in Greek epic. Alcmaeon rejects the belief that certain diseases possessed a separate existence and were ultimately subject to the whim of the gods and holds them to be the result of disturbances of the body's natural equilibrium. He thus regards them as a part of nature and, consequently, subject to the same rules that operate in the world at large. Just as Alcmaeon's Ionian predecessor, the Milesian philosopher Anaximander, had viewed the cosmos in terms of a balance or even a legal contract between equal opposed forces, so now Alcmaeon regarded the health of the human body as dependent upon the equilibrium (*isonomia*) of the powers within it, while the supremacy (*monarchia*) of any one of them caused disease. The influence of this medical theory was great. It was not only adopted within the Hippocratic *Corpus*, but was also combined by Empedocles with his four-element theory and given a physiological application when he sought to explain the composition of human flesh and blood upon the basis of an equal mixture (*isomoiria*) of his four world-components . and maintained that, whenever this gave way to inequalities, deviations from perfect health occurred. Its subsequent influence can be traced through the physician Philistion of Locri to Plato. Under the influence of the four-element theory the constituent humours of the human body also were limited to four—blood, phlegm, yellow bile, and black bile. The theory of the four humours, subsequently endorsed by Galen, exercised a powerful influence throughout the history of medicine and, like its philosophical counterpart, was subsequently linked with this view of disease as the result of disequilibrium within the body. As a consequence of this conception, dietetics, in its widest sense, was accorded a role of primary importance within Greek medicine. To restore health and redress the imbalance the doctors would prescribe for their patients not only a specific diet (in the modern sense of the word) but also a comprehensive regimen of life, recommending, according to the patients' individual requirements, baths, massage, gymnastic exercises, and even changes of climate.

Alcmaeon also had wide physiological interests and conducted pioneering investigations into the nature of the sense organs. His preoccupation with these matters stimulated the interest of later pre-Socratic philosophers in them. After Alcmaeon such physiological questions as the nature of the semen, the mode of nourishment of the embryo, and even the sterility of mules became almost standard topics of enquiry. This heightened interest in biology and medicine amongst philosophers in the fifth century BC had important influences upon the formation of their physical systems and, conversely, resulted in a still greater influence of philosophy upon medicine. In extending their views upon the world at large to man himself, the philosophers began in consequence to subordinate medical theory to their general philosophical standpoints. Thus philosophy again came to exercise a powerful influence upon medicine. From its continued connection with philosophy medicine derived certain important benefits. It became incorporated within self-consistent and tightly integrated systems. Rational modes of explanation based upon formal, deductive reasoning and sustained by logical argument were now employed to account for medical phenomena within an ordered world whose laws were discoverable. Man himself was regarded as part of that world, a product of his environment, made of the same substances and subject to the same laws of cause and effect that operate within the cosmos at large. Furthermore, the diseases to which he is prone were themselves defined strictly in accordance with the same natural processes and ran their course within a set time independent of any arbitrary supernatural interference. The debit side, however, was almost equally great, for, along with these benefits, medicine took over the pernicious legacy of a priori reasoning, the tendency to deduce explanations from a preconceived position, which resulted in the propensity to accommodate observation to pre-established conviction. This had an adverse effect upon the development of a more empirical method manifestly more appropriate for the advancement of medicine. Experimentation was seriously inhibited and such 'experiments' as were carried out were almost invariably employed to confirm preconceived standpoints.

The danger to medicine inherent in such an attitude is clearly recognized within the Hippocratic *Corpus*. The author of *Ancient Medicine*, for example, is clearly aware of the distinction between the dogmatic, a priori methodology of the natural philosopher and the more empirical approach required of the physician, and vigorously rejects attempts to advance 'new-fangled' hypotheses to explain disease. A similar attitude is displayed in *Nature of Man*, although this time the polemic is confined to those who hold the unitarian belief that man is composed of a single basic substance. But, despite this vigorous opposition to the intrusion of philosophy into medicine, the *Corpus* clearly manifests the continued influence of philosophy. Some treatises reveal the influence of a single philosopher; others are more eclectic. Some, while vehemently condemning the intrusion of philosophy, are themselves unconsciously influenced by it. Even the author of *Ancient Medicine* is himself vulnerable to the very charge he levels at his philosophical opponents in that he adopts as the basis for his own theory of health a conception that is hardly less arbitrary and can be traced back ultimately to Anaximander. *Nature of Man* similarly manifests

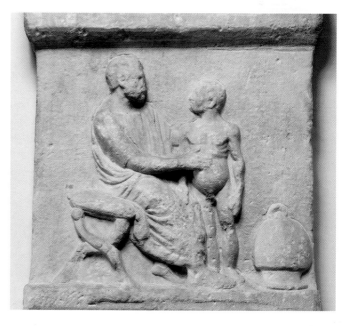

A physician at work. Portrayed seated upon a stool, he is palpating the swollen abdomen of his patient, who may be suffering from malnutrition. The outsize cupping-vessel on the right is included to symbolize his medical role. Detail from the tombstone of Jason, a physician from Acharnae in Attica, second century AD.

Apollo and Artemis killing the children of Niobe (*facing, top left*). Detail from the Calyx-crater *c*.445–50 BC from Orvieto.

The doctor's surgery (*iatreion*) (*top right*). Detail from the 'Clinic-painter' vase, a small Attic red-flgured *aryballos* (oil-flask) *c*.470 BC, showing the seated physician operating in his surgery upon the arm of a male patient. He seems about to incise a vein prior to the application of a cupping-vessel hanging on the wall behind him.

Erasistratus diagnosing the illness of Antiochus I as the result of the young man's passion for his stepmother, Stratonice (*below*). This tale, depicted here by the French artist, J.–L. David, became one of the most famous love-stories of the ancient world. Erasistratus, after much anxious thought, revealed to King Seleucus that his son was in love with his wife. The king, out of love for his son and to save his life, gave him his wife to marry.

Diagrammatic representation of the Hippocratic theory of the four humours, showing its development through the ages with accretions by Galen (tinted ring) and during the Middle Ages (white ring).

32

strong philosophical influence and, as a direct result, ironically puts forward a theory that, more than any other, contributed to the dominance of philosophy over medicine for the next two millennia: for the first clear statement of the classic theory of the four humours—itself the medical analogue of the Empedoclean four-element theory—appears in this treatise. *Nature of Man* presents a highly schematic and comprehensive system. Elaborate correlations are drawn between the four basic humours, the four primary opposites, and the four seasons. Each of the humours is associated with a particular season and with two of the primary opposites. Blood, phlegm, black bile, and yellow bile are held to predominate in turn according to season. Blood, the dominant humour in spring, is, like that season, characterized by the qualities hot and moist. In similar fashion, yellow bile, like summer, is hot and dry, black bile, like autumn, is cold and dry, and phlegm, like winter, is cold and moist. The symmetry and comprehensive nature of this theory, together with the support it derived from broad appeals to empirical phenomena, ensured its subsequent dominance. Its fourfold symmetry later embraced the four tastes, the four main organs of the body, the four ages of man, and, ultimately, after the arrival of Christianity, even the four Evangelists.

Philosophical influence upon medicine, however, was not limited to the adoption of philosophical postulates. Many of the pre-Socratic philosophers had keen interests in medicine and biology, and certain of the theories that

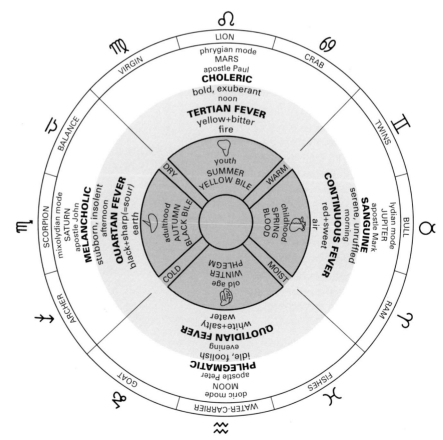

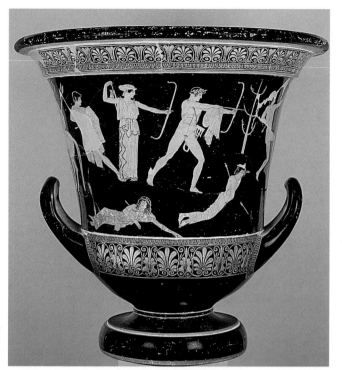

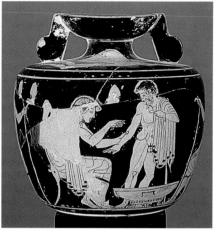

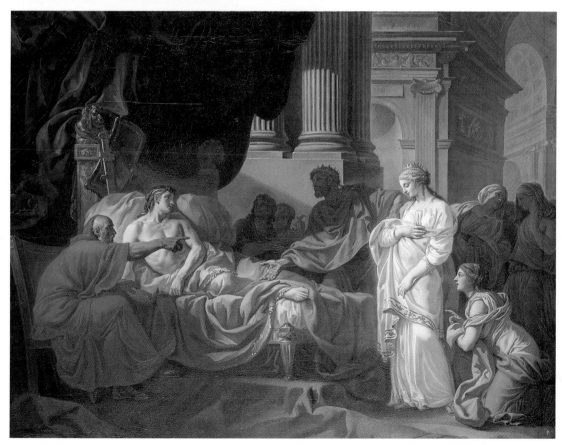

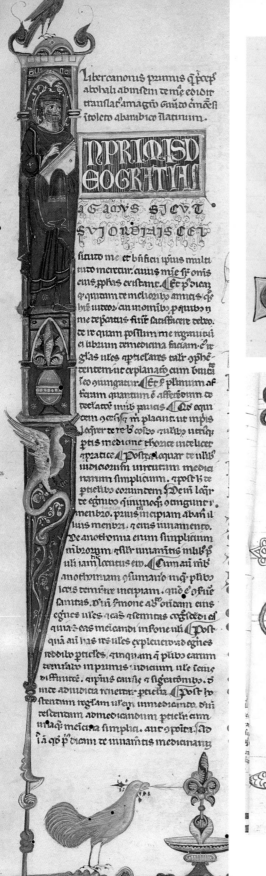

Liber canonis primus qz prcp
at abhali abinse in te me edidit
translat a magro gunto cremest
stolem ab arabico ŧ latinum.

NPRIMIS D
EO GRATIH[?]
AGAMVS SICVT
SVI ORDIS ICEI

sicuto me et bnficia ipius multi
tudo meretur. cuius nisi sz onis
eius, pphas eristant. Et p dicam
qz quantum te melioribz annexis/ cz
bne uixeroz, in monbz paribz in
me tepentuz fuit satisfacere retro.
te requam possum me regnirabi
et librum te mediana faciam. Et re
glas ules apticl ares tali yph e
rentem me explanatio eum bni
leo ourungatur. Et s plimum af
feram quantum e afferod mm co
trelatu mib puias. Et qz equi
cem ncesse in placuit. ut mpis
lasruz te re b cosz auxilib uteibz
ptis medicine thonce intelicer
apratice. Postea loquar te ulib
mdicioruz mueutum medica
naruz simplicium. qpost te
ptelibz cornndem. Denu lasru
te egmtoz simplicez otungter r
mentroz. prius incipiam abam il
ius menbr. q eius munamento.
De anothomia enum simplicium
mibroruz qsitur munantis mulib p
uli iam locutus eiv. Eum au mib
anothomiam qsumario mcz plib
icis reruire incipiam. quo e oxue
santas. q'ni simone ab oricam eus
eguies ules qeas eisentas cqsceoi es
qmas eas meicandi in sone uti. Postea
qua au has res ules expleueroz ad egnes
reddibo pticles/ sinquam q plib earum
rentsauo in puius mdicium ile seire
vi minute. eripius cause q sicontibz. o
mter admiciua renetur prtelia. Post h[?]
stentum reglam ulez mmediiateiter dui
resentiam ad medicandum prtelez eum
ursaq meiena simpla. aur qpiea. Se[?]
ta qo p dicam te munantis medianaruz

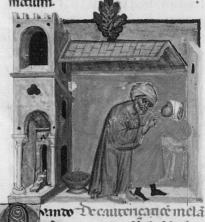

melu qz prcessit. Si aut infinuus est
puer tc pone cauteru subtile sin hunc
modum.

Qnando De cautericatice mela[?]
lei melancolie sut hui cohe
tates corrupte esta grossin. tc cauteri[?]
ipin cauterus que diri in bnte palis[?]
q si ca mlie. est supstuntates reduus r

they put forward, whether derived directly from their general hypotheses, or formulated in accordance with them, considerably influenced contemporary and subsequent medical theory. The two most influential philosophers in this respect were Empedocles, who based his medical and biological theories upon his four-element theory, and Diogenes of Apollonia, who had revived the unitarian belief originally propounded by Anaximenes that air is the first principle of all things.

Although the continued subordination of medicine to philosophy in this way brought about in several instances the very situation that the author of *Ancient Medicine* was at such pains to reject, and the logical satisfaction of an axiomatic system was frequently purchased at the cost of a diminished importance paid to observation, the empirical outlook that permeates other treatises and is most strikingly displayed in *Epidemics* I and III is highly impressive. The case histories cited here with their careful and systematic observations have come to be regarded as paradigms of clinical procedure. This empirical approach is considered to be an original characteristic of Greek medicine—a spontaneous growth engendered by the treatment of wounds, perhaps, or even the result of the development of dietetics for the training of athletes. But this assessment, though widely held, is surely too simplistic, and the relationship between philosophy and medicine in the late fifth and early fourth centuries is, in reality, of a greater complexity than has been generally realized, for the empiricism exemplified so impressively here in the *Epidemics* is manifested within a rational framework that is itself derived from philosophy.

Hippocrates and the Hippocratic *Corpus*

The Hippocratic *Corpus* reveals abundant evidence of the influence of philosophy upon medicine. Against this background, it is difficult to understand Celsus' puzzling remark that Hippocrates 'separated medicine from philosophy'. It seems doubtful that we shall ever know for sure what prompted him to make this assessment. Although the treatises of the *Corpus* generically bear the name of the 'Father of Medicine', sadly, insufficient evidence has survived of either Hippocrates' methodology or his doctrines to enable us positively to identify any individual treatise as having been written by Hippocrates himself. The heterogeneous subject matter of this collection, the variations in style, the diversity of dates, and the, at times, conflicting and even contradictory standpoints manifested within it make it self-evident that he could not have been the author of all of them. The collection has no inner unity except that all the treatises are in Ionic dialect, they are all connected more or less closely with medicine, and the *Corpus*, as a whole, is marked by a virtually complete absence of magic and superstition.

It has been suggested that the treatises composing the collection arrived anonymously at the Great Library at Alexandria, where the followers of Herophilus and Erasistratus developed the techniques of historical interpretation and set up Hippocrates as the 'Father of Medicine' by attributing to this historical figure an increasing number of these anonymous manuscripts. Other scholars believe that the *Corpus* is the remains of the library of the medical 'school' at Cos, which was at some subsequent date incorporated within

The *Canon of Medicine* (*facing, left*) written by Ibn Sīnā (Avicenna) in the eleventh century was known to Europeans through two translations. It was widely read and remained in use in medical schools at Louvain and Montpellier until the seventeenth century. This late thirteenth-century manuscript copy made in Italy has an 'author portrait' of Avicenna in the initial decoration along with other European decorative elements that are unrelated to the text.

Occasionally when copying the Latin version of Albucasis' 'Surgery' (*top right*) (a lengthy chapter from an Arabic medical encyclopedia), European artists introduced figures and interior settings into the illustrations. In such cases the instruments themselves were reduced to insignificance. In this fourteenth-century copy made in southern France the physician employing cauterization is represented as a Muslim wearing a turban, although the buildings are European.

Instruments for extracting teeth and interlacing loose teeth with gold and silver wire illustrated in an early thirteenth-century manuscript copy of Albucasis made in Italy (*below, right*). The instruments are treated as decorative devices on the page, with the result that they are no longer realistic or technically informative.

33

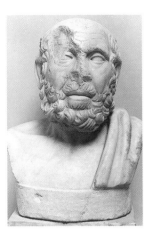

Bust of Hippocrates.
Roman copy of a
Hellenistic bust, com-
monly assumed to be of
Hippocrates, found on a
pedestal bearing the
Hippocratic Oath in front
of the tomb of a doctor at
Ostia.

the Library at Alexandria, where it was recopied and, perhaps, increased by the addition of volumes that had not belonged to the original collection. This latter hypothesis accords with the nature of the *Corpus*, since such a library would presumably have contained works of various dates derived from different sources together with some of little medical value that had been presented to the library or simply acquired by chance.

Notwithstanding the scant, ambiguous, and controversial nature of our evidence, scholars have long sought to identify the genuine works of Hippocrates himself. No consensus, however, has yet been achieved. Controversy still rages and disagreements remain as wide as ever. In 1901 Wilamowitz took a very sceptical view and described Hippocrates as 'ein berühmter Name ohne den Hintergrund irgend einer Schrift' (a famous name without the background of a single treatise). He later changed his mind, but this radically sceptical assessment has been subsequently repeated by Edelstein and by Lloyd. Yet, as Pohlenz originally pointed out, it would be something of a paradox if, when so many treatises have been attributed to Hippocrates, nothing of his genuine writings has survived. Accordingly, despite the forceful arguments of the sceptics, attempts to identify a genuine work continue to be made. The line of approach is generally the same: once the authenticity of one or a few treatises has been established—at any rate to the author's satisfaction—upon the basis of external evidence stemming largely from the Academy and the Lyceum, then the range of works that may be considered to be genuine is widened by using arguments based upon internal evidence. The ambiguous nature of our main sources of evidence, however, renders all such identifications dubious and suggests that scepticism in this matter is not misplaced.

Once the various treatises of the *Corpus* had been gathered together and ascribed to a doctor who had been mentioned with approval by both Plato and Aristotle, his fame so outshone that of all his contemporaries that 'Hippocrates' came to be regarded as the embodiment of all the medical virtues and this reputation was subsequently powerfully endorsed by Galen (AD *c*.129–216(?)), who regarded him as the originator of the medical synthesis which he himself adopted. Hippocrates established his predominance within the ethical sphere no less firmly than in the strictly medical one. The Hippocratic writings provide evidence of ancient Greek debate concerning medical ethics and etiquette. The so-called deontological works, the *Oath*, *The Physician*, *Law*, *Precepts*, and *Decorum*, all reveal attempts to establish codes of behaviour defining the role and duties of the doctor with regard to his patients and to society in general. The doctor is enjoined to ensure both that his medical knowledge is employed for good, and that his privileged relationship with his patients is not exploited in any way. Modern Western medicine still owes an abiding debt to these Hippocratic writings, not only for the ideal of the compassionate, dedicated, and discreet doctor presented here, but also for the explicit rules and implicit assumptions that still govern the doctor–patient relationship today.

After the abundant evidence afforded by the Hippocratic *Corpus*, our subsequent knowledge of Greek medicine again becomes largely dependent upon fragmentary remains and doxographical reports. Only fragments have survived of the works of Philistion, Diocles of Carystos, Praxagoras, and the

Alexandrians Herophilus and Erasistratus. However, both Plato and Aristotle display medical interests and their writings provide valuable information that enables us to set the development of Greek medicine within a historical perspective.

The 'Sicilian' Tradition in Greek Medicine

Although Philistion was a native of Locri, he was given the title 'Sicilian' because of the medical theories he adopted from Empedocles—namely, the four-element theory; the belief that diseases are caused whenever one or other of the elements becomes predominant; his belief in the concept of the innate heat; his belief that the purpose of respiration is to cool the innate heat, and (possibly) his theory that respiration 'takes place not only via the mouth and nostrils, but also over the whole body'. In adopting the element theory, however, Philistion apparently parts company with Empedocles in that he identifies each element with a single opposite, fire with hot, air with cold, water with wet, and earth with dry. It seems likely that it was through a direct acquaintance with Philistion that Plato became so influenced by 'Sicilian' medicine in his great cosmological dialogue, the *Timaeus*.

Diocles, called by the Athenians a 'younger Hippocrates' and described by Pliny as being 'the next after Hippocrates in time and fame', similarly reveals the influence of 'Sicilian' medicine and was accordingly originally held to be a contemporary of Philistion, active during Plato's earlier years—that is, during the first third of the fourth century. Subsequent research, however, has shown that Diocles' fragments reflect the philosophy and terminology of Aristotle, suggesting that the former flourished when the Peripatetic school was at its height. According to Galen, Diocles was the first to write a book on anatomy (i.e. animal anatomy) and it may well have been his influence that led to the introduction of systematic animal dissection and the consequent advancement of anatomical knowledge within the Lyceum. In physiology Diocles seems to have integrated his 'Sicilian' legacy with the Hippocratic tradition to form a comprehensive and integrated synthesis bringing the four-element theory into conformity with the humoral theory. He seems also to have exercised an important influence upon the theory of the *pneuma*, and upon the basis of these theories he put forward his explanation of disease. Like Philistion and Plato, he believed disease was due to an imbalance of one or other of the elements. He also shared with them the belief that diseases occur when the passage of the *pneuma* through the pores in the skin is impeded. These stoppages, he believed, were due to the influence of bile and phlegm upon the blood in the veins. The latter cooled the blood abnormally and compacted it, while the former caused it to boil and curdled it. In either event the *pneuma* was unable to permeate throughout the body and fever ensued.

The influence of 'Sicilian' medicine is also strongly in evidence in the fragments of Praxagoras of Cos, and Diocles is likely to have been the intermediary. For this reason, Jaeger claimed that the Hippocratic school at Cos had come under the dominant influence of the medical department of Aristotle's school. But elsewhere Praxagoras departs radically from 'Sicilian' theory. He holds, for example, that the purpose of respiration is not to cool the innate heat, but rather to provide nourishment for the psychic *pneuma*, and by propounding important and influential theories of his own he forms a vital link with the new medicine soon to arise in Alexandria. Having differentiated between veins and arteries, he stressed the diagnostic importance of the arterial pulse and took an important step towards the discovery of the nervous system made by his pupil Herophilus by conjecturing that certain attenuated arteries (*neura*—so called, presumably, because of their resemblance to sinews) served as channels for the *pneuma*, which transmitted vital motions from the heart to the extremities. His concept of bloodless arteries, however, subsequently taken up by Erasistratus, was to prove a less valuable legacy.

Alexandrian Medical Science

Despite the continuous influence of philosophy, one irrational taboo remained stubbornly entrenched. Religious scruples, veneration of the dead, and dread of the corpse had all combined to interdict human dissection and had seriously hampered advances in the knowledge of human anatomy. In the third century, however, Greek rational medicine was transplanted to Alexandria. Here two medical *émigrés*, working in this new and stimulating 'frontier' society with the support and provision of the first two Ptolemies, were able to dispense with inhibitions appertaining to the human corpse in vogue in mainland Greece and began the systematic dissection (according to some reports, even vivisection) of criminals provided from the royal gaols.

Herophilus, a pupil of Praxagoras, developing his master's work, discovered the nervous system. By transferring to the nerves the functions (as well as the name) which Praxagoras had attributed to certain arteries, he finally and triumphantly solved the problem that had long vexed philosophers and medical men alike and identified the means through which the soul participates in the processes of sense perception and bodily movement. Herophilus also drew more precise distinctions between veins and arteries than Praxagoras had done and pointed out that the arteries had coats six times thicker than those of the veins and did not collapse on death. Having distinguished between veins and arteries, Praxagoras had restricted pulsation to the latter. Herophilus developed his master's pioneering work and became the first to recognize the full importance of the pulse as a clinical sign in prognosis and diagnosis. He evolved a systematic (but largely fanciful) classification of different types of pulse employing the four main indications of size, strength, rate, and rhythm and is credited with making the first known attempt to measure the frequency of the pulse by means of a portable water-clock. Impressive advances in the anatomical knowledge of the brain, eye, liver, and vascular and reproductive systems were also made by him.

These anatomical interests were shared by his younger contemporary Erasistratus and evidence of the latter's researches into the brain, heart, and nervous and vascular systems has survived. In several respects his work reveals marked advances upon that of his predecessor. This is especially apparent in his description of the nervous and vascular systems and in his views upon the significance and structure of the human heart. He was probably the first to discover the coordinated function of all four main valves of the heart—even Galen remarks that his accurate account of them made it superfluous for him to describe them himself. Erasistratus also successfully traced the nerves into the brain. In physiology Erasistratus seems to have been much more innovative than Herophilus, who subscribed to the traditional humoral theory. He combined pneumatic theory with a corpuscular theory derived from the Peripatetic Strato and used it to explain such processes as respiration, nutrition, digestion, and growth.

Impressive results were achieved by these two Alexandrians, who had the imagination to realize the need to dissect and even vivisect humans as well as animals. Working within a new and stimulating cosmopolitan society, they were fortunate in having the protection and patronage of the Ptolemies that enabled them to overcome the deeply entrenched taboo that had inhibited human dissection in mainland Greece. As a result of the radical innovation of systematic human anatomy, they not only provided a basis and stimulus for the anatomical and physiological investigations of Galen more than four centuries later but also attained levels of accuracy and sophistication in their anatomy largely unsurpassed until the Renaissance. In physiology, however, as might be expected, they were less successful, although this study clearly benefited from being firmly based upon a more accurate knowledge of the structure and location of the internal parts of the human body.

The Medical Sects

Despite the individual achievements of these two Alexandrians, the rival 'schools' they founded seem to have largely dissipated their energies in fruitless sophistry and unrewarding sectarian strife. Nor did the practice of systematic human anatomy continue as a permanent legacy of Alexandrian medical science. By the second century AD it was already a thing of the past. Even Galen rarely had the opportunity to practise human dissection. His own dissections are based primarily upon the Barbary ape and later medical authors confined themselves to summarizing and commenting upon the views of their predecessors.

As well as the Herophileans and Erasistrateans, other medical groups, closely paralleling similar developments in philosophy, proliferated in the Hellenistic age. These sects derived their names from the views they held upon the correct methodology in medicine. Attitudes became polarized and the various factions frittered away their time in seeking to discredit the views of their rivals instead of fostering the progress of medicine. One of these sects, the so-called 'Dogmatists' or 'Rationalists', did not constitute a coherent movement and were united only in their commitment to theoretical principles and in their attempts to apply to medicine the methods of natural philosophy. Their principal rivals, the Empiricists, who had affinities with the Academic Sceptics, rejected such theoretical speculation into the hidden causes of health and disease and, making experience their guide, concentrated upon visible symptoms and causes. Unlike the Dogmatists, who approved of dissection since knowledge of anatomy aided the development of logical theories regarding the causation of disease, the Empiricists were opposed to it and maintained that it was neither legitimate nor necessary. The Methodists, who became

influential in Rome in the first century AD, and whose outlook corresponded
to that of the Pyrrhonian Sceptics, repudiated the standpoints of both these
older sects. Their *method* was based upon the simple and uncomplicated tenet
that disease depended upon the tenseness or laxness of the body, and their
treatment followed directly from this premiss: diseases of flux needed
astringents, whereas those of constriction required relaxation. A fourth
sect, the Pneumatists, founded by Athenaeus, a pupil of Posidonius, seems
to have conflated certain of the main doctrines of the Dogmatists with
elements of Stoic philosophy. According to them diseases were caused by
disturbances of the *pneuma* in the body produced by an imbalance of the
humours.

Greek Medicine Comes to Rome

These four sects, prominent in the two centuries immediately before and after
the birth of Christ, spanned the period during which Greek medicine established itself in Rome. Earlier contact, however, had been made. In 292 BC Asclepius was brought to Rome as he had been brought to Athens over 130 years
earlier at a time of emergency. If we can trust Pliny, the first Greek doctor to
settle officially in Rome was the wound specialist Archagathus, who came
from the Peloponnese in 219 BC. Initially he was highly regarded and given citizenship and a surgery at public expense; but subsequently as a result of his
savage use of the knife and of cautery he was nicknamed the 'executioner'
(*carnifex*), and his profession and all doctors became objects of loathing. Of
greater importance was the arrival of Asclepiades from Bithynia (died before
91 BC?). Although originally a rhetorician, he turned to medicine and, by substituting gentler means of treatment for the harsher remedies then in vogue,
he took the city by storm. As the basis for his medical practice he adopted a corpuscular theory, derived, apparently, from Erasistratus, and believed that diseases were due either to the particles being blocked in the pores through
which they passed or, conversely, to the excessive fluidity of their passage. This
theory influenced the Methodist sect, established initially by Thessalus of
Tralles but which traced its origins to Asclepiades' pupil Themison of Laodicea
(first century BC). Both of these Greek doctors practised at Rome amongst the
aristocracy.

According to Pliny, his Roman forefathers lived 'without physicians, but not
without physic'. Roman medicine was initially folk medicine. Cato the Elder
(234–149 BC) is recorded enthusiastically advocating traditional remedies and
extolling in particular the virtues of cabbage as a panacea. His hostility
towards Greek learning in general and to Greek doctors in particular is preserved in a diatribe to his son warning him that the latter conspire to murder
all foreigners and forbidding him to have any dealings with them. Pliny himself later echoes these sentiments in reaction against the continued intrusion
of Greek medicine into Rome during the reign of Nero. (It may be noted, however, that authors like Celsus and Seneca do not share this pronounced hostility towards Greek doctors.)

Cato died in time to be spared the inevitable. In 46 BC Julius Caesar introduced a decree conferring citizenship upon all who practised medicine at

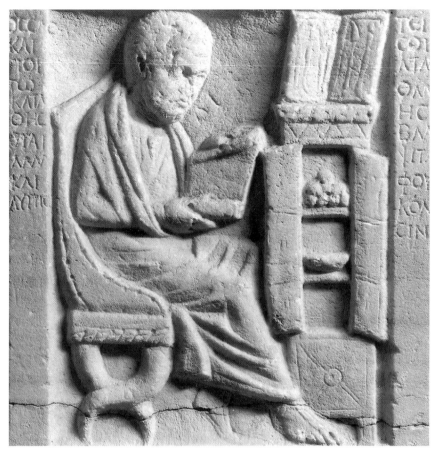

A physician reads from a scroll before a cabinet containing other scrolls and a bowl. His instrument-case is displayed open on top. Front centre panel of a Roman marble sarcophagus from Ostia, fourth century AD.

Rome, and by the first century AD Greek medicine was almost totally dominant at Rome, when, according to Nutton, of almost 180 doctors named only fifteen can be shown without any doubt to have come from citizen families. Significant Roman contributions to medicine were essentially practical—for example, improvements in public-health engineering and the invention of the military hospital. In AD 162 Galen arrived in Rome, where he produced a vast corpus of writings that ultimately became the chief authority on ancient medical knowledge. He was committed to the integration of philosophy and medicine and believed that to be a good doctor one had to be a philosopher; that medicine presupposed all parts of philosophy. The good doctor had to master the natural sciences in order to understand human physiology, anatomy, and pathology. He had to know logic in order to give proper definitions, to make the right conceptual distinctions, to analyse proofs, and to avoid fallacies. He needed training in ethics so that he could exercise sound moral judgement. In philosophy Galen was influenced primarily by Plato, Aristotle, and the Stoics; in medicine by the writings of Hippocrates (or what he conceived to be such), and by the anatomical and physiological researches of Herophilus and Erasistratus. The resulting tightly integrated and comprehensive system, offering a complete medical philosophy, came to represent the very embodiment of Greek and Roman medical knowledge and dominated medicine throughout the Middle Ages and beyond until the beginning of the modern era.

3 | Europe and Islam

EMILIE SAVAGE-SMITH

With us ther was a Doctour of Phisyk
In al this world ne was ther noon him lyk
To speke of phisik and of surgerye . . .
Wel knew he the olde Esculapius,
And Deiscorides, and eek Rufus,
Old Ypocras, Haly, and Galien,
Serapion, Razis, and Avicen . . .

So Geoffrey Chaucer wrote in his Prologue to the *Canterbury Tales*, naming the great physicians of the past that his fourteenth-century audience could be expected to recognize. In the list are five Greek figures: Aesculapius (or Asclepius), the focus of a Greek healing cult; Hippocrates (or 'Ypocras', as Chaucer called him), a fifth- to fourth-century BC physician whose name is associated with a fundamental collection of medical writings; Rufus of Ephesus in Asia Minor, a physician of the first century AD who composed over sixty Greek medical treatises; Dioscorides, whose treatise on medicinal substances written about AD 77 formed the basis of pharmaceutics for centuries; and, of course, Galen of the second century AD, arguably the most influential figure in the history of medicine.

Chaucer then goes on to name physicians from the medieval Islamic world: Haly, or more commonly Haly Abbas, a tenth-century medical encyclopaedist of Baghdad; a Syriac physician of the ninth century named Ibn Sarābiyūn, or Serapion, as he was known to Europe; the great clinician of the early tenth century al-Rāzī, whom Europe knew by the Latinized form of his name Razis or Rhazes; and Avicen, or Avicenna, as other Europeans called him, referring to Ibn Sīnā, whose early eleventh-century medical encyclopaedia was as important in Europe as it was in the Middle East. Just as early Greek medical teaching served as a common intellectual framework for professional medical practice in the Islamic Near East, so Arabic medical literature of the ninth to twelfth centuries, through Latin translations, provided late medieval Europe with ideas and practices from which early modern medicine eventually arose.

The earlier Greek medical teachings were welcomed and valued by an emerging Islamic empire which needed to find ways of dealing with medical problems common to all peoples: disease, pain, injuries, and successful childbearing. This heritage of medical theory and practice was assimilated and elaborated by a community of both Muslim and non-Muslim physicians speaking many languages—Arabic, Persian, Syriac, Hebrew, and Turkish, though Arabic became the lingua franca and Islam the dominant faith. From Spain and North Africa in the west through the central lands of Egypt, Syria, and Iraq, to Iran and India in the east, and over a period of roughly twelve centuries (from the middle of the eighth century to the present time), Islamic medicine has shown great variation and diversity. The medical care in the medieval Islamic lands involved a rich mixture of religions and cultures to be seen in both the physicians and the patients—a coexistence and blending of traditions probably unrivalled in contemporaneous societies. The medical profession in general transcended the barriers of religion, language, and country. Consequently, in this context, the term Islamic culture or Islamic medicine is not to be interpreted as applying only to the religion of Islam.

Military excursions as well as world trade routes provided ample opportunity for information and technology to be transported from one region to another. The expansion of Islam beyond the borders of Arabia began with the invasion of Syria and Iraq in AD 634, and by the middle of the eighth century Egypt, north-west Africa, Spain, Syria, Iraq, Iran, and Central Asia were subjugated, and in succeeding centuries Muslim rule extended over northern India. Also in the seventh century raids were begun on a number of Mediterranean islands. Cyprus was never fully subjugated, but for 250 years rule passed intermittently between the Muslim caliphs and the Byzantine emperors. Sicily was finally subdued in AD 847 and remained under Muslim rule until conquered by the Normans in 1072. The towns of Bari and Taranto on the Italian mainland were occupied by Muslims for several decades in the ninth century, and various points on the southern Italian mainland suffered repeated raids from the ninth through the eleventh century. With the Christian subjugation of the Muslim-ruled areas of Spain, from the eleventh century onwards, there was increased opportunity for Europeans to learn of medical and scientific literature written in the Arabic language. Throughout all these centuries, with occasional interruptions, there was considerable trade between ports rimming the Mediterranean.

Early in the ninth century, there was established in Baghdad a foundation called the House of Wisdom (*bayt al-ḥikmah*), which had its own library. Its purpose was to promote the translation of scientific texts, and placed at the head of this institution was a Syriac-speaking Christian by the name of Yūḥannā ibn Māsawayh (d. 857), a court physician with considerable influence among the wealthy and powerful. His writings, apparently all in Arabic, included a medical handbook which is the first to present the material in a diagrammatic format, as well as treatises on fevers, leprosy, poisons, melancholy, headaches, eye diseases, dietetics, the examination of physicians, and a collection of medical aphorisms. It is evident from his writings that certain diseases, such as an eye condition known today as pannus, were recognized and clearly described by him for the first time. It was reported that Ibn Māsawayh held regular assemblies where he discussed medical subjects with pupils and consulted with patients. At times he apparently attracted considerable audiences, having acquired a reputation for repartee. In Europe Ibn Māsawayh was known as

41

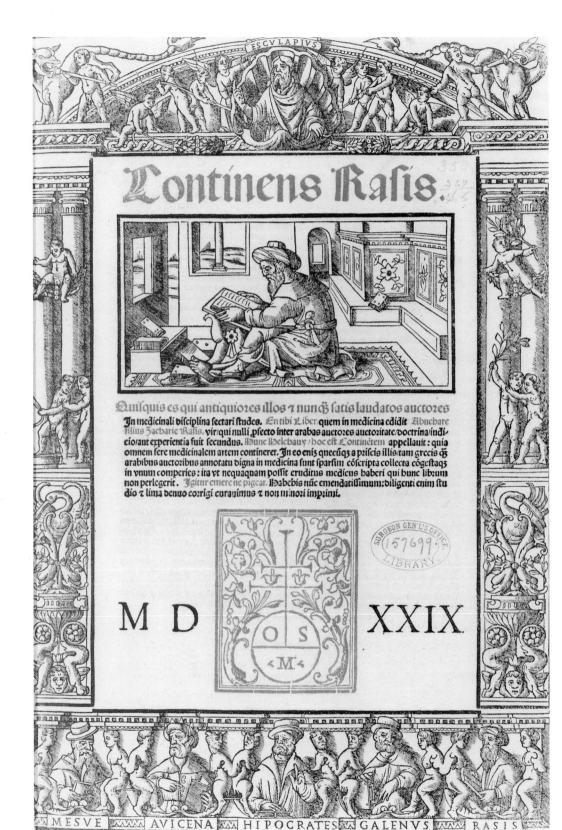

Continens Rasis.

Quisquis es qui antiquiores illos ⁊ nunc̄ satis laudatos auctores
In medicinali disciplina sectari studes. En tibi Liber quem in medicina edidit Abuchare
filius Zacharie Rasis, vir/qui nulli ꝓfecto inter arabas auctores auctoritate/doctrina/indi-
cio/aut experientia fuit secundus. Hunc Helchauy/hoc est Continẽtem appellauit: quia
omnem fere medicinalem artem contineret. In eo eniȝ quecũȝ a priscis illis/tam grecis q̄
arabibus auctoribus annotatu digna in medicina sunt sparsim cõscripta collecta cõgestaȝ
in vnum comperies: ita vt nequaquam possit eruditus medicus haberi qui hunc librum
non perlegerit. Igitur emere ne pigeat. Habebis nũc emendatissimum: diligenti enim stu
dio ⁊ lima denuo corrigi curauimus ⁊ non minori imprimi.

M D XXIX

ESCVLAPIVS

O S M

MESVE   AVICENA   HIPOCRATES   GALENVS   RASIS

Mesue, and a number of Latin medical writings are assigned to either an elder or a younger Mesue. The precise relationship of the various Latin texts with the Arabic treatises by Ibn Māsawayh (many of which are now lost) has yet to be settled. It is clear, however, that 'Mesue' was highly regarded in the West, and a 'portrait' of him was frequently included amongst the important early medical authorities. As late as 1474, Petrus Gulosius, a physician of Amalfi in southern Italy, stated that to read Mesue was as instructive as it was pleasant.

A pupil of Ibn Māsawayh, and the most famous of the translators of Greek medical literature into Arabic, was Ḥunayn ibn Isḥāq, a Syriac-speaking Christian originally from southern Iraq who also knew Greek and Arabic. He worked in Baghdad and was the author of several medical tracts that circulated in Latin versions in Europe, where he was known as Johannitius. His short treatise with the Latin title *Isagoge* was fundamental in establishing the basic conceptual framework of medicine in Europe, for it encapsulated the concepts of four elements, humours, and temperaments, the notion of natural and non-natural, and the polarity of theory–practice. Ḥunayn ibn Isḥāq is most often remembered, however, as a translator, an activity he began at the age of 17. He produced a prodigious amount of work before his death in about AD 873 (or 877), for he translated (together with his son and nephew) nearly all the Greek medical books known at that time, half of the Aristotelian writings as well as commentaries, various mathematical treatises, and even the Greek version of the Old Testament called the Septuagint. Ten years before his death he stated that, of Galen's works alone, he had made ninety-five Syriac and thirty-four Arabic versions. Accuracy and sensitivity were hallmarks of his translating style, and he was no doubt responsible, more than any other person, for the establishment of the classical Arabic scientific and medical vocabulary. Through these translations, a continuity of ideas was maintained between Islamic medicine and Roman and Byzantine practices.

Yet Islamic culture did not simply provide custodial care for classical medicine, serving as a mere transmitter of ancient Greek medicine and learning to medieval Europe. Islamic physicians produced a vast medical literature of their own, in which they imposed a logical and coherent structure on the earlier Greek (predominantly Galenic) medicine. They also added an extended pharmacology, more elaborate notions of medical pathology, a knowledge of new diseases (for example, smallpox and certain eye diseases), new therapies, and new surgical techniques and instrumentation.

By the tenth century it is evident that knowledge of Arabic astronomical treatises and instrumentation was reaching Europe, and in the eleventh century Arabic medical theories and practices began to filter into Europe. Medieval Islamic medicine influenced Europe by means of three conduits: through the written word (which is the easiest to document), through traders' transportation of commodities, and through the observations of travellers to the Middle East. The border areas of Spain and southern Italy, with their large multilingual communities, provided continuous points of contact between Europe and the Islamic Middle East. In these areas there arose two paths of translation from Arabic into Latin—that through Italy started by Constantine the African (d. *c*.1087), a monk at Monte Cassino whose lineage may well have been in the North African culture of Kairouan, and that through Spain, where

The title-page of this 1529 Venetian printing of Rhazes' *Comprehensive Book of Medicine* depicts a scholar seated on the floor at his desk. Only the turban marks him out as Middle Eastern, for the clothes and room are European. The central illustration is framed by a frieze supported by columns, with the figure of Asclepius at the top surrounded by putti, and at the bottom Hippocrates and Galen surrounded by three Islamic medical authorities: Mesue, Avicenna, and Rhazes.

Gerard of Cremona (d. 1187) was the most prolific translator, with sixty-eight works to his credit. Some translators, such as Stephen of Antioch and Philip of Tripoli, worked in Syria in the Outremer or Crusader kingdoms, though their output was considerably less than those in Spain and Italy. The translations into Latin occurred at the same time as the Crusades, though the role that the Crusades played in stimulating such activity is uncertain. Certainly the Crusades aggravated the relations between Christendom and Islam, but they also provided further opportunities to learn different technologies and practices. At the time of the Crusades, it was only Europeans who had much to gain intellectually and technologically from such encounters, for the medical and scientific knowledge then common in Islamic lands was vastly superior to that in Europe. Muslim physicians displayed considerable disdain for the medical practices (often quite lethal) they observed among the Frankish physicians in the Crusader states. The relationship between Christians in Europe and Muslims in Islamic lands, especially in the eleventh to thirteenth centuries, was a complex one, characterized (especially on the part of Europeans) by much hostility and ignorance. Medieval European scholars, while acknowledging their indebtedness to Islamic writers, tended to detach the Muslim scholars from their Islamic roots and to transform them into non-religious thinkers who functioned as passive agents for transmitting classical (and therefore European) learning to Christendom. European artists even portrayed Muslim scholars in the same dress and in the same buildings as Western ones.

A basic change in European learned medicine occurred following the translation into Latin of Arabic scientific treatises. Three of the early Arabic medical encyclopaedias soon came to dominate European medical theory through their Latin versions. Two of them were massive attempts at systematizing and synthesizing all available medical knowledge, and their sheer size gave them an aura of authority that was to prove stultifying rather than invigorating. All three of them had a permanent influence on the formation of Western medical theories and practices, as well as medical terminology—as seen, for example, in anatomical terms still in use today, such as saphena (from the Arabic *ṣāfin*) and pia mater (a translation of *umm raqīqah*, 'thin wrapping').

The first Arabic medical treatise to be translated into Latin was the large encyclopaedia by ʿAlī ibn al-ʿAbbās al-Majūsī, whom Europeans called Haly Abbas. He practised medicine in Baghdad in the mid-tenth century and served as physician to the founder of a famous hospital in that city, to whom he dedicated his only composition, *The Complete Book of the Medical Art*, also known as *The Royal Book*. In Europe this comprehensive and well-organized medical compendium was first known as the *Pantegni*, in a Latin paraphrase made by Constantine the African, who did not credit Haly Abbas as the author. It also circulated in a collection of translations of medical writings of Isḥāq ibn Sulaymān al-Isrāʾīlī, who died about 955. Thus Europeans initially associated the book either with Constantine himself or with Isaac Judaeus, as the Egyptian-born Jewish physician Isḥāq ibn Sulaymān al-Isrāʾīlī was known in Europe. It was not until a new Latin translation titled *Liber regius* was made in 1127 by Stephen of Antioch that Europe knew the encyclopaedia as a work of Haly Abbas.

One of the greatest names in medieval medicine is that of Abū Bakr

Muḥammad ibn Zakariyā' al-Rāzī, who was born in the Iranian city of Rayy in 865 and died in the same town about 925. Rayy, near present-day Tehran, was an important medieval commercial centre, though today it is an uninhabited ruin. The most influential of al-Rāzī's writings in Europe, where he was known as Rhazes, was his *Book of Medicine Dedicated to Manṣūr*, a relatively small general textbook on medicine in ten chapters which he had dedicated in 903 to the governor of Rayy. The treatise was translated into Latin in Toledo by Gerard of Cremona and was known as *Liber ad Almansorem*. It became one of the most widely read medieval medical manuals in Europe, while the ninth chapter, concerned with therapeutics, was frequently circulated by itself. In the Renaissance many editions of it were printed with commentaries by the prominent physicians of the day, such as the anatomist Andreas Vesalius. Among medieval Islamic physicians, the most sought-after of Rhazes' compositions was his *Comprehensive Book of Medicine* (*Kitāb al-Ḥāwī fī al-ṭibb*)—a large private notebook or commonplace book into which he had placed extracts from earlier authors regarding diseases and therapy, together with clinical cases he had recorded from his own experience. In it he was not adverse to criticizing the therapeutics recommended by Galen and other Greek authorities on the basis of his work in hospitals in Baghdad and Rayy. It was translated rather late into Latin, in 1279, under the title *Continens*, by Faraj ben Salīm, a physician of Sicilian–Jewish origin employed by King Charles of Anjou to translate medical works, and it was printed at Brescia in 1486 with repeated printings thereafter.

The third major Arabic medical encyclopaedia to be translated into Latin, and the most influential of all, was the *Canon of Medicine* (*al-Qānūn fī al-ṭibb*) by Ibn Sīnā, known in Europe as Avicenna. He was born in 980 in Central Asia and travelled widely in the eastern Islamic lands, composing nearly 270 different treatises. When he died in 1037 he was known as one of the greatest philosophers in Islam, and in medicine was so highly regarded that he was compared to Galen. His mammoth encyclopaedia was composed of five books, the first concerned with general medical principles, the second with *materia medica*, the third with diseases occurring in a particular part of the body, and the fourth on diseases such as fevers that are not specific to one bodily part, with the final book containing a formulary of recipes for compound remedies. The *Canon* was widely read by Europeans in the Latin translation of Gerard of Cremona made in the twelfth century. So great was the interest in this massive medical textbook that late in the fifteenth century Girolamo Ramusio attempted to improve upon Gerard of Cremona's Latin translation by comparing it with an Arabic manuscript, and in 1527 a new Latin version was published that had been made by Andrea Alpago (d. 1522), who had resided in Damascus for thirty years as a physician in the service of the Venetian Republic and had used his fluency in Arabic not only to translate it but also to append an Arabic–Latin glossary of terms. The *Canon*'s enormous size, in addition to its very title meaning 'codes of law', reinforced its authoritative nature. Between 1500 and 1674 some sixty editions of part or all of the *Canon* were published in Europe, mostly intended for use in university medical training.

Other early Islamic medical textbooks were also translated into Latin and had a profound effect upon late medieval and early modern European medicine. A lengthy surgical chapter from an Arabic medical encyclopaedia com-

An illustration of a vaginal speculum and two types of forceps for extracting a dead foetus (*below left*). From a 1271 Arabic copy of Albucasis' *Surgery* written in the tenth century. The speculum (on the left) operates by a screw mechanism at the top that opens and closes two blades at the bottom. The scribe has noted that the object suspended towards the right of the speculum is a double-edged scalpel and not part of the instrument.

The vaginal speculum from a fourteenth-century Latin copy of Albucasis (*below right*). The European artist not only drew the speculum upside down, but also did not understand the mechanical principle. The decorated bar at the top should be two blades which could separate and close by the screw at the bottom. The lantern-shaped device suspended at the right is a misunderstanding of the scalpel that in the original Arabic version was not part of the instrument.

posed about AD 1000 in Spain enjoyed great popularity in Europe through its Latin translation made in Toledo by Gerard of Cremona. Its author, Abū al-Qāsim al-Zahrāwī, was born in the town of al-Zahrā' near Córdoba. In the treatise he combined the surgical ideas from Graeco-Roman sources with his own observations and experiences as well as copious illustrations and descriptions of instruments. He modified many of the earlier instruments and designed some new ones, such as a concealed knife for opening abscesses in a manner that would not alarm the nervous patient, obstetrical forceps (though not for use in live births), and variations in the design of a vaginal speculum or dilator. This surgical chapter was copied and recopied many times in Europe, where the author was known as Albucasis. The translation of such an illustrated treatise offered two opportunities for misunderstanding—the rendering by the translator of the technical terms and procedures, and the illustration of instruments which would usually be copied by artists unfamiliar with their form or function. So inaccurate are the interpretations of some of the illustrations in the Latin versions of Albucasis that they could not have been used as guides for the making of surgical instruments in Europe. Moreover, Latin copyists often display a desire for a decorative pattern on the page, with the result that the instruments may be unrecognizable although the overall sense of design is pleasing. Occasionally when copying the Latin version, European artists introduced human figures and interior settings into the illustrations and reduced the instruments to insignificance. In such instances, the treatise lost its validity as a practical guide to surgery.

By far the most popular Arabic general treatise on regimen and diet was that written by Ibn Buṭlān, a Christian physician of Baghdad who in 1049 left Baghdad to travel to Cairo and Constantinople, finally settling in Antioch, where he became a monk and later died about 1075. His Arabic treatise, the *Almanac of Health* (*Taqwīm al-ṣiḥḥah*), presented hygiene and dietetics in a tabular format. In the course of forty charts, Ibn Buṭlān presented the properties and uses of 210 plants and animals and seventy other items and procedures useful for maintaining good health, such as the use of music, the regulation of sleep and

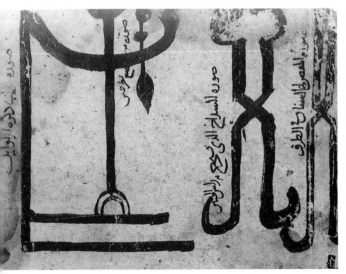

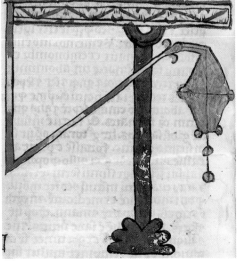

exercise, bathing, fumigations, the alteration of air quality, and seasonal changes. All 280 topics were accompanied by recommendations from various authorities whose names were represented by abbreviations. Its Latin translation, *Tacuinum sanitatis*, made in the thirteenth century probably in southern Italy or in Sicily, was very popular in Europe, judging from the large number of Latin manuscript copies preserved today. Most of the Latin copies, like the Arabic original, are in tabular format without illustrations. There are, however, a small group of Latin copies which are not in tabular form and which are illustrated with scenes showing the production of the medicament. All of these illustrated versions appear to have been produced in northern Italy, the earliest about 1380–90.

With some minor exceptions, no Islamic medical writers who lived after Ibn Buṭlān are represented by Latin translations of their writings. Consequently, Europe's knowledge of Islamic medical literature was basically restricted to a relatively few and comparatively early treatises. Yet medical ideas and practices continued to develop and change within Islamic lands. It is curious that, even though Europe had increased contact with Syria and Egypt in the thirteenth and fourteenth centuries, in part because of the Crusades but also through increased trade, so few of the important and innovative Islamic medical writings of the thirteenth century were available to Europeans. A subject of debate among historians is whether the commentary on the anatomical portions of the *Canon* of Avicenna, written in the thirteenth century by the Syrian physician Ibn al-Nafis (d. 1288), was available through translation to European physicians. In his commentary on the anatomical portions of the *Canon*, Ibn al-Nafis described the movement of blood through the pulmonary transit, explicitly stating that the blood in the right ventricle of the heart must reach the left ventricle by way of the lungs and not through a passage connecting the ventricles, as Galen had maintained. This formulation of the pulmonary circulation, sometimes called the 'lesser' circulation, was made three centuries before those of Michael Servetus (d. 1553) and Realdo Colombo (d. 1559), the first Europeans to describe the pulmonary circulation. It is known that Ibn al-Nafis's commentary on the last part of the *Canon*, concerned with compound drugs, was translated into Latin by the Renaissance physician Andrea Alpago (d. 1522), who had also prepared a new translation of Avicenna's *Canon*. The translation of Ibn al-Nafis on compound remedies was not published until 1547, when it was printed at Venice, but the possibility remains that other parts of Ibn al-Nafis's commentary might have been transmitted through unpublished translations.

In addition to formal written treatises, other avenues were available by which Islamic medical practices could influence Europe. Traders and travellers transported products and ideas that had a direct and indirect bearing on

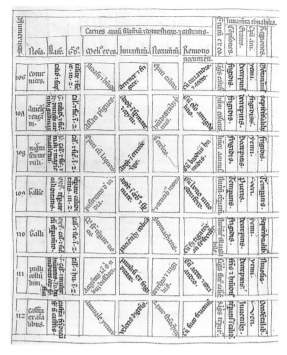

One of the forty tables comprising the *Tacuinum sanitatis*, or *Almanac of Health*, a popular handbook of diet and regimen based on an eleventh-century Arabic original by a Christian physician of Baghdad, Ibn Buṭlān. The page, from a copy made in Italy before 1326, discusses poultry, among other things, noting that it is good for those suffering from colic.

medical practices and care in Europe. The Middle East was an important source of medicaments—plant, animal, and mineral. In the field of *materia medica* and its applications, Islamic writers surpassed their earlier models, primarily because their broader geographic horizons brought them into contact with drugs unknown to earlier peoples, such as camphor, musk, sal ammoniac, and senna, as well as commodities previously unknown to Europe, such as cotton. The Greek treatise on *materia medica* written by Dioscorides in the

Islamic writers added new items to the fund of *materia medica* which had been inherited from classical antiquity. As their geographic horizons broadened, Islamic physicians introduced previously unknown drugs such as camphor and sal ammoniac, and these in turn were passed on to European physicians. This illustration of caraway and cumin is from an Arabic treatise written in Spain in the twelfth century by Aḥmad al-Ghafīqī.

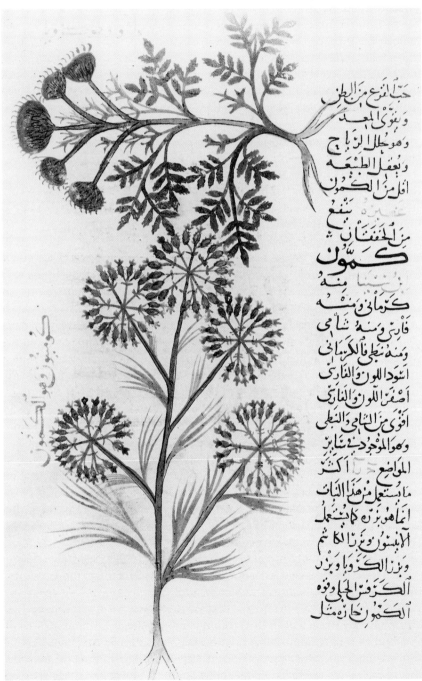

first century AD, through its Arabic translation, formed the framework of Islamic pharmaceutics. The Arabic translation, however, was not turned into Latin. Instead, the chapters on *materia medica* in Arabic encyclopaedias, as well as specialized Arabic treatises on medicinal substances, were translated into Latin for European readers. In the Arabic works, medicinals were used that came from as far away as China, South-East Asia, the Himalayas, southern India, and Africa. The largest and most popular of *materia medica* manuals was that by Ibn al-Bayṭār, who was born in Málaga in the kingdom of Granada towards the end of the twelfth century and became 'chief of botanists' in Cairo in the first half of the thirteenth century. His treatise covered over 1,400 medicaments in 2,324 separate entries and formed the basis of many subsequent manuals on medicinal substances. In addition to the Arabic guides to *materia medica* reaching Europe in a Latin format, many of the substances themselves were transported to Europe, along with numerous spices and herbs used in cooking as well as in medicine. The influence of Arabic treatises on simple and compound remedies, as well as the importation of drugs, can readily be seen in the first European official pharmacopoeia, written in Italian by Ludovico dal Pozzo Toscanelli, a physician of Florence, and published in 1499. Subsequent pharmacopoeias in European vernacular languages continued to show the influence of Islamic pharmacology until the beginning of the nineteenth century.

The form of drug jar most popular in Europe for storing herbs, roots, seeds, spices, and other medicinal substances also arose in the Islamic world. *Albarello* is the name given to drug jars having a contracted waist, allowing them to be easily removed from a row when set side by side on a shelf. The design employed by the pharmaceutical potters of Europe was taken directly from the medieval Islamic world, for the earliest examples were made in Syria in the twelfth and thirteenth centuries. Similarly, a distinctive style of mortar and pestle that was produced in Spanish-Islamic centres has been found at medieval sites in England and Wales, apparently transported by traders, and it can be seen to have influenced some of the earliest Italian mortars.

Of great potential influence in Europe was the model of the Islamic hospital. The hospital was one of the great achievements of medieval Islamic society. The relation of the design and development of Islamic hospitals to the poor and sick relief facilities offered by some Christian monasteries has not been fully delineated. The medieval Islamic hospital was a largely secular institution, although it usually included a mosque or some other place for prayer within the precincts. Many of them were open to all, male and female, civilian and military, adult and child, rich and poor, Muslims and non-Muslims. They tended to be large, urban structures and to serve several purposes: a centre of medical treatment, a convalescent home for those recovering from illness or accidents, an insane asylum, and a retirement home giving basic maintenance needs for the aged and infirm who lacked a family to care for them. It is unlikely that any truly wealthy person would have gone to a hospital for any purpose, unless taken ill while travelling far from home, for ordinarily all the medical needs of the wealthy and powerful would have been administered in the home or through outpatient clinics dispensing drugs. An association with a hospital seems, however, to have been highly desirable for a physician, and

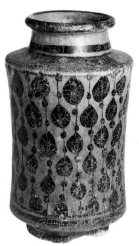

'Albarello' is the name given to drug jars having a waisted form with slightly concave sides, allowing them to be easily removed from shelves. The design arose in the Middle East in the twelfth century and became popular in Europe from the fifteenth century onwards, especially in Italy. This example is one of the earliest, made in Syria about 1200. It is painted in black under a transparent blue glaze.

bedside teaching was advocated by many physicians, such as Haly Abbas. Doctors made regular rounds in the hospitals and often used the patients as well as the attached libraries in their teaching.

The earliest documented hospital established by an Islamic ruler was built in the early ninth century in Baghdad, probably by the vizier to the caliph Ḥārūn al-Rashīd (of *The Thousand and One Nights* fame). In little more than 100 years, five additional hospitals had been built in Baghdad. In Egypt, the first hospital was built in the south-western quarter of present-day Cairo in 872, and by the end of the century two additional ones are said to have been built. In the twelfth century Saladin founded a major hospital in Cairo, although it was soon surpassed in size and importance by the Manṣūrī hospital in Cairo completed in 1284, which remained the primary medical centre in Cairo up to the end of the fifteenth century. In Damascus, the Nūrī hospital was a major one from the time of its foundation in the middle of the twelfth century well into the fifteenth, by which time the city contained five additional hospitals. Besides those in Baghdad, Damascus, and Cairo, other hospitals were built throughout Islamic lands. In al-Qayrawan, the Arabic capital of Tunisia, a hospital was built in the ninth century, and early ones were established at Mecca

The entrance to the hospital built in 1228 in Divriği in east-central Turkey. Pen and ink drawing by Michael Dols, 1988.

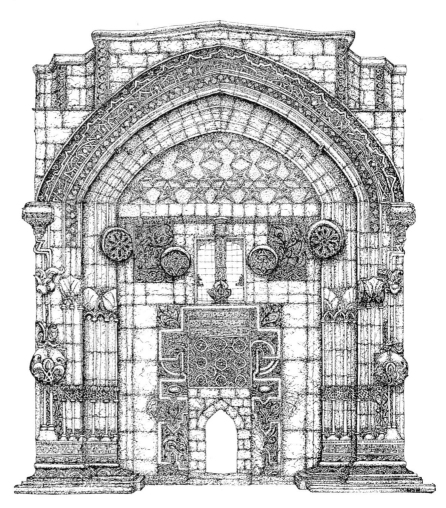

and Medina. Iran had several, including one at Rayy headed by Rhazes prior to his moving to Baghdad. Ottoman hospitals flourished in Turkey in the thirteenth century, and there were hospitals in the Indian provinces. The great Syro-Egyptian hospitals of the twelfth and thirteenth centuries, and those in Ottoman Turkey, were those most familiar to Europeans.

By the end of the fifteenth century the Islamic world was very fragmented, and the vitality and creativity evident in medieval Islamic medicine had disappeared. The hospitals were dependent upon charitable endowments for their maintenance, and with time these funds became insufficient to support them, or, not infrequently, the lands supporting the endowment were confiscated. As a result the hospitals tended to deteriorate and fall into disuse. The practice of medicine in general deteriorated to the point where it no longer represented the medieval tradition at its best.

In the latter half of the sixteenth century Islamic medicine became receptive to some of the ideas, techniques, and drug therapies developing in Europe. Modern European influence can first be seen in the earliest Islamic treatise on syphilis. This was written by ʿImad al-Dīn Masʿūd Shīrāzī, a physician at the hospital in Mashhad in north-east Iran. In his Persian treatise on syphilis, written in 1569, he followed the European practice of advocating for its treatment the use of China root (*chub-chīnī*), the rhizome of an Old World species of smilax found in eastern Asia. This new drug for treating a new disease was rapidly incorporated into Arabic medical writings. For example, Dāʾūd al-Anṭākī, a Syrian physician who died in 1599, included a similar description of syphilis and China root in his Arabic medical encyclopaedia. Dāʾūd al-Anṭākī also relied heavily upon medieval Islamic writers and earlier Greek sources, for which he learnt Greek so as to study them directly.

In the seventeenth century, early modern European medical theory had an impact upon Islamic medicine in the Ottoman Empire through the writings of the Paracelsians, followers of Paracelsus (d. 1541), whose 'chemical medicine' employed mineral acids, inorganic salts, and alchemical procedures in the production of remedies. Ṣāliḥ ibn Naṣr ibn Sallūm, a physician born in Aleppo, Syria, and later court physician in Istanbul to the Ottoman ruler Mehmet IV (ruled 1648–87), was greatly influenced by these writings. Ibn Sallūm incorporated into his book *The Culmination of Perfection in the Treatment of the Human Body* Arabic translations of several Latin Paracelsian writings, such as those of Oswald Croll (d. 1609), Professor of Medicine at the University of Marburg, and Daniel Sennert (d. 1637), Professor of Medicine at Wittenberg. Therapy was primarily a drug therapy, with diseases explained in terms of salt, quicksilver, and sulphur rather than the Galenic theory of the balance of humours. Many of the medicaments required distillation processes and plants that were indigenous to the New World, such as guaiacum and sarsaparilla. Ibn Sallūm's treatise not only reflected the new chemical medicine of the European Paracelsians, but also described for the first time in Arabic a number of 'new' diseases, such as scurvy, chlorosis, anaemia, the English sweat (probably a type of influenza), and plica polonica (an eastern European epidemic of matted and crusted hair cause by infestation with lice). By the seventeenth century it appears that Vesalius' Latin treatise *The Fabric of the Human Body* (*De humani corporis fabrica*) printed in 1542–3 was also known in the Ottoman Empire, for a number of preserved ink sketches from the seventeenth through to the nineteenth centuries indicate familiarity with illustrations from the *Fabrica*. The time lag evident in the introduction of early modern European medicine into the Ottoman Empire may have been due to its being mediated primarily through Jewish physicians migrating to Istanbul in the sixteenth century. The seventeenth-century Ottoman Greeks who studied in Europe, such as Alexander Mavrocordato, while returning to the Ottoman court to become personal physicians to the Grand Viziers, played no active role in bridging the gap between European and Ottoman medicine, even though they themselves had studied the latest European medical theories.

In the Renaissance many Europeans reacted against the anatomy and other medical teachings expounded in medieval Islamic texts, particularly the *Canon* of Avicenna. Leonardo da Vinci (d. 1519) rejected the anatomy, though by necessity he was forced to employ its terminology. Paracelsus (d. 1541) burnt a copy of the *Canon* at Basle, and in the next century the final blow was dealt to the medieval anatomy through the demonstration of the circulation of the blood in 1628 by William Harvey. Yet Harvey had read the *Canon* of Avicenna (probably in Gerard of Cremona's translation), and he knew secondhand the ideas of the twelfth-century physician/philosopher Averroes and cited them in his *Anatomical Lectures* to illustrate particular points. It was not until the time of Thomas Sydenham, who died in 1689, that the new science was sufficiently established that writers such as Sydenham made no reference at all to medieval Islamic physicians.

At the same time that Europeans were beginning to reject the medieval medicine transmitted to them through treatises from the Islamic world, they were also becoming interested in the actual medical practices, and particularly drug therapies, then current in the Islamic world. There was in Europe at this time a renewed awareness of Islam. New trading centres were established, and European states sent ambassadors and consuls to the Ottoman, Safavid, and Mughal courts. For example, Garcia d'Orta (d. 1568), a Jewish physician appointed physician to a Portuguese fleet setting out for India in 1534, prepared careful observations of medicinal plants that he observed in India. He published these in 1563 in his *Coloquios dos simples, e drogas he cousas mediçinais da India*, along with a description of what may have been Asiatic cholera, until then unknown in Western Europe. Many of the drugs he described were previously unknown, such as *Strychnos nux-vomica* L., from which strychnine is derived.

Slightly later in the sixteenth century Leonhard Rauwolf, a Bavarian Protestant physician for whom the genus of tropic plant *Rauwolfia* is named, travelled in Syria, Iraq, and Palestine from 1573 to 1575 and collected plant specimens of 364 species. In 1582 he published his botanical observations, along with descriptions of various customs he had observed (he was the first European to describe the preparation and drinking of coffee). Before travelling to the Middle East, Rauwolf had read Latin translations of Avicenna, Rhazes, Serapion, and Averroes.

Another example from the next century was Joseph Labrosse, who was born in Toulouse in 1636 and entered a Carmelite order, taking the name of Fr Angelus of St Joseph. In 1662 he went to Rome and studied Arabic for two years before travelling to Isfahan to study Persian. While in Iran, he used medicine as a means of propagating Christianity and in the process read many Arabic and Persian books on medicine and 'visited the houses of the learned people of Isfahan and paid hundreds of visits to the shops of the druggists, the pharmacists, and the chemists'. After returning to France in 1678 he published his *Pharmacopoea persica*, which consisted of a Latin translation of a Persian book on compound remedies written in the previous century by Muẓaffar ibn Muḥammad al-Ḥusaynī (d. 1556), with additional comments by Labrosse. A few years later, in 1684, he published *Gazophylacium linguae persarum*, a dictionary of Persian words with Italian, Latin, and French definitions, with much attention paid to medical terms and medicinal substances.

In the eighteenth century some European physicians again showed interest in the medieval Islamic medical literature and in particular in a small monograph on smallpox and measles written in the tenth century by Rhazes. His treatise was not the first on the subject (that honour goes to a ninth-century scholar in Baghdad named Thābit ibn Qurrah), but it was the best-known monograph on the subject within the Islamic world. Rhazes's treatise on smallpox and measles was twice translated into Latin in the eighteenth century, when there was much interest in inoculation or variolation for smallpox following the description around 1720 of the procedure in Turkey by Lady Mary Wortley Montagu, wife of the Ambassador Extraordinary to the Turkish court in Istanbul.

In the middle of the eighteenth century the plague befell Istanbul, and the traditional Islamic medicine seemed to do little to combat it. Consequently, the Ottoman sultan Muṣṭafá III ordered a Turkish translation to be made of two treatises by Hermann Boerhaave (d. 1738), a Dutch medical reformer and advocate of bedside instruction. The Turkish versions were completed in 1768 by the court physician Ṣubḥī-Zāde 'Abd al-'Azīz with the assistance of the Imperial Austrian interpreter Thomas von Herbert. Ṣubḥī-Zāde attempted not only to translate Boerhaave's ideas but to reconcile and harmonize them with traditional Islamic medicine.

In the nineteenth century profound changes occurred in the teaching of medicine in the Near East. In 1825 Antoine-Barthélemy Clot, a physician and surgeon at Montpellier, was appointed by the Egyptian ruler Muḥammad 'Alī to be surgeon-in-chief to the Egyptian army. By 1828 he had established a medical school near Cairo at which French, Italian, and German professors taught. In 1850 a military medical school, the Dār al-Fūnūn, was founded in Tehran in Iran, where the instruction was given in French by professors from Austria and Italy. A number of European medical texts were translated into Persian at this school.

Then, as now, however, aspects of traditional medieval Islamic medicine continued to coexist alongside the modern European medicine. While in Europe in the nineteenth century the Latin translations of medieval Arabic treatises were only read, if at all, by historians, in Cairo the medical treatises of Ibn Sīnā (Avicenna), al-Majūsī (Haly Abbas), and Ibn al-Bayṭār, amongst others, were printed because they continued to represent a vital tradition, which the Yunani medical colleges of Pakistan and India are continuing, at least in part, to maintain today.

4 | Medicine in the Latin Middle Ages

MICHAEL R. McVAUGH

THE Latin Middle Ages are sometimes explained as the gradual fusion, in the wake of a vanishing Roman Empire, of three cultures or traditions: classical, Christian, and Germanic. If the last of these is broadened to refer to a 'folk' or empiric element, the same analysis works not too badly as a characterization of medieval medicine, and helps us to understand the remarkable changes that medicine began to undergo about the middle of the eleventh century, when the classical medical tradition began to overshadow the other two.

From Rome (and so Greece) the early Middle Ages inherited first of all the sense that medicine was a rational art, so that diseases could be 'searched through to their causes in the light of reason', an achievement that Isidore of Seville (d. 636) credited first of all to Hippocrates. They inherited, too, a small collection of medical literature in Latin: Cassiodorus (d. 583) recommended that his community at Vivarium study 'the *herbarium* of Dioscorides . . . Hippocrates and Galen in Latin translation, namely Galen's *Therapeutics* written for the philosopher Glauco . . . Aurelius Caelius *De medicina*, Hippocrates *De herbis et curis*, and other works concerned with the art of healing'. Even though it is impossible to identify securely all these items, the list still suggests something of the character of the medical learning available to readers in the early Middle Ages. Caelius Aurelianus' *Acute and Chronic Diseases*, a guide produced in the early fifth century, represents a Latin-language medical literature at its most learned (though, admittedly, based on a second-century Greek text by Soranus), but several other far less sophisticated medical handbooks were in wide circulation. The reference to Hippocrates and Galen shows us that some of the Greek sources of that Roman literature were now also accessible in Latin, though we must not overestimate its amount or mistake its character: the most important, besides Galen's *Ad Glauconem*, were perhaps Hippocrates' *Aphorisms* and *Prognostics*, while Galen's longer, more theoretical treatises were missing. The early Middle Ages found most useful the texts with an immediately practical function, like the many herbals—often illustrated—that circulated under the name of Dioscorides or Hippocrates or Apuleius.

We can see in the surviving medical literature of Anglo-Saxon England one example of how classical medical thought could meld with folk or empiric practices and traditional beliefs. Some of those texts are Anglo-Saxon translations from the Latin of works like Dioscorides' *Herbal* or the *Herbarium* of pseudo-Apuleius. Others, such as Bald's *Leechbook* (*c*.900?), incorporate extensive citations from a considerable range of classical sources which alternate with remedies that appear to represent purely local practice. *Lacnunga* (11th century?), which has been described as a kind of medical commonplace book, prescribes both native English herbs and exotic Eastern ingredients and is revealing not only for its fascination with magical remedies, amulets, and charms, but for its acceptance of old folk explanations of disease—'elfshot', for example, caused by elves or witches or other spirits. A range of entirely comparable medical compendia can be found on the European continent as well; rather than a degeneration of classical medicine, this fusion of traditions in early medieval society might better be understood as a medicine increasingly reoriented towards an empirical practice and away from medical learning.

Christianity and Medicine

Early Christianity often expressed a certain ambivalence towards medicine of any kind, learned or practical. If God sends disease, to try to cure it can be seen as interference with His will, and it is only He who should be asked to heal; it may be a visitation for sin, and then repentance and prayer are the proper therapy. In this regard, the New Testament's many accounts of miraculous cures encouraged popular belief in the healing power of relics and shrines. St Augustine (d. 430) gave details of many such cures he had seen in his own day, often emphasizing that the physicians charged with the case had given up all hope of the patient's recovery. On the other hand, the physician can also be understood as God's agent for ministering to the sick, the practice of medicine understood as an exercise of Christian charity. In fact these attitudes seem to have coexisted: to visit a shrine in search of a cure did not preclude seeking medical care from a healer as well.

There was, of course, no professional medical corps in the early Middle Ages; even the institutionalized municipal practitioner of Roman times had disappeared from the cities of France and Italy by the seventh century. Nor was there any systematic medical education. Although occasionally at the courts of the Frankish or Ostrogothic rulers one finds reference to physicians with some claim to learning, most of the healers who served the public must have acquired their art as a practical craft—like Morigund, a Frankish woman who healed ulcers with prayers, the sign of the cross, and spittle mixed with leaves or fruit. If a written medical tradition continued to exert some influence, it was primarily within a Christian clergy. Monastic and cathedral libraries made elements of the classical medical tradition available to clerics, at least to some: John of Beverly (d. 721) chastised the nuns of Watton for not knowing that it was perilous to bleed a patient during the moon's waxing; the letters of Bishop Fulbert of Chartres (d. 1028) to his friends include a surprising amount of detailed medical advice and make clear that he was remarkably adept at compounding medicines. And the knowledge of such clerics was inevitably put to use outside as well as inside the church: a monk like Notker of St Gall (d.

975) tended his fellows within the monastery itself, as prescribed by St Bene-dict, but was often summoned away to attend laymen. Christian charity also encouraged the gradual spread in the West of hospices (their early name of *xen-odochia* reveals their origin in the Greek East) to care for the sick and needy, hos-pices often established by bishops or abbots as well as by the laity; though it would have been extraordinary to find them providing regular medical atten-tion.

Yet it would be difficult to insist on a sharp distinction between a learned and a popular practice in this period. Both kinds of practitioners offered simi-lar diagnostic, prognostic, and therapeutic procedures that might mix natu-ralistic with Christian or other ritual elements. Notker could tell a patient's condition simply from his or her urine, but monastic communities made much use of number magic as well as of Hippocrates' *Prognostics* in their con-cern to determine whether a sick brother would live or die.

A New Medical Learning

The relationship among these three traditions started to change rapidly at the end of the eleventh century, when a number of factors encouraged a new emphasis upon the classical, intellectual, strand in medicine. The process began when a North African named Constantine became a monk at one of the great European monasteries, Monte Cassino in southern Italy, and during the last three decades of the century prepared Latin versions of a long list of Ara-bic-language medical works—some originally Greek, like Galen's *Ars parva* (or *Tegni*) and his commentaries on the Hippocratic *Aphorisms* and *Prognostics*, and others composed in Arabic, like the encyclopaedic *Pantegni* of ʿAlī ibn al-ʿAbbās al-Majūsī (known in the West as Haly Abbas) or the *Viaticum* of Ibn al-Jazzār. With these works Western Europe now had available to it the details of the theoretical medical system—Galenism—developed in antiquity.

Constantine's translations had to be read and used in order to be of impor-tance; and only 100 miles to the south of Monte Cassino was the city of Salerno, whose medical practitioners had long enjoyed a certain fame. Here in about 1100 a tradition of medical instruction from standard texts began to develop, a tradition—paralleling the simultaneous development of arts education in the cathedral schools of the north—that seized avidly upon the new body of Graeco-Arabic medical literature. Over the next 100 years a series of Salernitan masters subjected Constantine's translations to intense study, in the process establishing the broad outlines of medical education as it would exist for half a millennium. They gradually fixed upon a canon of writings fundamental to students of medicine, known collectively as the *Articella* or *Ars medica*: this canon comprised the *Isagoge* or *Introduction to Medicine* of Johannitius (Ḥunayn ibn Isḥāq), Hippocrates' *Aphorisms* and *Prognostics*, Galen's *Ars parva*, and two originally Byzantine treatises explaining prognosis from urines and pulse. The Salernitans extended the evolving scholastic techniques of gloss and com-mentary to these texts, articulating the schematic outline of classical physiol-ogy and pathology comprised by the *Articella* with the much more comprehensive *Pantegni*, and in this way medicine at Salerno began to open the way to the development there of a broader, rather eclectic philosophy of

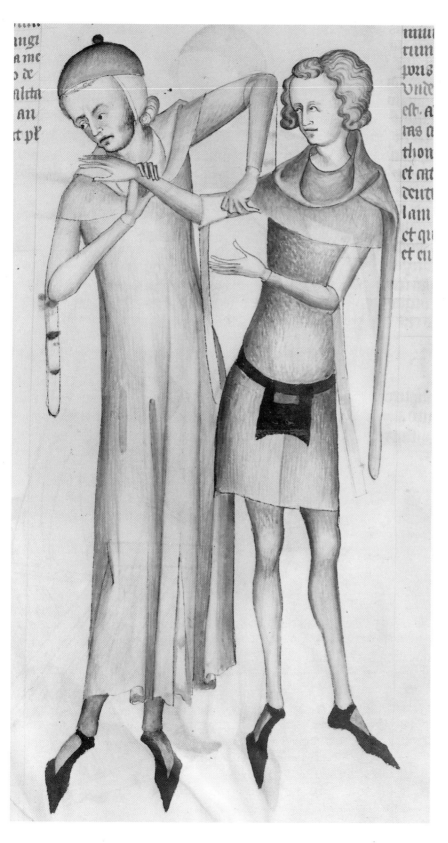

Taking the pulse at the
brachial artery. As the text
explains, this procedure is
a relatively late stage in
examining a patient.

nature; across the Alps, Fulbert's twelfth-century successors at the cathedral school at Chartres used the *Pantegni* as an authoritative source for their cosmological systems. In a gradual exchange, the term *physica*—which had originally applied to the study of nature and the cosmos—came in the twelfth century to be taken over as the name for a new kind of philosophically and rationally based medicine, and the term 'physicus' began to carry a connotation of learning that the older label 'medicus' could not.

The Beginnings of University Medicine

About the year 1200, groups of cathedral masters like those at Chartres began to receive legal recognition of their corporate status as universities, with authority over curricular and graduation requirements—first applied to the study of the liberal arts, but soon including the higher faculties of law, theology, and medicine. The thirteenth-century universities of Paris and Montpellier replaced Salerno as magnets for medical study, but they continued to base classroom instruction on the *Articella* texts. The new degrees of bachelor and master in medicine presumed not only study in the schools but practical training outside: by Montpellier's regulations of 1240, a practicum of six months' experience outside the city was a prerequisite for the master's degree, and the implication that students also followed their masters on visits to local patients seems obvious. For the teaching masters were practitioners as well—indeed, their practice was usually far more financially profitable than their teaching. The new textual genres of regimen and *consilium*—instructions aimed at a particular patient designed, respectively, for those who were healthy and those who were ill—were developed at the hands of thirteenth-century academic practitioners, such as Arnau de Vilanova of Montpellier (d. 1311) or Taddeo Alderotti of Bologna (d. 1295). But we must not suppose these early faculties to be mirrors of today's medical schools: they were still tiny—probably comprising no more than a few dozen individuals, masters and students together—and the essential core of their instruction remained the written word.

Constantine the African's works had been only the beginnings of a flood of translations produced during the twelfth century, from Greek as well as from Arabic, that had made virtually all the great achievements of earlier philosophy and medicine potentially accessible to Latin readers. While intellectually it was perhaps the philosophical works of Aristotle that were in the long run the most important of these new translations, treatises on medicine—mostly produced in the second half of the century—were more numerous. In Italy, Burgundio of Pisa rendered half a dozen works of Galen into Latin from Greek. In Spain, Gerard of Cremona translated some seventy scientific and philosophical texts from the Arabic (probably with the help of assistants), including Galen's *De complexionibus*, *De crisi*, *De creticis diebus*, and several others by the same author, and a number of the great texts of Arabic medicine: Rhazes' *Liber almansoris*, Serapion's *Breviarium*, Albucasis' *Surgery*, and, above all, Avicenna's *Canon*.

None of these new texts had been studied in Salerno, which was still trying to assimilate the Constantinian translations, and they made their way into the new university medical faculties only gradually, but by the 1230s Avicenna at least was being widely quoted. For teachers and students trying to master an intricate new intellectual world, the *Canon* was invaluable: it was authoritative, comprehensive, systematic, well organized. It gave medical faculties a first guide to assimilating the much less systematic works of Galen that the twelfth-century translation movement had produced. Then, from around 1300, we begin to find evidence that learned medicine felt ready to turn towards the study of Galen himself: evidence of new teaching aids, like the concordances to Galen and other authors drawn up at Paris; evidence of changing curricula, like that of Montpellier in 1309 which supplemented the old *Articella* with a wide range of Galen's own works; and evidence from one last wave of Galenic translations, some from Arabic but more than forty from Greek, the work of Niccolò da Reggio in southern Italy (fl. 1308–45). By the middle of the fourteenth century, a commitment to the breadth of classical medical literature characterized the new academic medicine, not only at Paris and Montpellier but at other schools like Bologna and Padua as well.

In the course of mastering these works, the new medical faculties sharpened their sense of what their intellectual world should comprise, in part at least by distinguishing it from natural philosophy. Some part of their subject, they insisted, should be recognized as *scientia* in the Aristotelian sense—true knowledge proceeding from first principles—but another part was *ars*, a term implying practical skill and experience. Their increasing familiarity with Galen's own writings revealed how often he and Aristotle were in disagreement on topics with medical implications (on the physiological role of the heart, for example). Pietro d'Abano's *Conciliator* (*c.*1310) is only the most famous of the many attempts to define the relationship between the truths of natural philosophy and those of medicine.

But the masters' continuing attention to niceties of detail did not materially alter the general outlines of either the theory or the practice of medicine. The basic elements of physiological and pathological theory remained the four humours and the four qualities (the latter fused in a patient's 'complexion'); their respective balance and temperancy were understood to be the objectives of health. Humoral imbalance or complexional distemperancy could be diagnosed easily through examination of the urine. Prognosis was assisted by the doctrine of critical days, days when illnesses were liable to take a decisive turn for better or worse. Therapeutic procedures followed the Hippocratic triad of regimen, manipulating not merely diet but sleep and activity, sex, and climate; drugs; and surgery, including bloodletting.

Such a system was at the heart of a widespread medical culture that was becoming broadly familiar to most inhabitants of medieval Europe in a variety of ways. Comprehensive works like the *Canon* can be found in the hands of practitioners who had no academic background, surgeons as well as physicians. The enormously popular therapeutic collection assembled by Peter of Spain (d. 1277), his *Thesaurus pauperum*, made the learned literature still more widely accessible by distilling it into a list of fifty diseases and the dozens of remedies that had been recommended for each; at least twenty copies of this work still survive from the period before 1350. In Germany, where no medical faculties existed and academic medicine was correspondingly rare, the vernacular handbook composed by Ortolf von Baierland (*c.*1280?) provided an

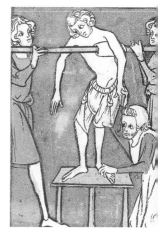

Reducing a dislocated shoulder by bracing the axilla and pulling down on the arm.

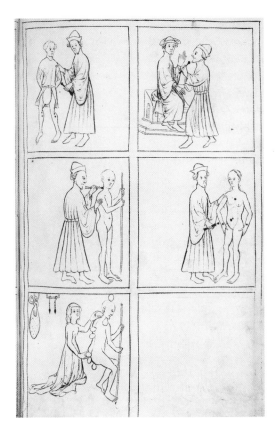

Cauterizing and cupping.
A physician applies cauteries for therapeutic purposes, a practice encouraged by Albucasis. At the bottom, a woman draws blood from a patient by cupping.

equally popular summary of physiology, pathology, and therapeutics. Vernacular translations of Latin medical works also appear in growing numbers during the later thirteenth century, with surgical texts an especial object of attention.

Medicine in an Urban Society

What made possible the dissemination of a learned medicine were the economic recovery of the Middle Ages, the rapid growth of the European population, and the revival of towns as centres of commercial and social activity—all features of the three centuries after AD 1000. The towns provided just the concentrated market necessary for the new medicine to flourish, and it is no coincidence that institutional changes in medieval health care regularly originated in the south, in the bustling Italian cities, and then gradually spread west and north. Yet academic medicine would not have developed and spread so widely if it had not been actively welcomed by the lay public. Medical learning had always been valued in some sectors of early medieval society—witness its patronage by the Frankish kings—but in the later Middle Ages it seems to have profited from a widening public perception that scholastic training led to both truth and a career: if university study made one more successful in the law or the church, should not the same be true of medicine? In the later thirteenth century, the growing European towns were beginning to prescribe that their practitioners have several years of formal education or else demonstrate equivalent preparation in a licensing examination—an unenforceable prescription, in fact, since only an insignificant number of physicians had received even a little university training, but one which shows that the public was an enthusiastic supporter of the new trend. So do the various legal procedures in which, again about 1300, lay authority was replaced by medical authority, in forensic testimony, for example, or in determinations of leprosy: individuals accused of being leprous felt more secure in entrusting this critical decision—one that might commit them for ever to a lazar house—to a physician than to their neighbours.

More broadly, municipal governments were beginning to express a concern for public health, motivated by charity as well as by social and economic self-interest. The classical institution of municipal physician began to be seen again, first of all in the larger cities of Italy and southern Europe, and it is notably the academically trained doctor who was most in demand. Arrangements varied widely, but as a normal minimum the municipal physician was expected, in return for his salary, to reside permanently in the city and to provide diagnostic and prognostic attention—sometimes free, sometimes for a small fee—to all citizens and their families; the prevention of illness by anticipating its signs in the urine or complexion and by prescribing an appropriate regimen was the ideal. Fourteenth-century Italian and Spanish cities also began here and there to provide support for hospices, institutions that had hitherto been exclusively ecclesiastical charities. The late-medieval hospices still ordinarily housed the indigent as well as the sick, but a few were served by salaried physicians and surgeons and developed an almost exclusively medical function: a prominent example is the hospital of Santa Maria Nuova in Florence, founded in 1288, which by 1313 had separate wards for male and female patients.

Academic versus Popular Medicine

Under these circumstances a correspondingly lower valuation came to be placed on popular or purely empirical medicine. University-trained physicians wrote dismissively—and perhaps sometimes a little defensively—about the practice of unqualified healers, the *vulgus*; they referred scornfully to the unscientific remedies and charms of old women (*vetule*). Though many expressed themselves as willing in principle to believe that such practitioners could make medical discoveries, they insisted that these discoveries had to be incorporated into an established scientific framework if they were to be truly useful. The *Antipocras* written *c.*1270 by a Dominican *medicus*, the empiric Nicholas of Montpellier, denied angrily that medicine should be controlled by reason and an élite and argued instead that God continually revealed the secrets of his creation's healing powers to the common people whom he loved; but Nicholas was fighting a battle that had already been lost.

In so far as such irregular medical practice was subjected to controls, it was controlled by municipal authority rather than a nascent medical profession, for guilds of medical practitioners of any kind were only slowly coming into existence. However, it was not in the civic interest to suppress a non-academic medicine entirely; the need for some kind of health care to be available to the public meant that a variety of medical occupations was tolerated everywhere, not just physicians but surgeons, barbers, and apothecaries as well. The apothecaries' separate responsibility for preparing medicaments was only gradually being defined during the early thirteenth century—municipal regulations trying to prevent collusion between them and physicians are a commonplace thereafter—and it seemed particularly natural to trust them as providers of routine medical advice. Indeed, even unlettered empirics, healers who offered medical care to their fellow villagers without claiming any formal occupational label, normally encountered no bar to their practice.

Such healers might include women as well as men, but increasingly women were being driven into the lower levels of this spectrum of medical learning. Rarely in the twelfth century women healers can be found sharing in the new literate medicine, like Salerno's shadowy Trotula, but this came to an end when that medicine became institutionalized in the universities, from which women were automatically excluded by their sex. However, they continued to offer medical care locally and, university trained or no, could even acquire a certain familiarity with the world of learning. In 1306 a woman named Geralda from a village outside Barcelona was questioned about her medical practice among her acquaintances: she admitted that she diagnosed

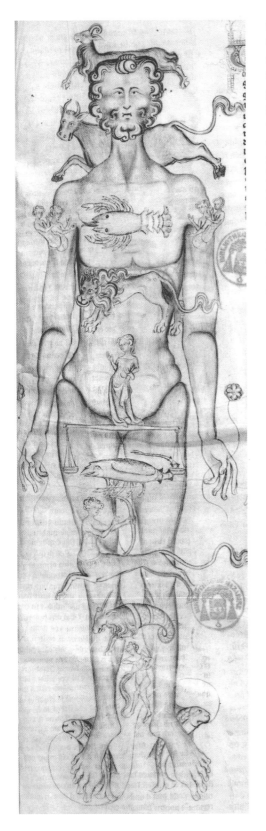

their condition by looking at their urines, but insisted that she never prescribed any medicines for them, and the senior physician in Barcelona agreed that under those conditions she could be allowed to continue to practise. Exceptionally in Paris, a woman empiric named Jacoba Felicie was prosecuted by the medical faculty in 1322 for unlicensed medical practice and, despite the testimony of numerous satisfied clients, was found guilty and fined sixty pounds; but Paris was the largest and wealthiest city in Europe, with an unusually powerful and assertive academic medical corporation.

Actually, between the practice of Jacoba, at one end of the spectrum of learning, and that of her learned urban practitioner-accusers, at the other, there was probably considerable common ground. Village healers eagerly assimilated scraps of medical theory when they could—Geralda had learnt her uroscopy from a physician passing through town—while academic physicians not infrequently felt free to incorporate empiric tradition into their treatments: Gilbertus Anglicus' recommendation (*c.*1240) to wrap smallpox victims in red cloth is an obvious example of this latter tendency, whether it foreshadows the Finsen red-light treatment for the disease or not. Still, the practice of all healers—including surgeons, apothecaries, and barbers—was subordinated more and more to the control of the learned tradition, at least in the urban centres of the Continent. The Parisian faculty required (1271) the city's apothecaries to administer medicines only in the presence of physicians; the kings of Aragon in eastern Spain ordained (1332) that the barbers of Valencia might bleed patients only on days determined by physicians to be astrologically favourable—astrology, if not yet at a particularly sophisticated level, was coming to be part of the baggage that physicians were expected to possess. As the surgeon Henri de Mondeville (fl. 1310) complained, the emphasis on learning was taking therapeutic and prophylactic phlebotomy out of the hands of barbers and surgeons and giving it to physicians.

The Growth of Surgery and Anatomy

Not surprisingly, therefore, we can detect the growing enthusiasm for learning affecting the internal development of even so determinedly empirical a subject as surgery. Originally a purely craft tradition, it began towards the end of the twelfth century to make itself over into a literate subject with pretensions to the scientific status its practitioners envied in medicine. The *Surgery* of Roger Frugardi of Parma, composed about 1180, launched this tradition; within fifty years it had been reissued with a commentary by Roland of Parma, which was in turn followed by a string of increasingly ambitious Italian surveys of surgery over the next 100 years—surveys which incorporated the new scholastic authorities, Avicenna and Albucasis, and which began to insist on the importance of anatomy as a necessary starting-point if surgery were to have a truly scientific character. The new literate surgery came to Paris about 1300 with Lanfranco, a political exile from his native Milan, and it is in France in the early fourteenth century that we find the most articulate defence of surgery's intellectual character in the *Surgery* of Henri de Mondeville, whose attacks on unlearned, untrained empirics are particularly fierce.

Mondeville had studied medicine in the universities, and perhaps surgery as well, for here and there in the schools of France, Spain, and especially Italy provision had been made for chairs of surgery. At the same time, but independent of that tendency, anatomical dissection was becoming a regular if occasional feature of medical education. Twelfth-century Salerno had already practised dissection on the pig as a way of illustrating the internal anatomy of humans, which it was supposed to resemble closely; the dissection of actual human cadavers in the universities seems to have grown out of forensic appeal to postmortem examinations in Italy, shortly before 1300, although Montpellier in France had provided for an annual dissection by 1340. In 1316 Mondino dei Liuzzi, professor at Bologna, produced an *Anatomy* meant as a handbook to accompany such dissections, which enjoyed popularity for centuries. Mondino's *Anatomy*, like the anatomies that surgeons incorporated into their texts, was not illustrated; Mondeville was unusual in having used pictures to teach the subject to students.

The Secularization of Medicine

The increasing importance of learning for medical careers corresponded with an increasing secularization of the discipline and a weakening of clerical involvement in it. In a sense, of course, academic medicine everywhere remained under ecclesiastical control, since universities were ecclesiastical institutions and their masters, by that token, in minor orders, but the old days in which bishops and abbots, priests and monks, might routinely be found offering medical advice and care were passing rapidly. In part this was the result of the Church's own decisions, growing out of the reform movement of the twelfth century. The new canon lawyers of the twelfth century had questioned whether churchmen could practise medicine for

Academic versus Popular Medicine

A zodiac man (*facing*), illustrating the parts of the body thought to be subject to the different zodiacal signs.

Surgical instruments from Guy de Chauliac's *Chirurgia magna* (1363). Drawings of surgical instruments often deteriorated in quality as a text was copied over and over, but these carefully drawn pictures of trepans, rasps, and other instruments for the treatment of head fractures are close in time to their originals.

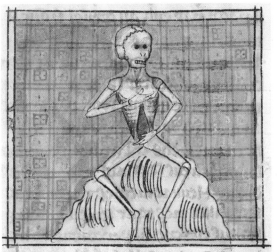
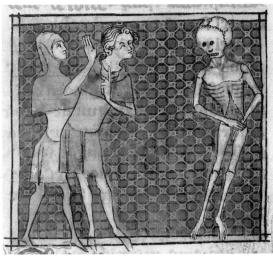

Anatomical illustrations. Though schematic, these pictures are among the earliest illustrations of a surgical text, in this case the *Chirurgia* of Henri de Mondeville, who had himself used anatomical illustrations in his teaching of surgery.

gain—indeed, whether one could function as a priest having been responsible for injury or death to a patient—and eventually the Fourth Lateran Council of 1215 prohibited those in major orders from practising surgery, at the same time restricting many clerics from leaving their posts for the purpose of studying medicine. The result was gradually to cut much of the clergy off from the kind of training that would increasingly be seen as a prerequisite for offering medical care, at the same time as medicine became an attractive secular occupation. There were still famous practitioners in the thirteenth century who held high ecclesiastical positions: the surgical author Teodorico Borgognoni (d. 1298), who was bishop of Cervia; or Petrus Hispanus, Peter of Spain, who was physician to Pope Gregory X before becoming successively archbishop of Braga, cardinal of Tusculum, and finally Pope (as John XXI). But in the next 100 years the importance of the clerical practitioner began to diminish, particularly in the south; further north—in England, for example—he remained a familiar figure much longer.

As time went on the Church's ambivalence about the value of secular medical assistance certainly diminished. In the twelfth century, St Bernard of Clairvaux (d. 1153) was still warning his brethren not to take special precautions for their health, but 100 years or so later prelates and their chapters were, with royalty, among the first patrons of the new academic medicine, providing the most famous learned doctors with a retainer to ensure that their services would always be available. Monastic communities still depended upon an infirmarer to provide routine health care, but by 1300 they regularly turned outside to the lay world in emergencies—not only in the south but in the north, as when the physician Robert de Renham was called to the dying Abbot of Westminster in 1307. The problem for the Church was now to keep medicine in its place, making sure that the health of the body was not valued above the health of the soul. It was again the Fourth Lateran Council that had tried to keep the two distinct by requiring physicians to get their patients to confess their sins to a priest before treating them, since 'anima sit multo preciosior corpore' (the soul is far more precious than the body) and—a conviction still deeply embedded—bodily illness might be the consequence of sin; but practi-

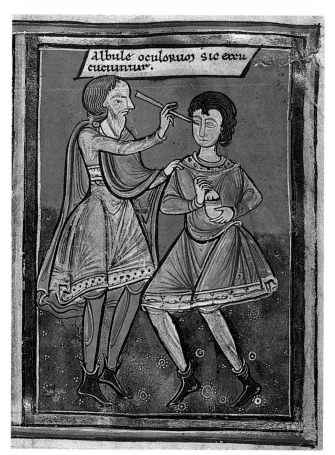

albule oculorum sic exeu cuciuntur.

An operation for cataract (*left*). The text says that it is being cut out, but the operation normally described in surgical texts was for couching, displacing the clouded lens from the axis of vision without removing it from the eye.

Examining a wounded patient (*below*). As in this case, physicians and surgeons were routinely accompanied by assistants in their practice.

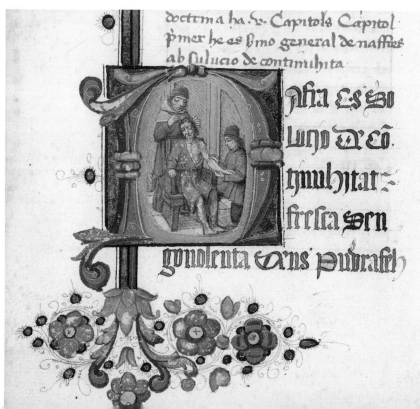

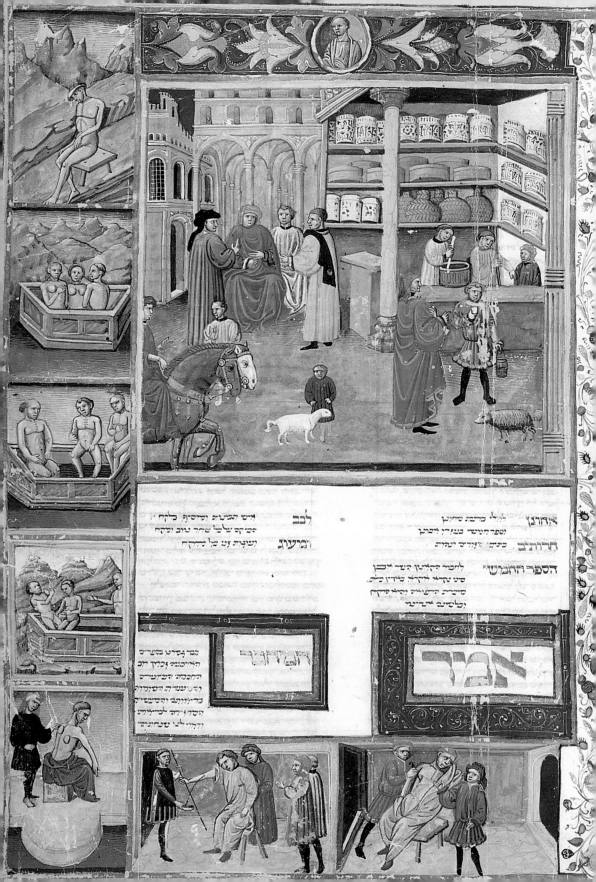

אהרן לַחֲלֵל מַרְבַּת שִׁחוּן לֵב וְיֵשׁ הַטֶּבַע וְהַיָסִיף כֹּלֶחַ
נַסְפַּר חִיוּרְשֵׁי בַּנַּרְיִן לְבַכַן הַבְקָה צָלוּל שַׁחַר טוֹב וְהָקַח
חַדּוֹתָב בָּיֵתֶם עַוְרַד יְשָׁחוֹת וּמֵעָט וְשָׁעוֹת צֵץ כֹּל סְחַח
הַסֵּפֶר וְהַחֹמֶשׁ לְחֵפֶר הַקָלוֹן הַצָּר אֲלֶבֶן
שֶׁנֵי נֶחֱלָא לִיקְרָא בֹּלדֵין כְּלָל
מֵהֲבַרָה הַשְׁמַעוֹת וְהֶלֵא סְרֵיחָה
יְהֹלְשִׁיעָא אֲרַהֲבִיטִי

נַבָּר בָּקְרֵת מֵחָרְרֵים
הַאֲיְהוֹנֵה וְכָּלֵף יֹב
הַהֲכַמֵה הַשְׁבַשֵׁירַם
וְהֵי צַשְׁחִיָה הַקִינִינוֹת
בַּרְ וְזַרַהַב וְהַהַבְשְׁלוֹל
הַהֵד יֵרַד לְבַילִימוֹת
וְהֵרִי לֵטָ שְׁכַחוֹבֵהּ

tioners worried that this would lead the sick to despair of their recovery, and, judging from the frequency with which the requirement was reiterated by the Church in the fourteenth century, it continued to be often neglected.

Religious motives also led Christian society to try to control, at least locally, the practice of medicine by Jews. The Jewish physician traditionally had a reputation for medical learning that appealed to the new Europe of the High Middle Ages, and in countries where Jews were tolerated Jewish physicians can be found treating Christians of all kinds, from peasants to kings. Yet at the same time Christian suspicion of the Jews (back to Gregory of Tours) hedged medical practice round with various restrictions or prohibitions: sometimes the Church forbade Christians to seek treatment from Jews at all; sometimes a municipality insisted that a Jew could only attend Christian patients in company with a Christian practitioner, who would administer whatever medicines were necessary. Again, the popular attractiveness of the new medicine was such that these restrictions were often ignored or left unenforced, though the very fact that they existed put Jewish practitioners at a competitive disadvantage. Jews could not attend the universities, of course, and, as medical graduates slowly increased in number, the importance of the Jewish practitioner in Christian society began correspondingly to decline.

At least in principle, the secular practitioner of the High Middle Ages was supposed to be guided by motives of Christian compassion just as much as the priest-physician of earlier centuries had been. Ideally, perhaps, the late medieval physician treated the poor without charge, but complaints about the avarice of medical practitioners suggest that charitable concern did not always come first. Perhaps more widely accepted as a norm for occupational behaviour were certain principles of occupational etiquette, based largely on passages from Hippocratic sources: the physician should avoid ostentation, should act with propriety towards his patients and their households, should be cautious in taking on dangerous cases, and should in general act as was necessary to maintain his psychological authority over his patient.

We should not be misled into believing, from the emergence of occupational guilds or from the sudden appearance of licensing, that a self-conscious and self-regulating profession of medicine had come into being by 1350. The practice of medicine was still so diffuse, so varied, that medical service might be better understood as a kind of contract between physician-sellers and patient-buyers in which the latter were often in the stronger bargaining position—a situation probably not very different from that current in Rome in Galen's day, almost 1,200 years earlier. Indeed, the medicine of the High Middle Ages could be thought of as a kind of fulfilment of the medicine of antiquity: a mix of traditions and approaches among which the rationalist enjoyed particular prestige. No doubt academic physicians felt themselves to be solidly in that tradition as they recovered and expounded the works of Galen. They certainly had not yet fully appreciated their age's institutionalization of medical education for what it was: a profoundly significant innovation, with the long-term potential for standardizing medical learning while conferring distinctive social power and status on its possessors.

A Hebrew medical manuscript. This fifteenth-century Italian manuscript of the medical textbook of Avicenna testifies to the continuing centrality of Arabic medical learning in the Renaissance and to the importance of Jews as medical scholars, teachers, and practitioners. The principal scene shows a physician (in red) holding a walk-in clinic in a pharmacy, while the marginal images demonstrate common therapeutic practices such as thermal baths, cupping, phlebotomy, and cautery.

5 | Medicine and the Renaissance

KATHARINE PARK

LIKE Giovanni Boccaccio's *Decameron*, the Renaissance period was overshadowed by plague. The *Decameron* begins with a vivid description of the Black Death, which had attacked the city of Florence four years earlier, in 1348. 'It started in the East,' Boccaccio wrote,

> either because of the influence of heavenly bodies or because of God's just wrath as a punishment to mortals for our wicked deeds, and it killed an infinite number of people. Without pause it spread from one place and it stretched its miserable length over the West. And against this pestilence no human wisdom or foresight was of any avail; quantities of filth were removed from the city by officials charged with this task; the entry of any sick person into the city was prohibited; and many directives were issued concerning the maintenance of good health. Nor were the humble supplications, rendered not once but many times to God by pious people, through public processions or by other means, efficacious.

Plague dominated the experience of Europeans from 1348 until well into the seventeenth century, returning repeatedly in a series of epidemics of varying severity. Its demographic consequences were devastating; between a third and a half of all Europeans died in the Black Death of 1348–53, and the population continued to drop catastrophically through the later fifteenth century, when the plague began gradually and intermittently to loosen its grip. In the 1490s, however, plague was joined by another frightening 'new' illness, in the form of syphilis, often known as *morbus gallicus* (French pox). Although syphilis never rivalled plague as a threat to collective health, its chronic character and the virulent and disfiguring form it took in its early years made it a special object of horror.

The prominence of plague and syphilis should not obscure the wide range of disease and other illness—endemic and epidemic, chronic and acute—that affected the inhabitants of both city and countryside in the Renaissance period. Rather, they stand as a reminder that pre-modern Europe was, by modern standards, a poor and remarkably unhealthy place—prone to famine and organized around crowded towns and cities strewn with rubbish and human and animal waste. These facts run counter to the common view of the Renaissance as an undifferentiated period of cultural progress and economic prosperity. Plague and syphilis challenged both the health of the population and the systems of healing that Europeans had inherited from their medieval predecessors. Although neither disease responded particularly well to contemporary medical techniques, both helped to encourage the foundation of hospitals, the development of elaborate public-health regulations, as Boccaccio suggested, and the creation of new institutions such as colleges of physicians, dedicated to protecting the practice and reputation of the higher levels of the medical profession.

At the same time, there was a great deal of continuity between medieval and Renaissance medicine, in the areas not only of therapeutics and systems of explanation but also of institutions and organization. The most dramatic developments in European health care belonged in fact to the thirteenth and early fourteenth centuries, when princes, universities, and municipalities began to develop the institutional, legal, and social frameworks that would structure the study and practice of medicine until at least the eighteenth century. By 1348 the emergent shape of those frameworks was clear, at least in the more highly urbanized parts of Europe such as northern and central Italy, southern France, and Spain. The succeeding three centuries saw significant innovations, such as the systematic humanist programme of searching out, editing, and retranslating ancient medical texts; the invention of printing,

Persecution and plague. This seventeenth-century Italian engraving records the torture and execution of two men—a public-health official and a barber—accused of spreading plague in Milan during the epidemic of 1630. After they had confessed, their bodies were burned and the house in which they had allegedly plotted was demolished and replaced by a memorial pillar, visible in the foreground on the right.

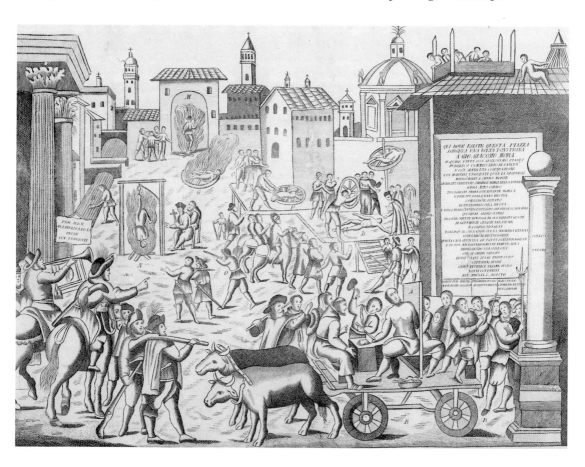

which allowed the diffusion of professional medical ideas and information
among a broader reading public; the appearance of new theories and systems
of healing, such as that proposed by the Swiss medical writer Paracelsus. But
for the most part, Renaissance medicine, in both theory and practice, represented a gradual development and refinement of techniques, ideas, and institutions inherited from the medieval past.

Sites of Healing and Types of Practice

In Renaissance as in medieval Europe, naturalistic medicine, whether practised by physicians, surgeons, or village herbalists, took its place in a loosely
integrated system of healing that also included religious and magical
approaches. This complex world of health care was embodied in a remarkable
variety of sites of practice and types of practitioner, especially in the larger
cities. All over Europe, however, the primary place where the sick were treated
was the home, and the principal nurses and healers, as numerous illustrations
and medical texts testify, were the women of the household—mothers,
daughters, wives, and servants. Because even professional medicine blurred
the lines between care and cure, the treatment given by these women
resembled in many ways that prescribed by physicians: they opened and closed
windows, burned aromatic substances, provided basic hygiene, prepared
what they considered appropriate food and drink, and administered medicinal preparations that used many of the ingredients found on pharmacists'
shelves.

Some wives and mothers, especially in rural areas where trained medical
personnel were in short supply, developed considerably specialized expertise,
particularly after 1500, when the printing press began to render accessible
medical knowledge previously restricted to professional physicians. Taking
advantage of this new technology, some wealthy women even compiled their
own medical libraries and private recipe collections. The Elizabethan gentlewoman Lady Grace Mildmay, for example, received some education from her
governess in herbal and astrological medicine, as well as minor surgery; she
supplemented this by consulting doctors and other acquaintances and by
reading in various vernacular medical books, and she developed an impressive
repertoire of remedies, both herbal and chemical, which she documented in a
series of manuscripts, manufactured in large quantities, and used to treat her
own family and needy tenants, as well as dependants.

In addition to domestic medicine, people received health care at home from
other practitioners—midwives as well as physicians and surgeons—who made
house calls. As early as the fourteenth century, however, in many European
cities, physicians also saw patients in the context of clinics held in the shops of
apothecaries, with whom they had regular contractual arrangements. There,
they examined ambulatory patients, diagnosed their illness, and made out
prescriptions. Like apothecaries, who provided medical advice as well as selling remedies, some surgeons also maintained their own shops, where they
stored the special tools and instruments required by their work. Like the contracts that often governed the relationships between doctor and patient in the
Renaissance period, formally specifying each party's obligations, the impor-

tance of shop-based practices testifies to the gradualness with which medicine evolved from a craft to a learned profession.

In addition to the more traditional sites represented by shops and private homes, the Renaissance saw the emergence and elaboration of a third, largely new, site of health care: urban hospitals, which were founded by princes and patricians as charitable institutions, intended to provide a range of free services, including medical services, to the poor. Although the first such hospitals were medieval foundations, established in the twelfth and thirteenth centuries, it was not until the mid-fourteenth century that some of these became exclusively devoted to treating the sick. At the same time, others began to combine specialized care of the sick with such activities as raising orphans, maintaining old and disabled workers, and lodging pilgrims and travellers. Some of the earliest and most highly developed of these hospitals were in the cities of central or northern Italy. Among the most famous were the Ospedale Maggiore in Milan, designed by the celebrated architect Filarete for Duke Francesco Sforza, and the hospital of Santa Maria Nuova in Florence, founded by Folco Portinari, father of Dante's Beatrice. The latter had its own fully staffed pharmacy, which dispensed medicines both to its hundreds of in-patients and to friends and relatives of poor people who were sick at home. In addition, it salaried a growing number of physicians and surgeons; some of these resided in the hospital, while others made daily visits to supervise the care of the patients. The fame of Santa Maria Nuova had become so great by the early sixteenth century that Henry VII of England took it as the model for his own hospital, the Savoy.

Hospitals of this sort were charitable institutions, dedicated to treating rather than confining the acutely ill, whose stays were generally short and whose discharge rate was high—approximately 90 per cent, in the case of Santa Maria Nuova. The pre-modern hospital of popular imagination—half warehouse and half prison—was for the most part a much later creation, reflecting an increasingly punitive and moralizing attitude towards poverty and a growing preoccupation with chronic disease. During the Renaissance, in contrast, there were only two specialized kinds of hospital that regularly confined their patients: leprosaria (though by the fifteenth century these were virtually empty, as leprosy gradually disappeared) and lazarettos, or plague hospitals, usually temporary structures built outside the city, particularly in the Mediterranean region, to isolate people suspected of being infected with plague. But many Renaissance hospitals for the sick—whether dedicated to the acutely ill, like Santa Maria Nuova, or the chronically ill, like the numerous hospitals founded to take in 'incurables', including victims of the new scourge of syphilis—were relatively effective and well-managed institutions that supplied the poor with free temporary medical care that might, in some cases, be at the highest level the medical profession could supply.

In addition to the naturalistic care offered by hospitals, physicians, surgeons, apothecaries, and other such healers, Europeans also looked to religious healing. Belief in its efficacy was not confined in the Renaissance to the poor and those with little formal education, but permeated the entire society. Just as Boccaccio could cite both natural and supernatural causes of plague (planetary influences and divine wrath), so his late fifteenth-century compa-

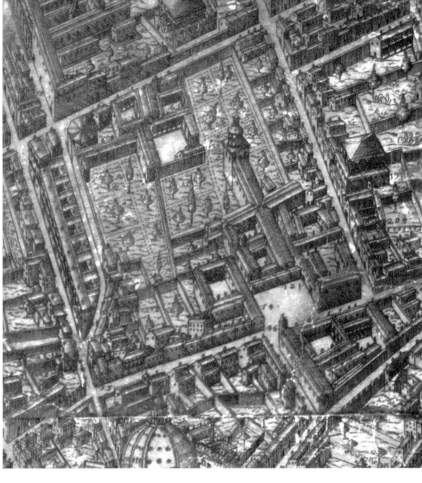

**The hospital of Santa
Maria Nuova**. This
woodcut, taken from the
1584 perspective plan of
Florence by Stefano
Bonsignori, shows the
men's hospital, with its
great cruciform wards, to
the north of the piazza,
and the more modest
women's hospital (marked
86 in the plan) to the
south. Santa Maria Nuova,
one of the first hospitals
to specialize in the
medical treatment of the
sick, became a model for
other such institutions.

triot, the Florentine physician Antonio Benivieni, included both kinds of healing in his work, *Some Hidden and Wonderful Causes of Disease and Healing*, published posthumously in 1507. Alongside the more usual cases described by
Benivieni, which were treated by purging, bleeding, herbal preparations, and
simple surgical procedures, he cited others, like that of his relative Giovannina
Benci, who had unsuccessfully consulted numerous doctors for her chronic
diarrhoea. Eventually, 'having abandoned all hope in the art of medicine', as
Benivieni put it, she went to the Dominican friar Domenico da Pescia, who had
a reputation for succeeding where natural means had failed and who immediately cured her by making the sign of the cross on her head. Benivieni saw no
contradiction between the two forms of healing: not only had he himself been
cured of dysentery by prayer at the age of 53, but he also understood that,
although God had endowed the physician's herbs and other preparations with
medicinal powers, at times He chose to dispense his cures directly, through
miracles in response to prayer.

This easy coexistence between natural and divine healing found its clearest expression in the figures of SS Cosmas and Damian, patron saints of medicine, who were reputed to have cured a petitioner in a dream by amputating his ulcerated leg and substituting for it one that belonged to a recently dead Moor. Although many early representations of this scene situate it in a private home, according to the most common version of the legend, it took place in an oratory attached to the Roman basilica of Santa Maria Maggiore. Thus sites of healing in the Renaissance period also included the churches frequented by devout Christians and the shrines that were the centres of particular healing cults. Some of these cults were local, like the devotion to the tomb of St Gineforte, the holy greyhound, near Lyon; others, however, like those of SS Sebastian and Roche, invoked in time of plague, or St Margaret, for childbirth, became common in the fifteenth century to most or all of Europe.

Institutionalization and Professionalization

The large number of hospitals founded in late medieval and Renaissance Europe are only one manifestation of what is perhaps the most novel and striking aspect of the medicine of the period: the increasing complexity and sophistication of the organization of health care. First in the western Mediterranean (Italy, Spain, and southern France), then in the more heavily urbanized areas of northern Europe (the Low Countries and southern Germany), and finally in England, we see the emergence of an elaborate network of new urban institutions and organizations that ultimately formed the foundations of the modern medical order in the West. These developments manifested themselves in three related areas: the elaboration of public-health measures, the professionalization and specialization of medical practice, and the increasing willingness of government officials to turn to formally trained and licensed medical personnel for aid and advice on matters related to health care. All three speak to a growing public confidence in medicine, an increasing willingness to submit to medical authority, and an enhanced recognition of specialized medical expertise.

The causes of these developments were various. On the one hand, they related to the assimilation and elaboration of a sophisticated written tradition of medical theory and practice derived from translations of Arabic and Greek medical texts. This body of learning enhanced public confidence in medical expertise. On the other hand, the new developments in medical organization reflected the consolidation of State and municipal authority. Although both conditions were clearly visible in the thirteenth century, the new system of health care predicated on them took shape only gradually, emerging to full visibility over the course of the Renaissance period.

The public-health measures adopted by Renaissance towns and cities varied significantly from place to place. Beginning in the thirteenth century, for example, some salaried physicians and surgeons began to attend to the needs of the local population, with an emphasis on the poor. In the later fourteenth and fifteenth centuries, these measures were supplemented by ones requiring much higher levels of institutionalization, such as the establishment of health boards, especially after the Black Death, to create and enforce special measures to control epidemic disease. In the beginning, these measures were traditional: providing for the autopsies of plague victims, promulgating recommendations for diet and prophylactic treatment based on those findings, enforcing pre-existing regulations designed to control pollution of water and the air. By the later fifteenth century, especially in Italy, increasingly stringent measures were developed to control the spread of plague: the compulsory confinement or segregation of the infected, including the establishment of lazarettos and isolation hospitals; the compiling of bills of mortality designed to track the course of epidemics; and the development of an elaborate system of health passes, quarantine regulations, and *cordons sanitaires*. The fact that these measures were all based on the assumption that plague was directly contagious, rather than transmitted most commonly by flea bites, does not detract from their historical significance.

Concurrent with these developments, we see an increasing investment by public authorities in establishing standards for medical practice and controlling who might legally lay claim to medical expertise. Thus in the early fourteenth century, Mediterranean towns began to establish systems of licensing,

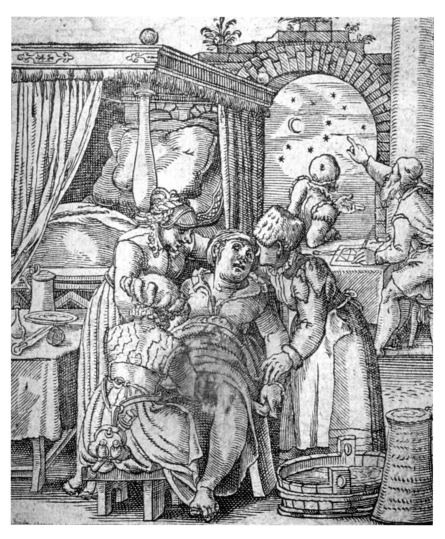

Birth scene. This woodcut from Jacob Rueff's obstetrical textbook, *On the Conception and Generation of Man* (1580), shows a midwife and assistants managing the last stages of childbirth. Meanwhile the male astrologers in the background determine the child's horoscope.

predicated in most cases on the demonstration of technical competence, either through evidence of formal training (an apprenticeship, for example, or a university degree) or through an examination. Here, as throughout Europe, medical practitioners were often organized in craft guilds, which established their own entrance criteria and standards of practice—criteria and standards that the State often merely ratified. Over the course of the fifteenth century, the model of licensing and regulation was in some areas extended to groups that previously had escaped formal organization, such as midwives.

As yet, relatively little is known about the practice of midwifery in the fourteenth and early fifteenth centuries, in part at least because the craft only gradually became visible as a specialized occupation, and then mainly in cities and larger towns. By the mid-fifteenth century, however, municipal councils began to institute formal licensing and oversight procedures for midwives, most notably in Germany. These procedures were intended to ensure minimum levels of technical competence and, especially, moral character. Thus, alongside the informally trained and unlicensed midwives who practised in both city and countryside emerged a recognizable group of specialized urban midwives who had been trained through formal apprenticeship, licensed, and in some cases employed by civil or ecclesiastical authorities to care for poor or needy women.

The increasing formalization of standards for professional practice inevitably affected the composition of the body of officially recognized health-care providers. In particular, it produced significant stratification, creating gaps between university-educated physicians (and very occasionally surgeons), surgeons and apothecaries trained by apprenticeship, and empirics with no documentable training at all. Equally inevitably, the higher ranks of the profession began to develop their own organizations and regulations, ostensibly aimed at establishing standards for practice, but in fact largely concerned with guaranteeing or expanding their own authority and market share. The most visible result of this impetus was the establishment, initially in Italy, of a new kind of élite medical institution, the college of physicians, with ambitions to oversee medical practice as a whole. (The English Royal College of Physicians was founded on the Italian model in 1518.) These bodies exerted increasing pressure on the lower levels of health-care providers, monitoring, controlling, and eventually attempting to limit their practice.

Among the groups most strongly affected by these changes were women practitioners—in many cases a distinct minority, outside a domestic context— who were typically trained by husbands or fathers and had little or no access to the kind of formal education increasingly taken as the touchstone of medical expertise. Although women do not seem initially to have been singled out from other empirics, the Renaissance saw an accelerating series of local and national regulations aimed at excluding female practitioners as a sex. In this, as in many other areas, there was clearly a gap between the ambitions of physicians and their ability to enforce them; in 1421, for example, the attempts of English physicians to exclude women from the practice of physic, under the pain of 'long emprisonment', came to nothing. By the sixteenth century, however, the number of women engaged in regular, licensed, commercial practice seems to have been in decline throughout Europe.

The case of Jewish practitioners was somewhat different, and efforts to exclude them were correspondingly less successful. Jews had a special claim to intellectual authority in the world of late medieval and Renaissance medicine, based largely on the familiarity of some, particularly in Spain, with the Arabic language and the Arabic medical tradition, which served as the core of learned European medicine. Mainly privately trained, in the late thirteenth and fourteenth centuries, Jews were regularly licensed in the cities of Italy, Spain, and southern France, and often admitted into medical guilds. (Jews had already been expelled from England and large parts of northern France.) But the rising tide of Renaissance anti-Semitism placed increasing restrictions on Jewish practice. The exile or forced conversion of European Jews continued, culminating in the Spanish expulsions of 1492. And even in those areas where Jews were allowed to live and practise, ecclesiastical and secular authorities attempted to prevent them from treating Christians, whom they supposedly sought to harm. As a result of these prejudices, Jews in many parts of Europe had been accused of an international conspiracy to spread plague during the Black Death, and a number of Jewish communities in Germany were massacred or exiled. The generalized prohibitions on Jews treating Christians were not broadly effective; Jews were sometimes salaried as municipal doctors—though at lower salaries than their Christian colleagues—and employed as personal physicians by princes and popes. None the less, the overarching structures of anti-Semitism created a persistent suspicion of Jewish doctors in the minds of the Christian population, engendering accusations of malpractice and sexual misconduct, as well as sorcery and poisoning.

Medical Learning

Up to about 1500, the most dramatic innovations in Renaissance medical culture came in the area of medical organization. At the same time, the late fourteenth and fifteenth centuries also witnessed changes in medical learning, as represented by Latin and vernacular texts written for both academic and lay audiences. In this connection, too, it is important to stress that medical learning continued to be organized around the work of the eleventh-century Persian author Avicenna, and it remained correspondingly static in the area of medical theory. But other areas of medical learning saw significant shifts in orientation and emphasis.

The first and perhaps the most pervasive such shift was the increasing prominence of the branch of learned medicine called *practica*. Whereas medical theory was organized around general physical and physiological principles—such as the prime qualities, the humours, and the ideas of form and matter—*practica* dealt with particular diseases and particular remedies. In this respect, medical learning followed general intellectual patterns within the culture. Just as the intellectuals known as Humanists subordinated more abstract areas of philosophy, such as logic and metaphysics, to those areas of enquiry most relevant to human life in society—the 'humanities' that gave them their name—so contemporary medical writers found most compelling those areas of medical learning that related to the actual diagnosis and cure of disease. Thus the fourteenth and fifteenth centuries saw the multiplication of works in this vein: *practicae* (encyclopaedic reference works relating to disease and treatment, classified by organ and ordered from head to foot); *consilia* (detailed descriptions of a single case, with prescriptions for therapy); regimens (short treatises with specific recommendations for food, drink, exercise, and other practices intended to maintain health and prevent disease); *experimenta* (proved remedies) and other collections of recipes for prophylactic and therapeutic preparations; herbals and other works of *materia medica*; and treatises devoted to a particular type of therapy or to a particular disease.

Most of the earlier examples of the last genre focused on plague, as might be expected. By the later fifteenth and early sixteenth centuries, however, doctors and other intellectuals were beginning to write on a number of specific illnesses, ranging from occupational diseases of miners and metalworkers, through illnesses of children, to the new scourge of syphilis. Ulrich von Hutten's treatise *On the French Disease*, for example, written in the 1520s, combined a dramatic first-person account of the author's own symptoms and sufferings with descriptions of a variety of cures. In this way, the new writing on practical medicine often shaded over into newly important literary genres such as autobiography, just as it drew on important innovations in the area of art.

This burgeoning practical literature, in both Latin and the vernacular, reflected a growing market for medical learning not only among practising physicians, but also among their princely and noble patrons, and, with the spread of printing, middle-class readers as well. It also reflected an increasing orientation on the part of medical researchers and compilers towards the particularities of medical practice: the symptoms of particular diseases; the intricacies of particular surgical procedures; the therapeutic properties of particular plant, animal, or mineral substances. Coupled with this was a growing emphasis on the direct observation and description of everything from specific anatomical structures to the smell, colour, and temperature of particular mineral springs.

This general orientation towards the particular was given new impetus in the late fifteenth and early sixteenth centuries by the work of a number of medical scholars who aligned themselves with the programme of classical revival first elaborated in more literary and philosophical disciplines by Italian humanists such as Petrarch and his friend Boccaccio. The members of this movement, led in the late fifteenth century by Niccolò Leoniceno, insisted on the direct study of ancient medical texts in the original languages. Their work produced a flood of new editions and Latin translations of the most important Greek writers, such as the pharmacological work of Dioscorides and the great Greek edition of Galen published in Venice in 1525.

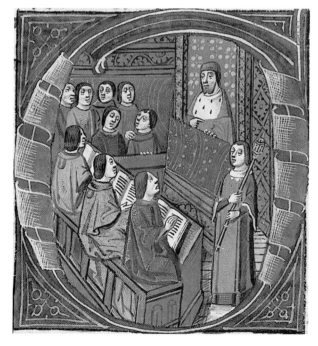

Although university medical teaching centred on reading and commenting on texts by ancient and medieval authorities, as shown in this fifteenth-century French manuscript, it was often supplemented by clinical training and attendance at human dissections.

Although Italian in origin, this movement spread and gained momentum north of the Alps during the first three decades of the sixteenth century, in the hands of scholars such as Thomas Linacre, Guillaume Cop, Leonhard Fuchs, and John Caius.

In addition to insisting on the direct study of ancient texts, Leoniceno and his followers also prized the direct study of nature—a method they identified with Galen himself. In his work *On the Errors of Pliny* (1492), for example, Leoniceno criticized contemporary physicians who, rather than concentrating on the all-important fields of anatomy, nosology, and *materia medica*, 'sit in school, discussing things of no relevance to life and men's fates, placing faith in others rather than themselves'. Although many humanist medical writers dramatically overestimated their independence from earlier sources—the anatomist Andreas Vesalius is a good example—their orientation towards direct observation none the less reinforced the emphasis on concrete particulars embodied in the fifteenth-century literature of medical practice.

By the middle of the sixteenth century, this new orientation had begun directly to affect the organization of medical teaching and research. Professors at Italian universities, most notably the University of Padua, refined and formalized the clinical component of medical education, while specialized new chairs were founded in *materia medica* (sometimes expanded to include all of natural history) and anatomy (which had previously been subordinated to the teaching of surgery). As these two areas of study became increasingly institutionalized, universities added innovative teaching facilities, in the form of the botanical garden, the natural history collection, and the permanent anatomy theatre. As in the case of medical humanism itself, the first examples were Italian, but they were soon imitated in other parts of Europe, first in Spain, where the physician Andres Laguna persuaded Philip II to establish his own botanical garden, and then in northern European universities such as Leiden.

One of the effects of this fascination with *materia medica* was the dramatic increase in the number of known species. Whereas late fifteenth-century European compilers were familiar with several hundred kinds of plants, a century later their repertoire included thousands. In part this expansion resulted from the more efficient cataloguing and exchange of information concerning native species. But it also grew out of the voyages of exploration and the colonization by Europeans of previously unknown parts of the globe. Even Columbus brought back reports of American plants and other *naturalia*; his interests were primarily commercial, and Asia—where he thought he had landed in 1492—had long been the source of expensive spices used more often for preparing medicines than seasoning food. By 1565, however, the Spanish physician Nicolas Monardes could claim in his *Two Books on All the Things Found in our West Indies* that America's plants were worth more than its gold. Monardes, who had never personally visited America, described a host of new and reputedly valuable medicinal plants, such as sassafras, coca, sarsaparilla, and tobacco, which he touted as a wonder drug. European writers reserved a special place in their exotic pharmacopoeia for guaiac wood, promoted by some as a new treatment for syphilis; the toxic properties of the old remedy mercury were well known to Ulrich von Hutten and others who had experienced them first-hand. Much was made of the fact that guaiacum came from the New World, as did (reput-

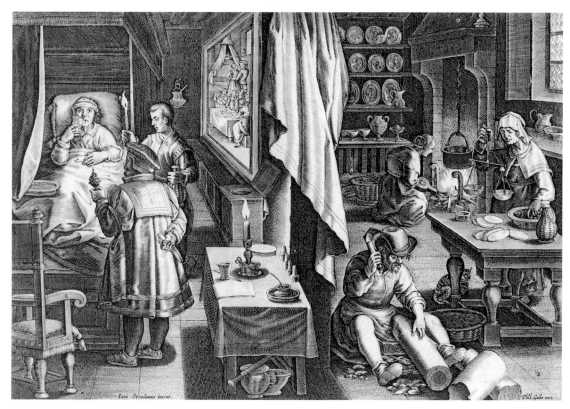

edly) *morbus gallicus* itself. The conjunction of the two was taken to be a sign of the providential order, which had ordained to each disease its cure.

Because it was both widespread and widely perceived as new—unknown to the ancients and therefore absent from their work—syphilis became one focus where old and new theories of illness and healing intersected. Some authors attempted to fit the disease into a traditional framework, attributing it to planetary conjunctions and the corruption of the air, or to sin, or to the malice of lepers, Jews, prostitutes, and other marginalized groups. Others used it to develop novel medical theories. These included the early sixteenth-century Italian physician Girolamo Fracastoro, who elaborated the idea of what he called 'contagion', based on the transmission of clinging and imperceptibly small 'seeds of disease', and his Swiss contemporary Theophrastus Paracelsus, who interpreted *morbus gallicus* as a mutable entity that invaded the body from outside.

Paracelsus was by any measure the most original medical theoretician of Renaissance Europe, in a period when medical creativity, as I have already mentioned, was focused overwhelmingly on problems of practice and therapeutics. For the traditional Galenic and medieval model of physiology and illness, focused on complexional and humoral imbalance and organized around the prime qualities of hot, cold, wet, and dry, Paracelsus substituted a model based on alchemical principles, which took the elements salt, sulphur, and mercury as the fundamental causal entities in both healing and disease. Combining these ideas with a radical spirituality and a deep animus against the medical establishment, Paracelsus elaborated a complex and often confusing

Treating syphilis. Widely perceived as a new disease when it appeared in epidemic form in 1494, this disease was quickly identified by many medical writers with sexual licence and the 'New World'. In this seventeenth-century print, after Jan van der Street, the patient is being treated with a decoction of guaiac wood, itself a product of the Americas, while the cautionary image on his bedroom wall reminds him of the promiscuous behaviour that laid him low.

77

theoretical cosmos that gained increasing influence over the next 100 years; studied and admired, particularly in later sixteenth-century court circles, it became the staging ground in the seventeenth century for an all-out assault on the core tradition of Renaissance medicine, rooted in the works of Hippocrates, Galen, and their Arabic followers.

Renaissance Medicine and Art

Just as medical writers drew on the intellectual movement of humanism, so they exploited the achievements of Renaissance artists, producing works in which the images were increasingly integrated into the argument and the text. The illustrated medical text was not a Renaissance invention. But, as the figures in both this and the preceding chapter indicate, medieval medical illustrations did not on the whole emphasize naturalistic description. Most images found in medical manuscripts were schematic, intended to help the reader assimilate and recall the information presented verbally in the text: locations and shapes of organs, characteristics of wounds, names of diseases, types of surgical instruments, correspondences between zodiacal signs and parts of the body, salient features of medicinal herbs. The principal exceptions to this generalization were the decorative treatises produced for princely patrons, like the famous northern Italian *tacuina sanitatis* (manuals of health) of the late fourteenth and early fifteenth centuries, with their lavish illustrations of domestic scenes and easily recognizable plants.

By 1500, however, with the establishment of the technology of printing, the images in medical works had begun to assume a new character; rather than being merely decorative or schematic (though these functions remained important), they increasingly moved in the direction of naturalistic description. Through the medium of printing, woodcut illustrations became the bearers of detailed and exactly reproducible information not easily transmitted in words. Early examples included the images in the famous illustrated herbals of Otto Brunfels (1530) and Leonhard Fuchs (1542). Most influential of all, however, was the *Fabric of the Human Body*, published in 1543 by Andreas Vesalius, which exploited to the utmost the new anatomical interests of contemporary Italian art.

As early as the first half of the fifteenth century, Italian art theorists had stressed the importance of a knowledge of anatomy for both sculptors and painters. Lorenzo Ghiberti included detailed information concerning the human skeleton in his *Commentaries*, and Leon Battista Alberti recommended first-hand study of the bones and muscles: 'as Nature clearly and openly reveals their proportions,' he wrote, 'so the zealous painter will find great profit from investigating them in Nature herself.' Initially, artists confined themselves to surface inspection, but by 1500 Leonardo da Vinci and Michelangelo Buonarroti had begun to perform their own dissections, in order to study the human body in detail.

Vesalius was the first medical writer to realize the full potential of a close collaboration between the anatomist and the anatomically informed artist, versed in the techniques of linear perspective. For his *Fabric*, he worked closely with an artist, probably Jan van Calcar, to produce the remarkable woodcuts

Vesalius and the New anatomy. Attributed to Jan van Calcar, the woodcuts from Andreas Vesalius' great anatomy text were based largely on human dissection and testify to the collaboration of author and artist in every phase of the project. Images like this one, based on the first-century Roman fragment known as the Belvedere torso, testify to the importance of ancient sculpture in shaping the presentation of the Renaissance body as both a visual and a medical object.

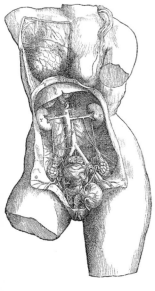

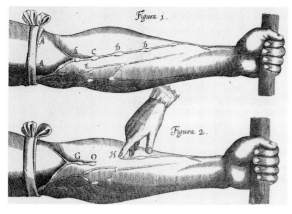
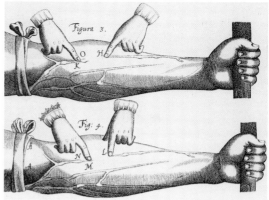

that accompanied the work. These images reflect many of the most important new preoccupations of contemporary medical academicians, including an orientation towards the first-hand observation of particulars and a deep-seated classicism that manifested itself in Vesalius' and Calcar's use of ancient sculptural models for many of the images in the text.

Vesalius' book achieved immediate fame; its splendid woodcuts were copied (often poorly) and disseminated throughout Europe in books intended for both lay and professional readers, and the study of anatomy flourished both in Italy and the north. It remained for an Englishman, however, to take the anatomical image as bearer of information and transform it into a kind of argument, as William Harvey did in his famous treatise *Anatomical Disquisition on the Motion of the Heart and Blood in Animals* (1628). Building on the work of Italian anatomists, which he had studied at the University of Padua, he presented detailed evidence in support of his conclusion that blood, rather than simply flowing outward from the heart and liver to the extremities, circulated through the arteries and veins, eventually returning to the heart. The famous figures in his treatise demonstrate not a structure but a process—the elaborate series of ligatures with which he determined that the blood passes in the extremities from the arteries to the veins.

The work of Vesalius and Harvey points forward into the modern period. It is important to emphasize, however, their links to the earlier tradition. Just as Vesalius, despite his many criticisms of Galen, remained tied to a remarkable extent both to the model of Galen's procedure and to the details of his work, so Harvey appealed to Aristotle in arguing the central role of the heart in human physiology. In its organization and institutional framework, the medicine of Renaissance Europe had evolved significantly over its ancient and medieval predecessors, but its links to earlier medical theory and therapeutics remained extremely strong.

The circulation of the blood. These figures from William Harvey's *Anatomical Disquisition on the Motion of the Heart and Blood in Animals* (1628) show a series of experiments demonstrating that the veins contain one-way valves that keep the blood moving towards the heart. Harvey argued that the rapidity with which the veins refill and the sheer amount of blood passing through them were proof of its circulation.

6 | From the Scientific Revolution to the Germ Theory

HAROLD COOK

FROM the publication of Harvey's work on the circulation of the blood in 1628 to Pasteur's formulation of the germ theory in the 1860s, European medicine changed dramatically. Three developments stand out: rapid growth in the number of formally educated and certified practitioners; development of medical theory and practice that assumed truth lay in investigations into chemistry and the material structure of the body; and, towards the end of the period, sudden population growth and urbanization, contributing to enormous alterations in the human environment. The development of a materialist outlook meant that medicine threatened established views even while it developed more precise ideas about the cause of disease; the rise of a formally educated medical profession meant harder times for women and alternative practitioners; and rapid urbanization brought about terrible living conditions for many people while increasing the need for governmental medical intervention. The consequence of these processes was that university-based medicine gained authority, a process sometimes termed 'medicalization'.

The Scientific Revolution in Medicine

Both human tragedy and promising developments marked the years from the 1620s to the end of the seventeenth century. War in Europe, and between Europeans and Asians, Africans, and Americans, erupted continually. The Thirty Years War (1618–48) devastated Germanic-speaking peoples and many of their neighbours, causing a 15–20 per cent population drop in central Europe (over 50 per cent in some places). Plague remained a threatening presence, frequenting Europe in the early part of the century. While plague declined in Western Europe later in the century, the virulence of smallpox apparently increased. Bad weather brought local famines or malnutrition. As a consequence, the seventeenth century generally saw a stagnation in European population gains of the previous century.

Yet there were organized attempts to relieve suffering humanity, limited as they were. Charity and ideas about collective good promoted development of medical institutions. When plague threatened, for instance, civil authorities imposed quarantines and local plague orders to minimize infection, often with the support of religious authorities. Perhaps the increasing ability of nations to seal their borders against people from infected places contributed greatly to the decline in outbreaks of plague. But other epidemic diseases— such as smallpox—were so common, and moved through communities so quickly, that nothing could be done to halt their spread. As the incidence of plague declined, smallpox became the most feared disease. Some evidence suggests that the virulence of this deadly and disfiguring fever worsened in Europe towards the end of the century, while in the Americas it continued to destroy hosts of indigenous people.

In Europe, both civil magistrates and Church governments organized regular parish relief for the local poor, who might sometimes number half the population. Some parishes or towns even provided doctors and nurses to visit the poor. On the Continent, the office of town physician (first reinstituted during the later fifteenth century) continued to develop, becoming in some places a provincial medical officer. The officially appointed, university-educated town and regional physicians cared for the sick poor and worked with local authorities to oversee medical practitioners and to develop and enforce rules for health. Duties of medical oversight included the establishment of plague orders, and inspection of apothecaries' and chemists' shops and food markets. To ensure that skilled assistants were available during childbirth, by the end of the century in some places midwives were instructed and supervised by (male) medical officials. Together with out-relief and medical oversight came institutions for supervised care of the sick poor. In Catholic lands, the Church still operated hospitals, sometimes in conjunction with local governments. Hospitals were indistinct from hospices, since they still provided the sick poor with food and shelter in a religious environment, and sometimes with medicine or surgery too. Although the poor might regard hospitals as places of last resort,

A depiction of the large wards, full of bustling activity, typical of eighteenth-century general hospitals, which imitated the interiors of big churches. On the left a tradesman or apothecary wearing a leather apron is accompanied by a dog, in the centre a woman carries food to the inmates while a cat begs for what just came from the containers, and on the right a group of nuns doles out food.

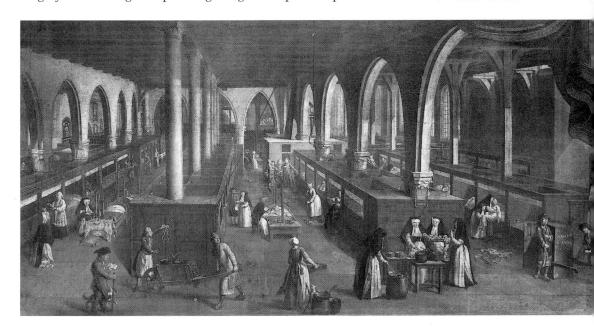

they did use them in great numbers: by the end of the century the Hôtel Dieu de Paris had added four new wings, even bridging the Seine. In Protestant lands, the Roman Church's dissolution tended to displace the religious orders who once staffed the hospitals, while rents that furnished hospitals' incomes were confiscated. Nevertheless, many municipalities, like London, took over hospital operation from the Church because they thought local hospitals essential to poor relief. Also, many places like the Netherlands continued to build municipal hospitals and small houses for the aged (*hofjes*), although these too were run mainly by local notables (both male and female) rather than by brethren and sisters. Governments, too, built hospitals, as throughout Europe admiralty boards established hospitals in major ports and staffed them with trained surgeons, and generals sometimes did the same for their garrisons. Louis XIV of France built and rebuilt general hospitals in Paris, and founded the Hôtel des Invalides in 1674 as a hospice for old and maimed soldiers; the English followed suit with the Greenwich naval hospital and the Chelsea Hospital for pensioned soldiers. While none of these various medical and semi-medical institutions hoped to care for everyone who needed help, they did shelter and assist many.

Most times, however, ordinary people relied on family, friends, and neighbours for medical help. The local wisewoman or wiseman who knew herbs and spells, the blacksmith who set bones, the person marked as a healer because of being born with the caul (a bit of the placenta sticking to the head upon birth), the seventh son of a seventh son, or grandmother and her best recipe: these were the medical resources of first resort for most people. Priests, ministers, and rabbis, and their wives, also visited the sick for solace and advice and sometimes to help with nursing. And ladies of the manor showed their *noblesse oblige* by visits to the homes of dependants, bringing food, medicine, and advice to the sick.

In such a world, many medical practices tended to remain traditional. People continued to have definite desires and expectations: for instance, even decades after learned physicians had attacked and ridiculed the idea that inspecting strangers' urine might help in diagnosis or prognosis, patients still insisted on uroscopy when visiting a practitioner. Many still demanded bleeding or purging for all kinds of complaints, or at the change of season. And in Venice most famously, apothecaries continued compounding thèriac, an ancient remedy with dozens of ingredients, during a grand annual public ceremony under the gaze of municipal authorities and learned physicians.

But increasingly it was possible to develop new remedies and to convince both the learned and the unlettered of their efficacy. Some new remedies introduced in accordance with new theories included cooling regimens for fevers and all kinds of chemically prepared medicines (including those made from heavy metals like mercury, and from various spirits like gin). Increasing numbers of the well-to-do frequented medicinal baths and spas, which attracted medical practitioners, hoteliers, and other entrepreneurs to spa towns. Other new medicinals were imported from the East and the Americas, such as tea, coffee, chocolate, and cinchona. Cinchona, commonly called 'Jesuit's bark', came from Peru in the mid-1600s, and countered the effects of intermittent fevers. (Quinine from the bark relieves malarial fevers.) By the

1660s the bark had obtained such a reputation that patients at European courts and elsewhere were demanding it of their (often sceptical) physicians, although no one knew why it worked. Needless to say, medical controversies raged over whether the new medicines were effective or even safe. Increasing numbers of ordinary practitioners depended on the monetary economy. Many itinerants sought custom by selling medicines or removing cataracts, bladder stones, or cancerous breasts, or repairing hernias. To attract attention, some pitched their medicines to market crowds or at busy intersections, mounting benches or wagons to be visible (hence the word 'mountebank'). Still others drew crowds by providing entertainment in the form of tightrope dancers, jugglers, drummers and musicians, or actors (the *commedia dell'arte* was closely associated with the entertainments of mountebanks)—followed by a harangue about the wonderful medicine on hand. The patter always seems to have included a recital of the ailments these medicines would surely cure. Such medical salespeople earned the appellation of 'quack' or 'quacksalver' (a word of obscure origin). The itinerants, who sold their remedies to strangers and then moved on, could seldom be held to account for whatever good or ill might be attributed to their potions, pills, or operations. Others, however, settled for a few weeks before moving on, and developed closer relationships with their

A well-to-do young female patient, in a late seventeenth-century painting, possibly suffering from love-sickness (a favourite subject for many painters). She is being treated by a physician (wearing a wig and taking her pulse) and a surgeon (who has drawn blood from the foot). She is sitting next to her covered bed.

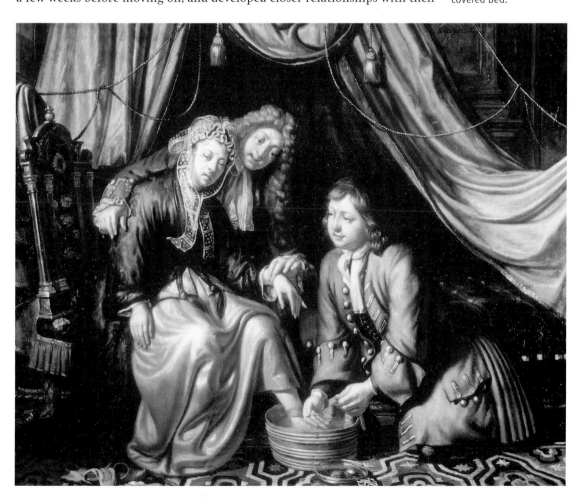

patients. Sometimes husbands and wives collaborated to attract patients of both sexes; women even sold medicines alone. In large cities many residents marketed medicines as their primary income source.

The number of ordinary practitioners who advertised in print grew. Practitioners composed handbills and broadsides (sometimes with woodcut illustrations) to distribute on streets, slip under doors, or post in markets, taverns, and coffee houses. The printed advertisements, like the oral pitches, recounted the expertise and reputation of the practitioner, listed the ills cured, and where the practitioner or medicine could be found. Literacy was common enough for many townspeople and some who dwelt in the countryside to be able to read to themselves or to others. The market for printed medical information grew rapidly. Some people made livings by writing for printers who produced almanacs and cheap pamphlets containing some medical lore. Other practitioners wrote signed medical pamphlets to advertise their practices and to increase their clientele. They wrote tracts on common diseases, little medical books of general interest, provocative attacks on rivals or defences of their own views, or accounts of their therapies—often said to be written in the public interest. With the growth of postal systems and newspapers carrying advertisements, medicines could be marketed and sold by third parties (such as innkeepers, booksellers, stationers, or pedlars) with the help of printed publicity. By the end of the century, the use of the vernacular for conveying medical information had become so common that even university-educated physicians might publish their books in the common tongue.

The number of university-educated physicians certainly grew over the course of the century, especially in the last half. Most universities prescribed a religious test for matriculation or graduation: Paris remained staunchly Catholic and Oxford and Cambridge strictly Anglican, for instance. But for tuition and for public service, some places made it easy for students to avoid religious tests. Still others (such as the famous medical school of Leiden) had no such tests, enabling Jews as well as Christians of various persuasions to study medicine there. The schools that held on to religious tests tended to have more traditional curricula and fewer students, emphasizing inner discipline and a deep appreciation of medical philosophy through lecturing and disputation; those with lower religious barriers tended to take in large numbers of students and to emphasize worldly learning and the acquisition of clinical skills and chemistry. The students and professors of each system stoutly defended their methods: the conservatively trained stressed deep knowledge and discerning judgement developed only through the discipline of long study, while innovators stressed a knowledge of the best methods of medical diagnosis and treatment.

Yet those who had medical doctorates shared much knowledge. Both new and old medical schools emphasized anatomy, not only for content but also for its moral connotations. Most notable schools built expensive anatomy theatres, with a central pit where the demonstrator would open and display the body, surrounded by circles of ascending benches for the audience. The theatres' expense was all the greater because they were used only for a few winter days (since bodies deteriorated less quickly in the cold). But the pre-Lenten season when the demonstrations took place also heightened the moral purposes of the lesson. In Bologna, public anatomies even took place at carnival. During the rest of the year, pieces of art, skeletons, and natural-history specimens might be displayed in the theatres to edify visitors, for the anatomy lessons not only showed the wonderful means by which God and nature constructed the human frame, but also reminded the public about mortality, a basic step in moral instruction. To the wider public, anatomy lessons came to be associated not only with the lessons of death but also with the lessons of the gallows. Judges made the public dissection of a criminal after execution a further and more horrible sentence, and sometimes postponed hearings on capital offences until the proper season for an anatomy. The moral significations of anatomy accompanied a growing emphasis on investigation of nature; both educated and ordinary practitioners took part in demonstrating the significance of these methods. Many ordinary practitioners insisted that simple experience (sometimes coupled with intuition) provided the foundation for all medical knowledge; learned physicians usually argued that such experience must be grafted onto reason to yield demonstrable knowledge. A notable result of new investigative methods is the discovery made by William Harvey (1578–1657). In his *De motu cordis et sanguinis* (1628), he announced that the blood coursed from the heart through the arteries and back through the veins to the heart—that it moved in a circle (which the ancient philosophers held to be perfect motion). Harvey had learnt exacting anatomical and vivisectional techniques and the latest philosophy while a student at Padua. By probing various questions about the motions of the body (including the relationship between the motions of the heart, the lungs, and the pulse) and by contemplating recent discoveries like the valves in the veins, and by executing careful investigations on living animals as well as on dead ones, in the early to mid-1620s Harvey asserted that the blood circulates. He employed anatomical, physiological, philosophical, and even quantitative arguments in his book. Harvey undoubtedly expected that his theories would be challenged, because he undercut Galenic physiology, which postulated a one-way system of motion that digested food into flesh.

Various medical parties quarrelled vigorously. Some philosophically minded doctors promoted mechanical explanations of physiology. For example, the Italian follower of Galileo, Giovanni Alfonso Borelli (1608–79), treated locomotion, digestion, and respiration in animals in a rigorously mechanical manner; Giorgio Baglivi (1668–1706) pushed mechanical analogies even further to account for all bodily actions and functions. But others—not all university-educated—gave chemistry precedence. Among the most important medical theorists was Jan Baptiste van Helmont (1577–1644), from Flanders. He emphasized how active agents (*archei*) work in the body through chemical processes rooted in fermentation. Van Helmont's ideas were adapted for learned medicine by people such as the Leiden professor François de la Boë Sylvius (1614–72) and Thomas Willis (1621–75) at Oxford.

For people like Sylvius and Willis, chemical physiology was melded with anatomical study. Others, such as Gui Patin (1601–72) in Paris, objected to medical chemistry as a form of charlatanism. Still others, such as Marchamont Nedham (1620–78) in London, ridiculed anatomical studies: he thought that anatomy had become the physicians' equivalent of the mountebanks' stage tricks. By and large, then, many if not most medical investigators adopted physiological theories eclectically; but some were rigorous in preferring anatomical to chemical study (or vice versa), or in preferring mechanical explanations to vitalistic ones (or vice versa).

The Enlightenment

Intense intellectual debates continued throughout the eighteenth century, an era often referred to as 'the Enlightenment'. The term was used by some eighteenth-century intellectuals—often referred to as *philosophes*—to describe a self-conscious international movement. Their intent was to use reason against what they saw as the ignorance and superstition of both the entrenched politico-religious establishment and folk traditions. Many dreamed of a new society in which human well-being and freedom were founded on a search for truth. A few became rigorous philosophical mechanists and atheists, more were vitalists and deists, and even more remained pietists or even religious traditionalists. But all believed that they could change the world through the gospel of Reason. This outlook accompanied new opportunities for gaining a living by the pen. In the bourgeois coffee house, gentleman's club, and aristocratic salon, people met to discuss news and recent developments in literature and science, reading newspapers, pamphlets, and even entire books. Eighteenth-century doctors, surgeons, apothecaries, and ordinary practitioners participated fully in the increasingly dense print culture. They still published their own works, advertising their medicines and practices, publishing more in the vernacular than in Latin; they also attended coffee houses, clubs, and salons as witty intellectuals, even seeing patients in such places. The number of educated doctors increased, even in the countryside, where the doctor and curate ruled literate village society.

Changes on the supply side fuelled this growth. New medical schools were opened and old ones transformed. Early in the century, the famous Leiden medical school became even more renowned for chemical, botanical, and clinical teaching under Hermann Boerhaave (1668–1738); in France, the University of Montpellier developed an equally strong reputation for natural history, chemistry, and medical theory. When in the early eighteenth century the city fathers of Edinburgh decided to open a medical school, they modelled it on Leiden's medical faculty, and ensured that chemistry and clinical and surgical skills were taught as well as anatomy and the rudiments of medical philosophy. In Vienna, Gerhard van Swieten (1700–72), helped by the Empress Maria Theresa, also established a medical school modelled after his Alma Mater, Leiden. The Vienna school, too, became famous for its clinical teaching.

Places in clinically oriented medical schools increased, along with the number of private medical teachers. Newspapers often advertised anatomy and chemistry courses. Students received a certificate upon completion of a course (which could run from days to a few weeks). In most such courses, students learned by doing, experimenting, or performing anatomies under an instructor. In London, some private anatomy teachers such as William Hunter (1718–83) became famous, while in Paris at the end of the century clinical teaching on large hospital wards drew students from all over Europe.

The Catholic Church, municipalities, and military forces continued to build and support hospitals for the sick poor, which grew in size and number. In places like England, sentiments of humanity, social patronage, and moral reform helped promote the foundation of 'voluntary' hospitals for the deserving poor, named because of the voluntary nature of the annual contributions that supported them. Gentleman contributors earned the right to admit a certain number of people each year depending upon the amount of their donation, thus neatly combining personal with institutional charity. Most European hospitals remained general, but some specialized—treating venereal diseases, for instance (so-called 'lock' hospitals). By the end of the century almost every hospital focused on admitting the curable and discharging the well or incurable: they increasingly supplied treatment. The physicians and surgeons took more responsibility for admission and care, sometimes to the dismay of lay governors or religious sisters, who heard the medical staff demand that their own interests govern the institutions.

With a supply of impoverished patients having little say about care, hospitals became the foci for development of new medical knowledge. This was in part because clinical teaching by attending physicians and surgeons became increasingly common. In some places, universities had arranged with local hospitals to allow professors to bring in pupils; in most places, hospital teaching was private, with pupils paying the hospital and teachers to walk the wards and view (and sometimes treat) the sick. Both pupils and instructors prodded the bodies of hospital patients in ways that they could seldom have done in their private practices. Hospital inmates were consequently subjected to various kinds of investigations, even after death. One result was that medical and surgical knowledge could be readily developed and passed on in the hospital setting; another result was that hospitals increasingly became viewed by the poor themselves as places of discomfort and sometimes of mistreatment.

The sense that diseases resulted from a defect of material physiology became ever more pervasive. Attempts to classify diseases as ontological entities with stable sets of symptoms resulted in the development of the science of 'nosology', or the systematics of disease. For instance, the great Swedish physician and naturalist Carl von Linné, or Linnaeus (1707–78)—who introduced the modern binomial system of biological classification—published a nosological work, *Genera morborum* (1763), organizing diseases into 325 genera. Even more famous is the *Nosologica methodica* (1768) of François Boissier de Sauvages de la Croix (1706–67), which organized diseases into ten classes, with subordinate orders, 295 genera, and 2,400 species.

Developments in pathological anatomy revealed the materialist notions of disease that lay behind much of this thinking. The custom of performing clinical post-mortems—following the course of a hospital patient's illness and then opening him or her up after death to correlate the outer symptoms with inner pathological changes—had already been common at places like Leiden in the seventeenth century. But in the eighteenth century, as philosophical materialism spread along with clinical teaching in hospitals, the number of post-mortems rose dramatically. The large collection of post-mortem observations and their systematic correlation that Giovanni Battista Morgagni (1682–1771) published in his *De sedibus* (1761) helped shape the study of pathology, and dealt a blow to humoral theory. The belief that symptoms expressed underlying pathology in the body's structure also informed diagnosis. Most important was the development of auscultation, or percussion of the chest, by Leopold Auenbrugger (1722–1809), physician-in-chief of the Hospital of the Holy Trinity in Vienna. Auenbrugger developed this method of thumping the chest and noting the resulting sound by working on cadavers and then on hospital patients.

Surgical techniques developed rapidly alongside medical materialism in the burgeoning hospitals. One of the most dangerous operations was amputation. But the most dramatic successful intervention for an internal disease involved removing bladder stones. Men especially suffered from bladder stones, which were painful and sometimes fatal. Even in the pre-anaesthetic and pre-aseptic era, however, skilled surgeons could remove stones and heal the patient. The entire operation might take only a minute or less. The Paris surgeons, who had large hospitals in which to train, stand out as some of the most skilful operators of the century. But even a monk, Frère Jacques de Beaulieu (1651–1714)—the Frère Jacques of nursery-rhyme fame—demonstrated his techniques on hospital patients. And Charles-François Félix (1650–1703) operated successfully on Louis XIV for an anal fistula in 1686 only after practising on numerous hospital patients, which not only enriched Félix but gained the surgeons new medical authority. Under Louis XV and Louis XVI, the Paris surgeons rivalled the physicians in power. The growth of medical materialism may owe much to the surgeon's outlook.

Eighteenth-century physicians also attributed the efficacy of medicine to some material cause. For instance, several eighteenth-century theorists proposed that all living tissues inherently responded to stimuli, a proposition some (such as Georg Ernst Stahl, 1660–1734) used to argue for vitalism. Others, like William Cullen (1710–90), made life into a form of nervous energy. Cullen's Edinburgh colleague John Brown (1735–88) developed from this a medical system that suggested life was the result of the action of external stimuli on an organized body. This led him to assert that diseases were caused by too much or too little stimuli, which could be corrected by stimulants (especially alcohol) or depressants (especially opium). Brunonianism, as Brown's doctrine came to be called, had strong advocates in North America, Italy, and especially Germany. The most faddish medical treatment of aristocratic Paris—Mesmerism—had a similar kind of explanation. Franz Anton Mesmer (1734–1815) experimented with magnets and became interested in the magnetic influences of the human hand. He believed that animal fluids, like the recently discovered electrical fluid, could be channelled to effect cures. The channelling of this animal magnetism took place in séances around a tub holding his magnetic fluid, from which iron conductors protruded. Many experienced a 'crisis', during which they convulsed or fainted. In Britain, James Graham developed a similar method at his 'Temple of Health', where patients watched dancing girls and experienced mild electrical stimulation.

One of the most famous new medicines from materialist principles was digitalis, developed by William Withering (1741–99), who published his *Account of the Foxglove* in 1785. He described how he had obtained a complex recipe for dropsy from a woman in Shropshire. On the premiss that some material property of one of the herbal ingredients was responsible for the cure, Withering tried them each out on animals and then on patients, finally settling on foxglove (*Digitalis purpura*). The general conclusion by many was that a well-educated natural historian and physician could sift truth from superstition using the principles of reason and experiment, to benefit humanity.

Withering's example shows, too, that physicians of the eighteenth century were willing to begin their investigations by probing and reforming folk customs. Two of the most prominent examples of this tendency involved new treatments for the dreaded smallpox. The first was inoculation, imported in the 1720s by Lady Mary Wortley Montagu (1689–1762) from the Near East and Africa. While in Constantinople in 1718, Wortley Montagu had her 3-year-old son inoculated, and three years later, after her return, she insisted that her English doctors perform the procedure on her 5-year-old daughter. Inoculation thereafter became a widespread if controversial practice in English-speaking lands—including in the American colonies—with people like the Sutton family travelling the countryside inoculating thousands for a fee. Many French Anglophiles, such as Voltaire, advocated its use elsewhere. In the late 1790s Edward Jenner (1749–1823) also used a folk tradition to develop a superior method of escaping the disease. He noted that the dairymaids of Gloucestershire believed that those who had contracted cowpox (a mild illness) would not get smallpox. Jenner used cowpox matter from the arm of a milkmaid, Sarah Nelmes, to 'vaccinate' a young boy (so called after the Latin word for cow, *vacca*). The boy, James Phipps, contracted cowpox; later Jenner inoculated Phipps with smallpox matter, but Phipps remained healthy. Jenner experimented with the same process on a number of other people, publishing the results in *An Account of the Causes and Effects of the Variolae Vaccinae* (1798). Despite early opposition, Jenner's vaccine for smallpox proved to be a powerful tool.

A case of cowpox. From Edward Jenner's book on the experiments on vaccination he began in 1798. This is a depiction of Sarah Nelmes's case of cowpox ('case xvi'); the careful hand-colouring suggests that Jenner kept a very exact record of her symptoms.

Not only individual investigations undergirded medical developments in the Enlightenment: humanity and Reason were often linked to collective institutional changes within the framework of *raison d'état*. In a period of mercantilist economic theories, many argued that a state's wealth depended on the size of its productive population. Governments needed large and rising populations to wage successful wars and to produce taxable goods. Ideas about how the health of the body depended upon harmony of its parts were easily transported into political theory through the notion of the body politic. In France, several economic thinkers called physiocrats, such as François Quesnay (1694–1774), were physicians. They wanted to bring harmony to the body politic so that it remained healthy. Consequently, political thinkers successfully urged the French monarchy to enact several measures. One was to lower infant mortality by educating mothers and midwives, building orphanages, and otherwise keeping women and children healthy. Madame du Coudray travelled France as an official instructor of midwives, reaching perhaps 5,000 of them. A second was to control epidemics. A commission on epidemics, established in 1776, became the new Royal Society of Medicine two years later, a body to which medical correspondents wrote from all over France. A third area of effort was military medicine. The French, Prussians, and Russians were among those who spent time and effort training military surgeons and developing policies to keep troops healthy.

England produced the most famous eighteenth-century studies of military medicine, where Sir John Pringle (1707–82) and James Lind (1716–94) published important works on military hygiene in the 1750s. They advocated measures that amounted to public-health campaigns: burning the clothes of new recruits, washing and delousing them, and giving them clean uniforms to prevent the introduction of 'camp fever'; locating latrines away from camp kitchens; and regulating diets to avoid scurvy and other chronic diseases. By the third quarter of the century, ships could circumnavigate the world with hardly a soul lost to disease—a far cry from previous unsuccessful attempts to blockade ports when the sailors died within a few weeks. It would be a long time before civilian public-health authorities could successfully institute the lessons learnt in the European armed forces.

But try they did. The merging of medical reason and public policy that developed so clearly in autocratic monarchies came to be called 'medical police' or (as we would now say) 'medical policy', a phrase adopted from German. The most notable formulation of this vision came from Johann Peter Frank (1745–1821), who published his *System einer vollständigen medicinischen Polizey* ('A Complete System of Medical Policy') in four large volumes from 1776 to 1788. It set out systematic policies for governments to adopt to further public hygiene. Not even the rulers of the Empire could enact Frank's plans, but the ideal of a strong government devoted to humanity through public hygiene appealed to many and came to have a growing influence.

The Age of Revolution

At the end of the eighteenth century, revolutionary developments swept Europe and its colonies. Population exploded, urbanization raced ahead, and many places—notably England—underwent an economic transformation termed the industrial revolution. Intellectuals continued their worship of Reason, but some feared the materialism of contemporary science, focusing their attention instead on the spirit. At the same time, the modern nation state fully emerged, accompanied by painful changes. Rebellion in the English colonies of North America led to the foundation of the USA; French aid to that rebellion helped to bring on a fiscal crisis which helped to bring on the French Revolution of 1789; consequent terrible wars convulsed Europe up to Napoleon's defeat in 1815; wars of revolution followed in the Spanish colonies of America; the revolutionary democratic Chartist struggles emerged in the UK during the late 1830s, and popular revolution again swept the Continent in 1848. Radicals also began public agitation against slavery, and advocated women's rights, temperance, and an end to animal experimentation. In such conditions, medical institutions were also transformed.

Near the end of the eighteenth century, new medical societies took root outside the old guild and university structures that had divided regular practitioners into surgeons, apothecaries, and physicians. The new societies often grew from hospital dining clubs composed of all medical staff members, no matter their branch of medicine. Some societies opened membership to practitioners outside the hospital, and also published medical journals. During the French Revolution and the French occupation of Europe, guild structures were torn down, throwing together all kinds of educated medical practitioners. At the Revolution's height, a new kind of practitioner emerged: the *officier de santé*, state-educated for work among the public and the armed services but without association with any of the old medical groups. Although some older institutions—such as the Paris faculty of medicine and the Society of Medicine—returned after the Terror, the French medical profession had been changed for ever, with the old division between surgeons, apothecaries, and physicians no longer crucial. In the UK, while the old corporations survived, they had to respond to agitation for reform, which resulted in the Apothecaries' Act of 1815. This Act gave the London Society of Apothecaries the responsibility for educational standards for regular medical practitioners. Groups and individuals, such as the medical agitator Thomas Wakley (1795–1862), who published the *Lancet* (founded in 1823), continued to attack the old corporate system. The British Medical Association began in 1832 when a physician to the Worcester Infirmary called a meeting to press the demands of provincial doctors against the London élite. The gradual development of a single medical profession through the agitation of ordinary doctors marked the period everywhere in Europe.

Reasons for disestablishment of old structures were political and social, but the development of a common education also furthered the process. The requirement that all practitioners have some formal medical education spread throughout Europe in the laws of states and the ordinances of medical

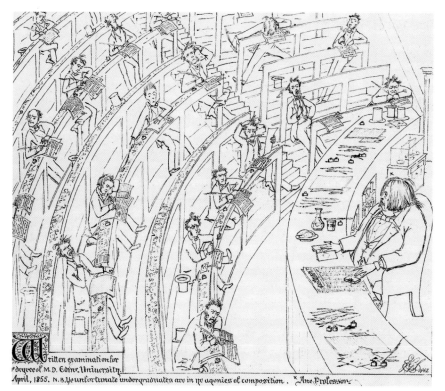

Written examination for degree of M.D. Edinr. University.
April, 1855. N.B. ye unfortunate undergraduates are in ye agonies of composition. Ane Professor

Professor invigilating a medical examination at Edinburgh University, *c.*1855. The students are shown in the common day dress of the period, sitting in an amphitheatre-like hall in which they would have both heard lectures and seen surgical and anatomical demonstrations. The drawing may well be a self-portrait of Sir James Young Simpson, the famous professsor of obstetrics most noted for his use of chloroform in labour in 1847. The original is captioned: 'Written examination for ye degree of M.D. Edinburgh University April 1855. N.B. ye unfortunate undergraduates are in ye agonies of composition'.

91

societies. The newly legitimated practitioners increasingly squeezed out traditional ones. They not only took private fees, but earned salaries from local governments for caring for the poor, and they worked with Friendly Societies and
other similar insurance schemes, although many faced economic hardship.
Since medical schools continued to refuse women, the newly developing profession became an all-male bastion. Elizabeth Blackwell was admitted to
Geneva Medical College in rural New York state in 1847, but that college was
closed to women afterwards. In the early 1850s a few women entered the Western Reserve College in Cleveland, Ohio, before it, too, excluded them. Women
would have a long struggle for admittance to medical school before some
small successes at the end of the century.

At the heart of the common education that doctors received lay medical
materialism. One famous example is the work of Marie François Xavier Bichat
(1771–1802). A military surgeon who went to Paris for further medical training
as an *officier de santé* in 1794, Bichat studied at the Hôtel Dieu and stayed on as
a medical teacher. In his *Treatise on Membranes* (1799), Bichat argued that
lesions of the basic tissues from which the organs were all made caused disease: the nervous tissue, vascular tissue, mucous tissue, connective tissue, and
so on. Physiology and pathology of these elementary tissues, Bichat argued,
could explain all diseases.

An important result of this continued emphasis on the fine material structure of the body was the increasing importance of physical diagnosis made by
the doctor to supplement visible symptoms, and oral histories reported by
patients. The invention of the stethoscope by René-Théophile-Hyacinthe Laënnec (1781–1826) exemplified the process. Laënnec studied in Paris under
Napoleon's physician, Jean Nicolas Corvisart (1755–1821), who popularized
direct auscultation among his pupils and associates. Laënnec took physical
diagnosis a step further with his invention of the stethoscope for indirect, or
'mediate', auscultation. It amplified the sounds of the chest, and allowed private patients privacy: they did not have to bare their chests or be subject to a
doctor's thumping. With such an instrument, physicians could hear into the
patient's body, and could be trained to make fine aural discriminations that
helped in diagnosis, most importantly in bronchitis, peritonitis, emphysema,
pneumonia, and pulmonary tuberculosis (of which Laënnec himself died). In
attempting to discern the physical state of the tissues of the body while the
patient was still alive, Laënnec and his successors made physical diagnosis into
a critical component of the physician's art.

New clinical entities developed from the new orientation towards disease.
For example, the collection of outward signs popularly known as 'phthisis'
(wasting of the body, often accompanied by discomfort in the lungs, coughing,
and fever) became supplemented by a group of inward symptoms discerned by
a doctor's physical diagnosis, labelled 'tuberculosis' (a disease of the tissues
caused by the growth of tubercles). Various kinds of 'fevers' became sorted
according to the kinds of tissues involved, resulting in new diagnoses such as
typhoid, typhus, and diphtheria. Even mental illnesses were attributed to
pathology in the brain's tissues. Among those who thought this was Philippe
Pinel (1745–1826), who removed the insane housed at the Bicêtre from their
chains in 1798. Others in Europe shared the belief that mental patients should

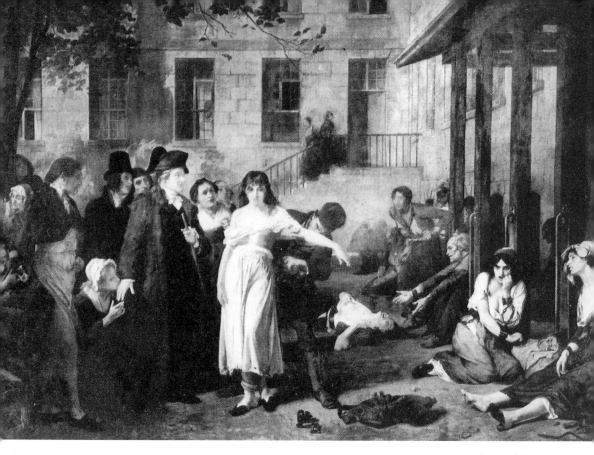

be given supportive care rather than incarceration: the Quaker Retreat in York, England, founded in 1794 by William Tuke, is a famous example. Long into the nineteenth century, physicians like Wilhelm Griesinger (1817–68) clung to the belief that madness was caused by physical changes in brain tissue, despite their inability to locate such changes in post-mortem dissections.

As a consequence of rising demand for medical education in the material structure of the body, the need for teaching material in the form of patients and cadavers also rose. Paris became famous for clinical education, both because of the fine Parisian teachers and because of the large numbers confined in the hospitals there whom the students could study. Moreover, in Paris hospitals and elsewhere, the bodies of the poor could be opened after death to teach diagnosis or gross anatomy. Where hospitals were less common, held fewer patients, or prohibited staff from dissecting, demand for anatomical instruction presented problems of supply. Publishers and professors published anatomy books and atlases. Instructors also used anatomical models made from papier mâché or wax. Some of these wax models are examples of exacting artistic mimicry of the body's material structure coupled with vivid contemplation of the living human frame.

Professors and students still demanded that some anatomical material be from the human body. Consequently, body-snatching from graveyards became common in England and elsewhere. The Burke and Hare scandal of the late 1820s helped bring about new regulations in England for the supply of bodies to anatomy professors. William Burke (1792–1829) and William Hare (fl. 1829),

A grand memorial of Philippe Pinel's famous gesture of 1793, in which he released forty-nine insane patients from their bonds (with the permission of the National Assembly). Pinel believed that all diseases, including mental diseases, were due to lesions in the tissues of the body. In a manner typical of the early nineteenth century, the painting celebrates Pinel in heroic style, the diseased patients in the foreground being represented as lovely female innocents kissing his hands for this act of humanity.

who ran a poor lodging house in Edinburgh, sold anatomists the bodies of those who died in their house; when no deaths occurred naturally, they smothered at least sixteen people. Among those who surreptitiously purchased cadavers from Burke and Hare was the noted anatomy professor Robert Knox (1791–1862), Bichat's chief advocate in Britain. When students identified anatomical specimens as having been healthy poor lodgers just a short time before, rioting broke out against Knox (whose reputation was destroyed), and Burke and Hare were tried and hanged. A few years after, Lord Warburton's Anatomy Act of 1832 helped remedy the problem by assigning all unclaimed bodies to the dissectors. No wonder that Mary Wollstonecraft Shelley formed the results of this materialist medicine into the nightmare world of *Frankenstein: Or, The Modern Prometheus* (1818).

Accompanying the growing medical materialism was the use of statistics to analyse cases numerically. The assumption behind this 'numerical method' contrasted with the medical assumptions of classical medicine: the new medicine assumed that diseases were due to material changes that would result in the same set of symptoms and signs—and in the same reactions to treatment— in anyone, no matter what their individual constitution may have been. In the Parisian hospitals, especially, doctors began to keep statistics on patients there.

New emphasis on physical diagnosis accompanied by statistical measurements had implications for therapy. Notably, Pierre Louis (1787–1872) advocated both correlating symptoms numerically with signs of pathology after death and accounting for therapies given to patients with various symptoms and their outcomes, grouping these observations into tabular form. His *Recherches sur les effets de la saignée* (1835) gave statistical evidence about the number of cases venesection had helped and the number it had impeded, showing that, while bloodletting was of some use in some diseases when done in moderation and at the beginning of the disease, it had no efficacy when done in other diseases or at other times. Debates raged for many years between supporters and opponents of the numerical method in the French Academy of Sciences and the Academy of Medicine, especially over purging instead of bleeding in typhoid fever; eventually, Louis and his supporters established their own Society of Medical Observation to promote statistical investigations of therapies. Such methods led to a period of 'therapeutic nihilism' or 'expectant therapy', in which the doctor merely waited for nature to take its course, simply supporting the patient with food, warmth, and rest.

Other methods of treating disease also developed along the view that the doctor must assist nature, not fight it. Perhaps the most influential was homoeopathy, which taught not that diseases should be treated by opposites (as was customary) but that they should be treated by minute doses of the poisons that gave rise to the disease in the first place. The homoeopathic movement was founded by Samuel Christian Friedrich Hahnemann (1755–1843), who had had trouble establishing a medical practice despite an excellent education and powerful patrons. In 1790, while translating William Cullen's *Materia medica* into German for money, he tried out Cullen's therapies. After taking cinchona, he felt himself developing a very slight fever, the same symptom that it worked against. His conclusion was *similia similibus*: like cures like. But

The tradition of caricaturing doctors and their methods continued. This lithograph by Honoré Daumier is captioned: 'The Doctor, "Why, the devil! does it happen that my patients end up thus? ... Yet I bleed them, I purge them, I drug them ... I simply cannot understand!"'. By the 1830s, the increasingly widespread view that many well-established remedies, such as bleeding and purging, were actually useless or worse made it easier to poke fun at old-fashioned doctoring. At the same time, Daumier gives one a sense of the timeless sadness of doctors, who are unable to conquer death despite their best efforts.

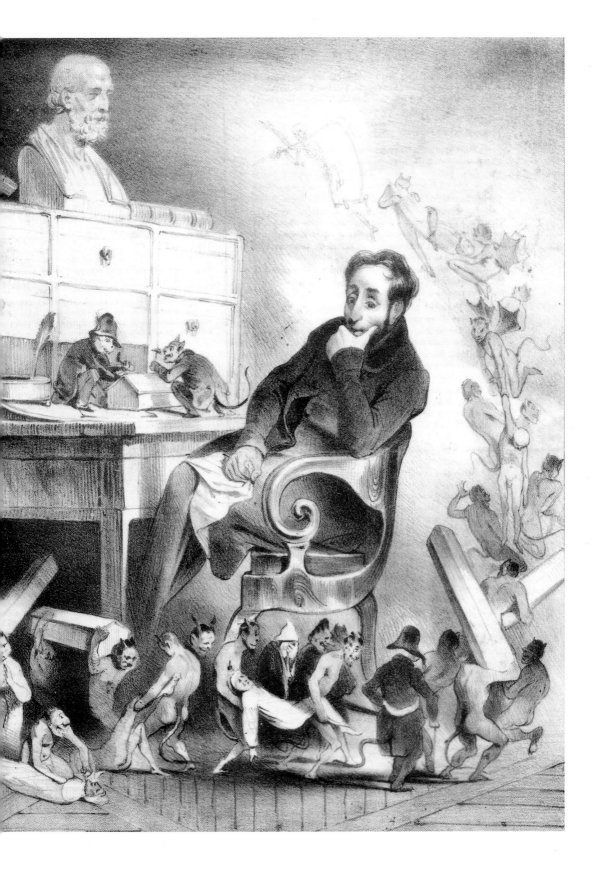

The third-century martyrs,
Casmas and Damian, were
the patron saints of
medicine. Attributed to
the Spanish artist Alonso
de Sedano, this painting
(*c*.1495) shows the
miraculous operation in
which they cured a
Christian by appearing to
him in a dream and
replacing his diseased leg
with one from a Moor who
had recently died. The red
robes and hats of the
saints recall those of
contemporary physicians.

**The development of
surgical anaesthesia**.
A growing faith in material
progress was building in
the new industrial age.
A belief that radical trans-
formations were a natural
part of medical improve-
ment encouraged people
to take note of each new
step. Consequently, the
first successful operation
using ether, in Boston in
1846, was immediately
proclaimed as one of the
great medical break-
throughs, and the scene
was recreated for a
photographer shortly
afterwards.

he coupled this finding with the principle of administering medicines in very small doses, shaken vigorously in water to impart their vital structures to the whole liquid. He expanded his views by experimenting on himself, his family, and friends, and published several books, most importantly the *Organon of Rational Healing* (1810).

Water cures also enjoyed great popularity. By the later eighteenth century, towns with medicinal baths (such as Bath, Spa, Baden-Baden, and Aix-les-Bains) were frequented by the well-to-do, who came to socialize as much as to drink and bathe in the waters. Such places became even more popular after the mid-century railroad made access easier. An early nineteenth-century variation was the development of hydrotherapy by Vincent Priessnitz (1799–1851), which used cold, pure water in various mechanical ways to tranquillize and stimulate the nervous system and so to effect cures. From the late 1830s, hydrotherapy became popular with central European aristocracy, and by the middle of the century the practice had spread even to England, where James Wilson (d. 1867) and James Gully (1808–83) established a fashionable treatment centre at Malvern. Many took the cure there, including Charles Darwin, Tennyson, and Carlyle.

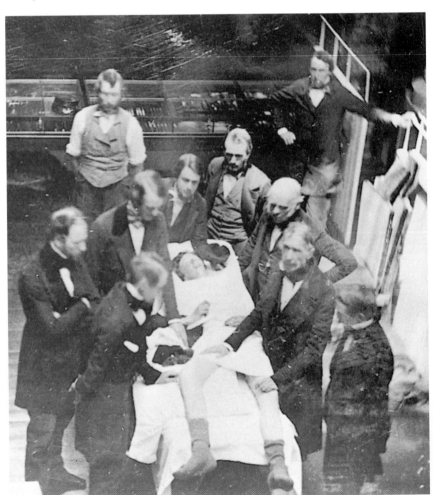

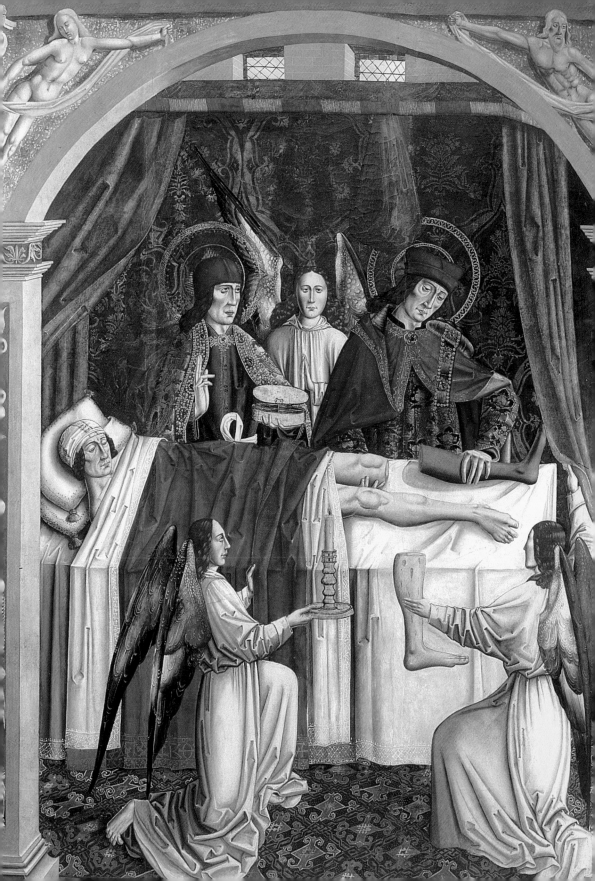

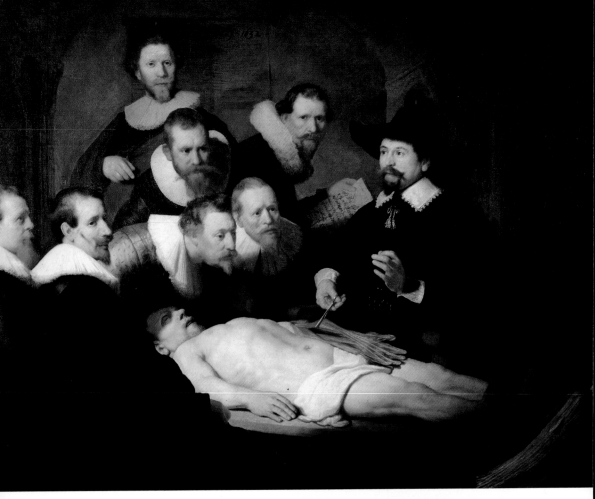

Rembrandt van Rijn, *The Anatomy of Dr Nicolaes Tulp.* The most famous example of a genre depicting anatomical demonstrations before private groups. Here Dr Tulp, *praelector anatomiae* of the Amsterdam surgeons' guild, is shown demonstrating the structure of the hand to seven surgeons. Paintings of anatomical lessons carried not only social connotations about the people who paid to be portrayed in them (like other group portraits), they also conveyed moral messages. The moral lesson here is double and paradoxical: we are but dust, but also created in the image of God.

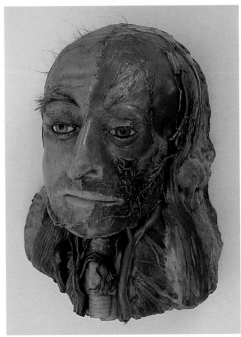

An anatomical wax head. In the eighteenth and early nineteenth centuries, richly detailed anatomical figures and parts were produced in wax and used for teaching. In the tradition of Vesalius, the artists portrayed flesh and blood people—eyes open, skin almost palpable, every hair plain to be seen, and the whole stripped layer by layer to reveal underlying structures. Such models remain unsettling reminders that anatomy was meant to reveal the fabric of life.

While supportive treatments were popular with many, other new medicines came from laboratory research. For instance, François Magendie (1783–1855) performed ingenious animal experiments to study the toxic action of several drugs of vegetable origin in 1809. He could produce similar effects from drugs of different origin, and argued that the similarities must be the result of the same chemical substances. He tried to isolate these substances in their pure states. He and Pierre-Joseph Pelletier (1788–1842) pioneered the use of mild solvents and isolated a wide range of biologically active alkaloid compounds in plants (including caffeine, cinchonine, colchicine, strychnine, and quinine) which were introduced into medical practice in Magendie's *Formulaire* (1821). Accurate dosing and the elimination of impurities now became possible. One of Magendie's pupils, Claude Bernard (1813–78), developed yet further techniques for experimental medicine, finding ways to produce diseases artificially in animals in order to study both disease and treatment in the living system. (He was, however, attacked by antivivisectionists, and required the protection of a friendly police commissioner.) And the famous chemist Justus von Liebig (1803–73) argued that most organic processes (if not all) could be reduced to chemical processes, especially to fermentation—a strictly mechanical view that provoked some of Louis Pasteur's later researches. Liebig established a chemical laboratory at the University of Giessen in 1826, and trained many medical students there.

A more empirical line of chemical experimentation resulted in anaesthesia. Following the work of Joseph Priestley (1733–1804), various kinds of gases had been used in 'pneumatic' medicine, especially through the efforts of Thomas Beddoes (1760–1808), who treated diseases with inhalation of gases. Dr Crawford Long (1815–78) of Georgia noticed the anaesthetic effects of ether on a slave, and subsequently used it to remove a tumour from a patient's neck in 1842—but he published nothing about it at the time. Following the suggestion of one of Beddoes's assistants, Sir Humphry Davy (1778–1829), Horace Wells (1815–48), a dentist of Hartford, Connecticut, began to use nitrous oxide to remove the sensation of pain from his patients in 1844. Before a patient died under his hand and put an end to Wells's practice, he told his friend William Morton (1819–68) about its use. Morton used at least two varieties of the new chemical compound ether to perform painless dentistry, and persuaded John Warren, of the Massachusetts General Hospital, to try his gas on a patient, from whom a neck tumour was removed on 16 October 1846. In a month, Henry Bigelow announced the discovery to the world. Within a year, James Young Simpson (1811–70) used chloroform as a substitute for ether. With ether and chloroform surgical technique was transformed because it could proceed with deliberation rather than speed.

Moreover, shortly after 1839, cell theory—the idea that organisms are composed of cells—became widely accepted. Mathias Schleiden (1804–81), studying the microscopic structure of plants, published a paper in 1838 announcing that all plants were communities of cells, with growth due to an increase in the number of cells; his colleague Theodore Schwann (1810–82) looked for and found cells in all animal tissues, even in the embryonic stage, publishing his paper in 1839. He regarded even non-cellular elements (like teeth) as arising from cells. Rudolph Virchow (1821–1902) took this further in

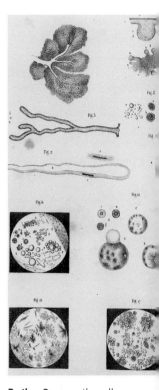

By the 1830s, as the cell theory was being developed, anatomical atlases were publishing illustrations of the microscopical structure of the body. In this example from Marc Jean Bourgery's *Traité complète de l'anatomie de l'homme* (1833–54), Bourgery's illustrator, N. H. Jacob, used a new technique of printing illustrations: lithography. This process enabled many finer effects to be achieved, and therefore chimed well with the efforts to depict the smallest anatomical elements.

97

the mid-1850s by developing the concept of cellular pathology. According to Virchow, all pathology could be defined as what happens to cells (thus ending humoral pathology, in his view): the seat of disease was always to be sought in the cell, and signs of disease were due to reactions of cells to causes of disease.

The consequences of all these investigations for disease theory were many. One of the most important was the connection between organic dirt and disease. In Vienna, Ignaz Phillip Semmelweis (1818–65) demonstrated that cleanliness could prevent the spread of disease. But Semmelweis was not the only person to draw a connection between dirt and disease. The first decades of the nineteenth century saw the proverb 'cleanliness is next to godliness' rise to popularity, while upper- and middle-class people began to separate themselves from the odours of the labouring population. Many people argued that particles produced from organic decay—miasmatic vapours—caused diseases, and that these vaporous miasmas could be identified by their foul stench. Florence Nightingale (1820–1910), a believer in miasmas, became famous for her war against dirt and disease (see Chapter 12). She became a figure of great public authority as a result of her expedition to the British hospitals during the Crimean War (1854–6). She not only offered aid and comfort, but restructured many military hospital services, waging her own war on disorganization and dirt. Together with others, Nightingale's efforts paid off handsomely. When Nightingale's party first arrived at the Scutari base camp in November 1854, the soldiers there were suffering a 60 per cent mortality rate. But at the end of the period of Nightingale's reorganization of the hospitals there and at Balaclava, the mortality rate dropped to just over 1 per cent, with an overall drop in British military hospitals from 42 per cent to 2.2 per cent. While many factors contributed to this drop, the cleaning and scrubbing she organized undoubtedly helped. From her time at least, the cleansing and whitewashing of up-to-date hospital interiors left its own chemical scent on the staff and inmates.

Rapid population increase and migration to the cities (with an accompanying migration to the European colonies and Americas) made fighting contagious disease by fighting filth difficult. The demographic revolution, which began towards the end of the eighteenth century, was probably caused mainly by higher fertility rates (apparently largely due to a falling marriage age), although falling mortality rates also helped contribute to the rising population. European population more than doubled from about 120 million in 1750 to about 265 million in 1850. At the same time, new systems of land tenure and efficiencies in farming required fewer rural labourers, causing migration to the cities. With an abundance of cheap labour and new steam technologies, industrialization often accompanied this intensive urbanization. If the shortening height of British working men is any indication, the health of large segments of the population subsequently declined. Systems meant to help the destitute and the working poor could not cope. In England and Wales, the 'New Poor Law' replaced the old in 1834, creating central authorities in the persons of Poor Law Commissioners (after 1847, Poor Law Boards), who enforced a uniform system of poor relief for the 'deserving' poor along the principle that recipients of relief should be cared for at a level below that of the lowest labourer. The Poor Law Boards unified tax-gathering, built workhouses, organized outdoor relief, and oversaw public medical assistance.

In the cities, mortality rates continued to be very high. Most medical commentators believed that the high rates were due to the unsanitary conditions in which most people lived. And everyone felt threatened by the kinds of contagious diseases that were believed to breed in the cities, spreading through both poor and rich neighbourhoods. Cholera was among the most feared contagions, first appearing in epidemic form in Europe and America in 1830. A second major outbreak occurred in 1847, a third in 1853, and others in the 1860s and after. During these epidemics, mortality rates shot up dramatically, with all segments of the population affected (although the poor were hurt the most).

Attempts to understand the course of infectious outbreaks and their solutions proceeded on all fronts, but especially statistically. In France, for example, Louis Villermé (1782–1863) began studying public hygiene with numerical methods developed in studies first of the army, then of prison and penitentiary populations, and finally of urban society. He was interested especially in numerical investigation of mortality differences among social groups. He showed that clear differences existed in the mortality rates of different urban neighbourhoods, and he correlated those differences with the wealth of the inhabitants. He made a strong case that the higher mortality of poor neighbourhoods was caused by 'filth diseases', and that these diseases were due not to environment but to impoverished living conditions. He believed, however, that the conditions would gradually improve along with the rising wealth of France, urging people in the meantime to take steps on their own to amelio-

Urban life as many of the labouring poor experienced it: crowded and insanitary. New methods of cheap print made it possible to reach large parts of the public through popular newspapers and magazines, and for social and medical reformers to carry their messages to the middle classes and even to the poor themselves. Coupled with the information of trades unions and mass political parties, public debate about the health conditions of teeming urban neighbourhoods gathered momentum in the early twentieth century.

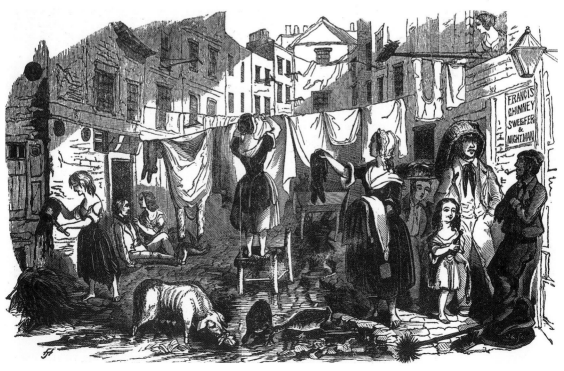

rate their conditions by using clean water for bathing, for washing clothes, and for carrying away waste.

In England, William Farr (1807–83), appointed Compiler of Abstracts in the Registrar General's Office in 1839 (because of nepotism he never achieved the post of Registrar General), believed in a miasmatic account of disease, and showed statistically that contagious diseases were worse in low-lying areas than on higher ground, therefore proving, he thought, that the morbific particles had weight. The solution was to remodel urban neighbourhoods and buildings, allowing for a better circulation of air and removal of organic wastes. Farr's fellow reformer, Edwin Chadwick (1800–90), who had been secretary to the founder of utilitarianism, Jeremy Bentham, became chief of the new Poor Law Commissioners in London. In 1839 he commissioned three doctors to look into connections between disease and poverty, who concluded that poverty contributed to disease and that disease could turn the poor into paupers. Perhaps one-fifth of all poverty in London was due to disease, they argued. Controlling disease would therefore benefit the economy and hold down the poor rates.

Chadwick followed the initial study with the *Report on the Sanitary Condition of the Labouring Population of Great Britain* (1842), based on evidence sent in from 1,000 Medical Officers of Health (who were attached to local Poor Law Boards). It was a detailed and scathing report on the inner cities of England, examining the connections between mortality rates and the physical conditions of dwellings, their occupancy, their external services (water and sewage) and internal services (air, light, and so on), the diet of their inmates, food adulteration, and other factors. The *Report* exposed the connections between living conditions and shorter lifespans, reduced working efficiencies, and increased crime and violence among the poor. Chadwick and his followers argued that the solution was to reduce illness mainly by removing filth through sanitary works, plumbing, and better buildings. Taxes would have to pay for the new sanitary infrastructure, and central government involvement was necessary to force local governments to meet their obligations to their citizens. The relationship between polluted water and cholera became even clearer after John Snow (1813–58) had the handle removed from the Broad Street pump during the London epidemic of 1854, after which the disease in the neighbourhood declined dramatically.

But others went further, concluding that the need for change demanded more. Friedrich Engels (1820–95), for instance, drew heavily on Chadwick's *Report* in drawing up his own manifesto on *The Condition of the Working Class in England in 1844* (1845). In it he argued that, since society now knew that the conditions under which it made people live brought them to premature and 'unnatural' deaths, their deaths had been as premeditated as in murder. Engels, too, used scientific arguments to prove his point: the millions of lungs and hundreds of thousands of coal fires concentrated in the four square miles of London, for instance, consumed an immense amount of oxygen while producing large quantities of carbon dioxide, at the same time that decaying organic matter generated poisonous gases. For Engels, who had just met Karl Marx, a radical transformation of society would be necessary to allay the murderous conditions of the working class.

Conclusion

The example of the uses Engels made of contemporary medical theory in his examination of the condition of the English working classes is a reminder that the medical materialism of the period might be dangerous to the establishment. From the time of Harvey to that of Bernard, priests and poets, ordinary people and princes, had worried about the potential atheism inherent in investigations into the living body, investigations that assumed that physical structure and electrical and chemical fluid could explain all the properties of health and disease. Medical materialism became associated in the minds of many with the radicalism of the French Revolution, and with the medical agitators who were trying to reform the profession; these associations may have kept Charles Darwin from publishing his views on evolution for many years. Yet others, including those who were trying to move their societies towards less cruelty towards both animals and other people, saw the medical establishment as an enemy that promoted unfeeling mechanism. On the other hand, many profoundly religious spirits—whether contributors to hospital projects or reformers like Florence Nightingale—sometimes made common cause with the latest medical thinking. Given the complex texture of the cultural fabric from 1620 to 1860, the variety of opinions about medicine should come as no surprise. Controversy raged both within the medical establishment and between it and other practitioners and publics.

But the growing power of medical materialism would have had much less influence had the number of medical practitioners with a formal education not increased at the same time. These men, organized into new professional groups, were increasingly able to shoulder aside other practitioners, although they did not yet hold a monopoly on medical practice. From Harvey's time onwards, they made their way in the market economy all the while trying to maintain a view of medicine as something more than simply the sale of procedures or drugs. They defended their learning, diagnostic skills, and scientific outlook as superior to what any others possessed. They had Reason on their side, and the encouragement of governments, who required their assistance in meliorating the living conditions of their citizens. Throughout the period, medical men gave authoritative advice on good government. That advice became ever more important as national governments took on more authority and responsibility and as the conditions of the working poor worsened. Taken together, these processes add up to something called 'medicalization': greater numbers of medically educated practitioners gaining greater authority over others while also viewing more and more problems as rooted in the material structures of the human frame. Even by the middle of the nineteenth century, these processes were far from complete. But they do suggest that the development of medicine has been intimately connected to the forces that have helped to create the modern world.

7 From the Germ Theory to 1945

E. M. TANSEY

THE latter half of the nineteenth century was characterized by exploration and change, both physical and intellectual. The appearance of *The Communist Manifesto* by Karl Marx and Friedrich Engels (1848) and *Origin of Species* by Charles Darwin (1859), both of which were to have enormous impact and influence, epitomize that intellectual reform, and social and scientific revolution. At the same time, expeditions to remote regions, tropical and polar, to high altitudes or bathyspheric depths, coincided with explorations into new microscopic and atomic worlds, as techniques and instruments increasingly revealed the physico-chemical determinants and mechanisms of living material, and promoted investigations into disease causation. The records of these enquiries and explorations became ever more visual, especially after the announcement of Daguerre's discovery in 1839 of photography. Images as diverse as photomicrographs, X-rays, and physiological tracings not only began to be used as techniques of record and note, but also became increasingly incorporated into routine practice and research as integral components of the conduct of medicine and medical science.

Cell Theory and Germ Theory

Microscopic visualizations played a large part, during the mid-part of the century, in developing and supporting concepts of normal and abnormal structure and function. The work of the German physiologist and histologist Theodor Schwann (1810–82) and his compatriot Jacob Schleiden (1804–86) emphasized that living matter was composed of units called cells. Cell theory was elaborated into a theory of disease causation by the German pathologist Rudolf Virchow (1821–1902), whose *Die Cellularpathologie* (1858) proclaimed 'omnis cellula e cellula'—that all cells originated from cells and that all disease was a disease of cells. The further idea that micro-organisms, 'germs', were responsible for many common, often fatal, diseases, such as diphtheria, measles, tetanus, typhoid, and cholera, gained credence and acceptance from the work of many people. Foremost among these were the French chemist

Louis Pasteur (1822–95) and the German pathologist Robert Koch (1843–1910), often regarded as the fathers of bacteriology. Pasteur's investigations into the practical problems of fermentation in the brewing and viticulture industries led him to study the related phenomenon of putrefaction. His classic experiments, in which nutrient broth was placed in swan-necked flasks from which dust but not air was excluded, clearly demonstrated that putrefaction relied on the presence of micro-organisms.

By the 1860s Pasteur's theories about the roles of micro-organisms were further extended when he investigated a disease of silkworms that was severely affecting the French silk industry, and revealed that bacteria were responsible. In 1876 Robert Koch published a major work on the life cycle of the anthrax bacillus, demonstrating that the disease was caused by the active spread of the bacterium, which could lie dormant for many years, thus appearing at intermittent intervals, an aspect of the disease that had baffled many investigators. In 1882 Koch isolated the tuberculosis-causing bacillus, and developed a culture medium in which the micro-organisms could be grown *in vitro*. This was an important technical and theoretical contribution, and Koch suggested four experimental criteria that should be satisfied to prove the causative relationship between a micro-organism and a disease. The micro-organism had to be isolated from infected animals, cultivated and identified in the laboratory, and then reinjected into healthy animals which subsequently became ill. These three stages, with the additional proviso that the same micro-organism was further isolated from the host animal, became codified as 'Koch's postulates'. Koch and his associates subsequently discovered the causative bacteria of many diseases, and thus diagnosis, treatment, and prevention became increasingly possible by understanding, and controlling, the inductive micro-organisms. In particular, efforts were made to produce vaccines, preparations of attenuated or killed bacteria, which were able to stimulate a mild form of the disease and hence confer immunity. Although there were considerable debates about the mechanisms by which such immunity was created, Pasteur, Koch, and others attempted to produce reliable prophylactics. Pasteur developed, with limited success, vaccines and therapeutic protocols against anthrax and rabies; Koch developed tuberculin, a partial vaccine against tuberculosis that failed to live up to its curative expectations, and actually caused fatalities. Tuberculin did, however, become a useful diagnostic and epidemiological tool, as it stimulated an allergic reaction in persons or animals already harbouring the bacillus, allowing them to be clearly identified.

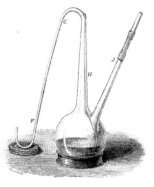

One of the irregular-necked flasks used by Louis Pasteur in experiments on spontaneous generation. He showed that culture medium in the flask did not putrefy because dust, including micro-organisms, failed to contaminate the broth, which was continuously open to the atmosphere.

Antitoxins and Pharmaceutical Beginnings

A major breakthrough in the treatment of infectious diseases came in 1890, when two former assistants of Koch's, Emil von Behring (1854–1917), collaborating with Shibasabura Kitasato (1842–1931), developed serum antitoxins to counter diphtheria and tetanus. In this technique, the toxin from the disease-causing bacillus was separately cultured and treated, and then it, rather than the bacillus, was injected into an experimental animal, initially a sheep or goat. The host animal's immune system then manufactured circulating antitoxins against the specific poison injected into it. After a period of time, blood was collected from the host animal, and a therapeutic serum, rich in specific antitoxins, prepared for injection into human patients suffering from the disease. Although the mechanisms by which the antitoxins were produced, or were effective, were not understood (it was not until the work of MacFarlane Burnet and other immunologists in the 1950s and 1960s that antibody production was construed), the technique opened up a major therapeutic possibility. This potential was increased in 1894 by the French bacteriologist Émil Roux (1853–1933), who raised antitoxins in horses, which greatly increased the yield of usable, and marketable, therapeutic serum.

So far, we have seen that during the late nineteenth and early twentieth centuries there was an extraordinarily rapid increase in new ways of treating and preventing many bacterial diseases with antitoxins and vaccines. These therapies were of biological origin, derived from animals, and were the practical outcome of cell theory and germ theory. They continued to be used and refined well into the twentieth century and provided a major stimulus to the development of the pharmaceutical industry. At the same time, the demand for 'wonder drugs' encouraged the production of new chemical agents, and these two lines of research, into biological and chemical therapies, continued hand in hand.

There was already, especially in Germany, a well-established chemical industry that developed and exploited these new therapies. This industrial development had resulted from the growth of the coal-tar and associated dyestuff industries, and from synergistic advances in both organic and inorganic chemistry. The first synthetic dye, 'mauve', had actually been developed in Britain, but it was German, and to a lesser extent Swiss, industrial machinery that extended the technical know-how into producing synthetic chemical therapeutic agents.

Many large pharmaceutical companies such as Hoechst, Bayer, Ciba, and Sandoz originated from the dye-stuff industry. Commercial companies and some academic institutes, such as the Pasteur Institute in Paris, attempted to produce Roux's therapeutic serum on a large scale. In Britain the London-based pharmaceutical firm of Burroughs, Wellcome & Co. and the Brown Animal Sanatory Institution, a small research laboratory associated with the University of London, first produced diphtheria antitoxins towards the end of 1894.

The search for new *synthetic* chemicals for treating disease accelerated towards the end of the nineteenth century. The potions, pills, and nostrums of the quack began to give way to rational, mass-produced, and mass-marketed therapies. The impact of biological therapies, animal-derived products such as vaccines and antitoxins, did not, however, deflect the burgeoning pharmaceutical industry away from synthetic chemistry. 'Aspirin' was produced at the very end of the nineteenth century by the Bayer company, and Paul Ehrlich, working in association with Meister, Lucius, and Bruning in 1909, developed Salvarsan, the potent anti-syphilitic drug.

Paul Ehrlich (1854–1915), one of the outstanding figures of twentieth-century medical science, made important contributions in several areas of research, and most notably fostered the science of chemotherapy, the use of chemicals to destroy disease-causing organisms. After early studies of the diphtheria bacillus and the generation of antitoxins, he began, at the turn of the century, to consider broader issues of experimental therapeutics. From a study of the differential staining properties of bacteria to dyes available from German industry, he proposed that some dyes could act as therapeutic agents. Ehrlich's experimental work was strongly influenced by, and in turn was influential upon, his theoretical concepts of cell–cell and cell–drug interactions, his so-called 'side-chain theory'. From this proposal arose major advances in understanding immunological and chemotherapeutic mechanisms, and concomitant technical advances in the treatment of some diseases. Ehrlich, for instance, proposed that it would be feasible to produce a therapeutic 'magic bullet' precisely targeted for the causative agent of each disease. Unrelated work, in the Cambridge Physiological Laboratory by John Langley (1852–1925), on the effects of poisons on elements of the autonomic nervous system led Langley to propose that the precise effects of toxins were associated with 'receptive substances' on the cell walls. These two theories coalesced during the early decades of the twentieth century into the receptor theory. This theory, which postulated that there were specific sites on cell membranes which interact with endogenous and exogenous agents, had a major impact on the discovery, design, and utilization of medicinal drugs and on the understanding of basic control mechanisms within the body.

Medical Research and Research Institutes

The provision of facilities for the support of medical research gradually increased as the nineteenth century progressed, and scientific endeavour moved from the domain of the interested and talented amateur into the realm of the professional. In continental Europe, the success of preventive techniques and bacteriology was epitomized by the creation of purpose-built institutes focused on practical applications. In Germany, Koch, Ehrlich, and Behring all had laboratories built for them, often financed by both private and public money. Ehrlich's institute received financial support from the commercial company Meister, Lucius & Bruning (later Hoechst). In France, Pasteur Institutes were established in Paris (1888), and other cities on mainland France and in French colonies, principally endowed by private subscriptions. Work less directly associated with disease mechanisms also developed: the physiological research of Claude Bernard (1813–78) at the Collège de France laid the foundations of experimental medicine and became internationally renowned. Amongst many contributions, Bernard investigated the function of nerves that control the dilation or contraction of blood vessels, discovered glycogen from experiments on the liver, studied the effects of drugs such as opium and curare on the nervous system, and examined foetal physiology and the function of the placenta. The work of such men as Bernard in France, and Johann Purkinje (1787–1869) and Carl Ludwig (1816–95) in Germany—systematic investigations of natural functional processes involving the use of recording and measuring equipment—laid the foundations of physiology as an experimental discipline.

The establishment of experimental physiology during the final decades of the nineteenth century was of vital importance to the development of sci-

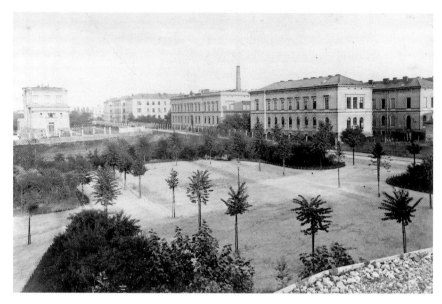

**Carl Ludwig's
Physiological Institute** at
Leipzig, c.1880. To these
laboratories students
travelled from all parts of
Europe and North America
to learn the techniques
and concepts of the new
experimental physiology.

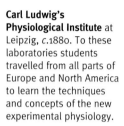

entific medicine in the twentieth. Physiology, the study of the basic normal
functioning of the body, underpins not only the study of the abnormal, pathological processes seen in disease, but also the development of rational therapeutic strategies to treat disease. The reputation of innovative investigative
scientists like Bernard and Ludwig, and their institutes, attracted students
from across Europe and North America, who travelled to learn new attitudes
and methods for the promotion of preventive and experimental medicine. The
further growth, diversification, and vigour of the new medical sciences were
contingent upon several factors, as these visitors returned to their homes to
agitate for the same facilities and salary support that they saw in foreign
laboratories. In Britain in particular this coincided with public concern about
the 'made-in-Germany' phenomenon, and some recognition that the inadequate funding and promotion of science severely handicapped manufacturers
and industrialists in applying what limited scientific knowledge they had
acquired. This was acknowledged as being particularly acute with regard to
the chemical industry, and the development of new therapeutic pharmaceuticals.

The situation was the same in the development of experimental medicine.
Physiology in the UK, for example, relied on the efforts of men directly
influenced by the continental experiences. William Sharpey (1802–80) at University College London did much to establish an infrastructure for physiological research and teaching. Michael Foster (1836–1907) left University College
in 1870 for Trinity College Cambridge, the first definitive step towards the
creation thirteen years later of the University's Physiological Laboratory.
Similarly, Foster's colleague and successor at University College, John Burdon-
Sanderson (1828–1905), moved to Oxford in 1883 to establish physiology at the
university, whilst Edward Schäfer (1850–1935) remained at University College
London until 1899, when he became Professor of Physiology in Edinburgh. In
much of Europe, and in the USA too, physiology was established and spread by
those directly influenced by continental developments, and many physiolo-

gists working at the turn of the twentieth century had had a formative period in a French or German research laboratory.

Despite agitation and concern about the financing and promotion of scientific enterprises, widespread state patronage for such endeavours was not rapidly forthcoming, and the promotion of research, laboratory or bedside, experimental or preventive, depended greatly on the initiatives of individual scientists and practitioners in persuading their universities or wealthy philanthropists or organizations to support their causes. In the UK, a public collection in acknowledgement of Pasteur's rabies work raised over £2,000, which led to the establishment in 1891 of the British Institute for Preventive Medicine (later called the Jenner, and later still the Lister, Institute). With an endowment of £250,000 from Lord Iveagh, a member of the Guinness brewing family, it acquired a purpose-built site on the Chelsea Embankment in London.

Charitable contributions from the general public were the basis of the Imperial Cancer Research Fund, established in 1901 to support laboratory research focused on that one particular disease. In contrast, the Beit Fund established in 1908 by the South African diamond and gold magnate Sir Otto Beit provided a major injection of support for professional medical research in the UK. The fund furnished ten annual scholarships, each of three years' duration, in medical research, and most unusually women were eligible to apply at a time when women's access to higher education was severely restricted. A far more conspicuous development in the promotion of scientific medicine, however, was the opening in 1901 of the Rockefeller Institute for Medical Research in New York, under the directorship of Simon Flexner (1863–1946), and supported by the oil-generated wealth of the Rockefeller dynasty. This institute, with a research hospital attached, quickly gained a reputation as a major player in US medicine, not only for the strength of its scientific research, which included serum and vaccine development, but also as an educational institute. Rockefeller money funded medically related projects worldwide, especially through its Sanitary Commission (later International Health Board), and Rockefeller money was vital for the resurgence and reconstruction of medical research after the First World War.

New Equipment and Technologies

Institutional and professional expansion during the final decades of the nineteenth century was accompanied by demands for specialized equipment as physical measuring and analysing techniques began to take their place in the research laboratory, clinic, and hospital ward. Several instruments to measure dynamic events were produced by the pupils of the German physiologist Johannes Müller (1801–58). Hermann von Helmholtz (1821–94) invented the ophthalmoscope to facilitate his research on the physics of vision; he also measured the speed of conduction along a nerve fibre, and developed a law of the conservation of energy—that energy could neither be created nor destroyed—which delivered a body blow to the theory of vitalism. Carl Ludwig (1816–95) devised several items of apparatus, including most notably the kymograph, a recording instrument that enabled the graphical representation of a variety of physiological phenomena such as the blood pressure, heart rate, and muscle contraction. These instruments did not remain as exclusive items of laboratory equipment. Improvements, adaptations, and alterations provided a new generation of instruments for use in clinical diagnosis. Ludwig's technique for measuring blood pressure depended on the insertion of a tube into an artery to allow blood to flow into a manometer. This was hardly suitable for clinical practice, and a reliable sphygmomanometer, to measure blood pressure without puncturing a vessel, was developed just before the turn of the century.

In contrast to measurements of dynamic functional parameters, improvements in microscopes for static observations and measurements were also made, especially after the invention of the achromatic lens by Joseph Lister (1786–1869), father of the surgeon Joseph (Lord) Lister. These were matched by advances in the techniques of preserving, cutting, and selectively staining sections for histological examination. An especially valuable staining technique for the nervous system was developed by the Italian Camillo Golgi (1843–1926). The beauty of his method was that it impregnated, with silver nitrate, just a few nerve cells in a slice of brain tissue, thus allowing them to be clearly identified and studied against a bland background. Golgi claimed that these nerve cells were connected together forming a net or reticulum. The Spanish anatomist Santiago Ramón y Cajal (1852–1934) used Golgi's own staining technique but arrived at a different conclusion, that the nerve cells, or neurons, were discrete units. Ironically perhaps, the two men shared the Nobel Prize in 1906, still wedded to their separate, contrary, hypotheses. By then, however, Cajal's views were increasingly accepted, and the British physiologist Charles Sherrington (1857–1952) had coined the word 'synapse' for the gap between nerve cells.

Sherrington made numerous contributions to the study of the structure and, most notably, the function of the nervous system, in addition to being one of the first to produce diphtheria antitoxins in Britain, in 1894, at the Brown Animal Sanatory Institution in London. His active career began in the 1880s, when neurological research was a part-time interest of medical practitioners, and ended during the 1930s, when it was a full-time professional activity, often of non-medically qualified scientists.

Sherrington used electrophysiological recording methods in anaesthetized animals extensively, and also developed detailed histological analyses to augment his studies. He described the reciprocal innervation of antagonistic muscles, by which the activity of one set of excited muscles is coordinated with another set of inhibited muscles, from which he proposed the existence of inhibitory mechanisms; he studied sense organs extensively, especially the distribution and mechanisms of proprioceptors; he mapped the motor areas of the cerebral cortex of mammals; and he described the functional unit of the nervous system, the reflex arc, consisting of at least two neurons. Sherrington postulated two major concepts from his investigations. 'The

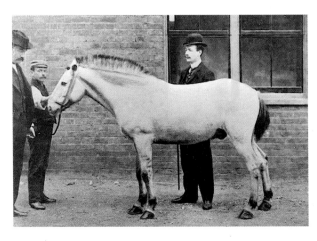

Tom, the horse in which diphtheria antitoxins were first raised in 1894, at the Brown Animal Sanatory Institution in South London. To the far right of the picture is Armand Ruffer, and standing behind Tom is Charles Sherrington, then the Professor-Superintendent of the Institution, and winner of the Nobel Prize in Physiology or Medicine in 1932 for his contributions to neurophysiology.

final common pathway' referred to the convergence of reflex arcs from several sensory inputs onto one efferent (output) neuron, which thus formed a final pathway, for all the inputs, to the effector muscle.

Sherrington's second major concept was summarized in *The Integrative Action of the Nervous System* (1906), which expanded his experimental observations into a conception of nervous system function, coordination, and connectivity that established the basis of modern understanding of the mechanisms by which the nervous system integrates and controls information from, and responses to, the external environment.

The nervous system was being subjected to a variety of different investigations at the turn of the twentieth century. Physiologists were probing the living brain of anaesthetized animals to correlate anatomical localization with behavioural function; neurologists and neuropathologists associated the effects of head injuries, often the result of industrial accidents, with deficits during life and post-mortem pathology; and in Vienna the psychiatrist Sigmund Freud (1856–1939), trained as a neurologist, divided the mind into the realms of the conscious, preconscious, and subconscious and developed the theory and practice of psychoanalysis.

Perhaps the most extraordinary discovery of that period, however, was that of X-rays in late 1895, the result of an unexpected observation by the physicist Wilhelm Röntgen (1845–1923). The potential of X-rays was recognized immediately, and they were rapidly integrated into hospital practice, heralding a move towards non-invasive diagnostic procedures that would grow throughout the twentieth century. The therapeutic and research possibilities of X-rays were picked up very quickly, the US physiologist Walter Cannon (1871–1945) examining the passage of radio-opaque food down the gastrointestinal tract of animals as early as 1897, and his technique was put to clinical use almost immediately. Many of the early X-ray workers, unprotected because of their ignorance of its dangers, developed ulcers, lesions, and even cancers from their exposure. Therapeutically, the burning power of X-rays was used to treat proliferative diseases, as were the emanations of radium, discovered in 1898, often as radium needles implanted into tumours.

Specialization

The development and use of specialized techniques and equipment in turn encouraged specialization within the medical profession. To examine just one clinical arena, the use of graphical registration methods in the laboratory, especially in the London physiological institute of Augustus Waller (1856–1922), encouraged the development of the clinical electrocardiogram (e.c.g.) in Holland by Willem Einthoven (1860–1927). The procedure not only facilitated understanding of normal cardiac physiology but also revealed a means by which abnormal pathology could be formulated and diagnosed. The provision and use of the recording equipment and the interpretation of the results encouraged practitioners to specialize in the diagnosis of heart disorders, and during the course of the twentieth century the e.c.g. became a routine part of clinical diagnosis, and the equipment and procedures involved in its preparation were increasingly clarified and simplified. Professional spe-

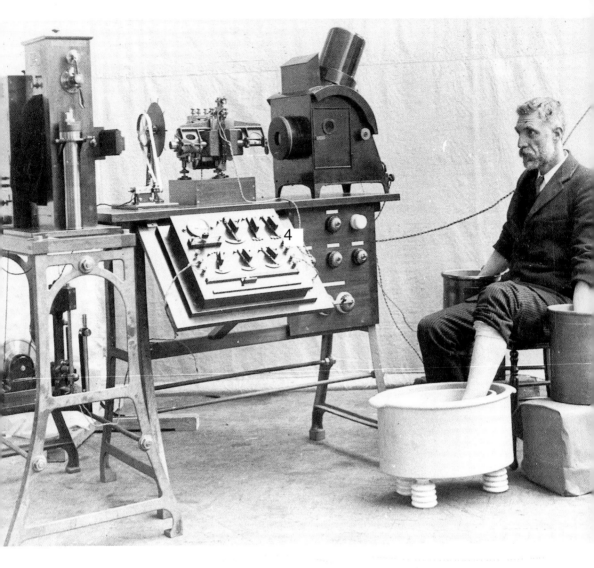

4

Electrocardiograph manufactured by Cambridge Scientific Instruments in association with Willem Einthoven in 1912. The electrodes were tubs of electrolyte solution (usually saline) in which the patients immersed their limbs.

cialization fostered the development of societies and journals devoted to specific fields of research and practice, and dedicated training schemes and qualifications became important in defining and reinforcing the boundaries of such specializations.

Therapeutic specialization was encouraged by the impact of antitoxins in the late 1890s, because their arrival coincided with, and exacerbated, concerns about the purity of drugs and the role of quacks and pill pedlars in the medical market place. In the UK, calls for an 'ethical pharmacy' from some medical practitioners and pharmaceutical manufacturers were reinforced in 1896 when the *Lancet* investigated the diphtheria antitoxins from nine European manufacturers, and pronounced many of them to be deficient or contaminated. UK procedures were heavily criticized, and increased demands for standardization and purity controls were voiced. In the USA such concerns received readier acknowledgement, and in 1906 the Food and Drug Act was passed to ensure minimum standards of preparation and to counteract adulteration, in US and imported food and medicinal products. In 1938 this was repealed, and largely replaced by the Food, Drug and Cosmetic Act, and was to lead, shortly after the Second World War, to the creation of the Food and Drug Administration of the USA, probably the largest, most demanding, and most comprehensive government watchdog in the world for the control of new foods and drugs. In contrast, it was not until 1926, after the discovery of insulin, that very limited legislation, the Therapeutic Substances Act, was enacted in the UK and not until the impetus of the thalidomide tragedy, after the Second World War, that broad legislation, the Safety of Medicines Act, came into being.

Further research on antitoxins led to the development of more prophylactic measures, and the trial development of serum therapies and vaccines against several types of diseases, including cancer. However, many of these products were unsuccessful, and the routine administration of antitoxins began to reveal an array of adverse effects, loosely categorized as 'serum sickness'. Further investigations into the mechanisms of immunity showed that a second injection of a foreign protein, such as antitoxin, into a body oversensitized by a first injection, could promote an enhanced, sometimes fatal, reaction by the body's natural defence mechanisms of the immune system. Experimental work on this phenomenon, named anaphylaxis, revealed a great deal about allergic responses in general, and laid the groundwork from which effective therapeutic strategies were developed for an array of allergic conditions, including hay fever and asthma, after the Second World War.

Surgery

The impact of the germ theory was especially profound in the practice of surgery. Joseph (later Lord) Lister (1827–1912) developed an array of antiseptic techniques, constructing a phenol spray to cover the wound and surrounding areas during operations and using dressings soaked in phenol to diminish post-operative infection. Later still, the surgical instruments, which both Pasteur and Koch had recommended boiling, and the hands and clothes of surgeons became incorporated into aseptic regimes, as did the use of protective gowns, masks, and gloves. The US surgeon William Halstead (1852–1922) first introduced rubber gloves because his fiancée, a theatre nurse, developed a sensitivity reaction to the antiseptic then in regular use. As the twentieth century progressed the more widespread use of stainless steel provided surgical instruments that were resistant to corrosion and easier to sterilize. Operative practice was further facilitated by the routine use of anaesthesia, introduced almost simultaneously in the USA and the UK in 1846. The increasing use of general and local anaesthesia stimulated the search for new and safer chemical agents for inhalation anaesthesia, and for new techniques and routes for anaesthetic administration, and laid the foundations for the development of the medical speciality of anaesthetics.

The increased ease and safety of surgery afforded by improved antisepsis and anaesthesia permitted surgeons to go into anatomical regions previously unexplored, thus stimulating the beginnings of surgical specialization. During the early part of the twentieth century, abdominal, neurological, endocrine, thoracic, and gynaecological surgery all began to move away from the province of the general surgeon, and into distinct and separate territories that would flourish after the Second World War. To take just one example, gastrointestinal surgery was strongly dependent on the work of surgeon Theodor Billroth (1829–94), to whom his close friend Brahms dedicated two string quartets. Billroth's technical developments, patient management, and follow-up strategies, including detailed post-mortems, influenced surgeons across Europe and the USA. He was a firm believer in Lister's methods, without which his own work would not have been possible. He developed operative procedures that are still, with modifications, in use today for surgery of the stomach, intestine, and thyroid gland, and did pioneer work on removing cancerous and diseased tissue, including the perforated appendix, the cause of often fatal appendicitis. The British surgeon Sir Frederick Treves used the technique of appendectomy with notable success, and much publicity, in 1902, when the coronation of King Edward VII was postponed because of his acute appendicitis.

Although Edward VII's operation took place in Buckingham Palace, the growing sophistication of surgical procedures encouraged the creation of special places—namely, properly equipped operating theatres in a hospital—where such techniques were performed. Hospitals, previously seen as the refuge of the sick poor, became increasingly accepted as places of specialized medical care for a wider section of the community. This was particularly marked in the USA, which in 1873 had fewer than 50,000 beds in less than 180 hospitals, including mental institutes. By 1910 over 420,000 beds were available in nearly 440 hospitals, and on the eve of the Second World War almost 7,000 hospitals provided over 1.1 million beds. Similar trends towards hospital-based medical and surgical facilities occurred in most Western European countries as the twentieth century progressed.

Another component of the growth of hospitals was that of the development of ancillary medical professions. Nursing had been revolutionized by the British nurse Florence Nightingale (1820–1910), who founded a Nursing School at St Thomas's Hospital in London in 1860. This improved the training and enhanced the status of the profession worldwide, although it was not until 1919 that Britain enacted licensing legislation with a Nurses Registration Act, eighteen years after the first such state registration in New Zealand.

Public Health and Hygiene

The astounding scientific advances of the late nineteenth century, characterized by antisepsis, anaesthetics, antitoxins, and X-rays, were accompanied by equally, if not more, important measures in hygiene and public health. Growing industrialization and overcrowding in city slum accommodation promoted sanitary and industrial reform, especially in the UK. Initiatives by John (later Sir John) Simon (1816–1904) resulted in the Factory Act (1867), the Workshop Act (1867), the Sanitary Act (1866), the Vaccination Act (1871), and the Artisans' and Labourers' Dwellings Act (1868). Minimum standards of public hygiene and workplace safety, the provision of clean water, recreational green spaces in public parks, and adequate sanitation all became increasing concerns as the twentieth century opened. Such social advances coincided with worries about infant mortality, stimulated in the UK by the poor physical condition of recruits for the Boer War. In particular, the attention of researchers and practitioners was focused on improving maternal welfare and education, and an especial interest became the improvement of domestic hygiene and nutrition.

Opposition to Scientific Medicine

The advances in medical science and practice that occurred through the final years of the nineteenth century were not without their critics, however. In the UK especially, the use of animals in medical experiments attracted attention from anti-vivisectionists. As early as 1875 a Royal Commission on the practice of subjecting living animals to experiments had taken evidence from opponents and proponents of the practice, and recommended that legislation was appropriate. The following year the 1876 Cruelty to Animals Act was passed, the first such legislation in the world, which allowed *bona fide* experiments to be performed by properly qualified individuals in premises registered with the Home Office. The procedures thus regulated included surgical operations, experiments controlling the type or amount of food or drink given to an animal, and the administering of injections. However, demonstrations and campaigns continued to vilify individual research workers. Apart from occasional isolated protests, such concerns were not consistently mirrored elsewhere in Europe or North America.

The wrath of British anti-vivisectionists was particularly targeted on physiologists. One such was the English surgeon Victor Horsley (1857–1916), whose work on the function of the thyroid gland and its importance in disease, on cerebral localization, and on rabies all depended on experimental animals, all of which attracted the opprobrium of anti-vivisectionists. Much of Horsley's experimental work was done in the Physiology Department of University College London, in which, in 1894, Edward Schäfer (later Sharpey-Schafer) and George Oliver (1841–1915) first isolated the active principle of the adrenal gland, a substance later, but not uncontroversially because of trade-name implications, called adrenaline in the UK (epinephrine is the common word in the USA). Eight years later, in the same department, Schäfer's successor, Ernest Starling (1866–1927), and Starling's brother-in-law, William Bayliss (1860–1924), discovered a substance they called secretin, a chemical messenger carried in the bloodstream, a class of substances they called 'hormones'. The importance of the therapeutic possibilities of these substances, as treatments for deficiency diseases, and their roles in understanding physiological control mechanisms of the normal body, extended far beyond their immediate discovery. The synthesis, understanding, and manipulation of hormones, the speciality of endocrinology, was to become an important component of twentieth-century medical science.

In addition to anti-vivisectionist activity, there were also protests, again articulated with particular force in the UK, against the practice of vaccination. These protests overlapped to some extent, because vaccine preparation required living animals. In 1871 district Public Vaccinators were appointed, doctors who would provide vaccination free of charge to all local children. Much of the opposition to the practice focused on the tricky issue of compulsion, and the arrival of serum antitoxins stimulated a fresh wave of anti-vaccination campaigning, which gained considerable momentum during military operations in South Africa and then the First World War. During these the British Army authorities tried to achieve 100 per cent vaccination of their troops, moves which caused outrage from opponents. Such opposition seems to have been non-existent or muted in other countries: during the First World War Germany had a policy of compulsory vaccination, which was used as pro-vaccination propaganda in the UK, both during and after the hostilities, with some success.

The First World War and Medical Research

The First World War created medical problems that dictated the course of research for the years of hostilities and for some time afterwards. In the UK the Medical Research Committee (which was founded in 1913 and became the Medical Research Council (MRC) in 1920) epitomizes some of these responses. At its very first meeting in 1913 members had recognized the need for a central research facility, modelled on the Rockefeller Institute, but their plans were frustrated until 1919, when the Committee established the National Institute for Medical Research in north London. Committee members identified a number of conditions, including tuberculosis and occupational diseases, which they wished to include in their research programme, and agreed on the need to develop the use and study of statistics. In the conditions of war, most of these plans were disrupted, but the collecting and analysing of statistics relating to casualties, treatment, and disease became of considerable importance. These developments were an integral part of the synergistic growth, and perceived importance, of epidemiology. After the war the use of statistical methods in designing and analysing proper trials of new therapies was greatly improved under the guidance of Austin Bradford Hill (1897–1991), and after the Second World War detailed protocols were evolved for the proper scientific evaluation of the therapeutic efficacy of new medications.

In the battlefields of the first war, the pre-eminent medical problems were the control of infections, the advancement of surgical techniques, and wound control. During that period, the management of compound fractures, wound infection, and the development of plastic, reconstructive surgery all advanced. Anti-vaccination campaigns in the UK subsided; and antitoxins against typhus and tetanus were in great demand in all combatant nations, thus stimulating the growth of pharmaceutical companies. Simultaneously, British manufacturers were under pressure to produce synthetic substitutes for medicines previously obtained from German companies, especially for Ehrlich's anti-syphilitic 'Salvarsan' or arsphenamine, and its more effective derivative, neo-arsphenamine, as treatments for infected troops. The need for effective therapeutic measures against tropical diseases, such as malaria, amoebic dysentery, and sleeping sickness, all concerns of pre-war colonial medical practice, also became exacerbated in wartime. The discovery by Ronald Ross (1857–1932) in the late 1890s of the dual-host (human and mosquito) life cycle of the *Plasmodium* parasite that caused malaria accelerated the search for therapeutic strategies and the development of eradication programmes. And indeed by 1927 the worldwide incidence of malaria was half that at the turn of the century.

However, the effect of disease in the battlefield can be gauged from statistics of the final year of the war—two-thirds of the fatalities amongst the British army were from disease, double the number who died from wounds. Those who survived the battlefields displayed new types of injuries: shell-shock and other psychiatric disturbances lasted for many years, often a lifetime, as did physical disabilities such as limblessness, blindness, and the effects of gassing. The medical care and social rehabilitation for injured servicemen provided fresh challenges to the caring professions, challenges that re-emerged after the Second World War.

The First World War was the first major battlefield on which the Red Cross (later, in Muslim countries, the Red Crescent), founded by five private Swiss citizens in 1863, acted. In 1919 the International League of Red Cross Societies was formed, and calls for peace around the world resulted in the formation of the League of Nations, of which a Health Organization subdivision was established. It was disappointingly ineffectual and collapsed at the onset of the Second World War, and it was not until the aftermath of that later carnage that a World Health Organization was created under the auspices of the United Nations.

Cessation of the hostilities of the First World War did not end medical needs: epidemic typhus spread through the former Russian Empire, riven already by revolution, civil war, and famine. A worldwide pandemic of influenza, of three waves beginning in 1918, may have caused as many as 15–20 million deaths, more than double the total casualties calculated for the preceding war. Not surprisingly, research efforts into influenza and its causative organisms intensified.

Viruses had first been recognized by a pupil of Pasteur's, who had developed a physical filter that allowed the passage of the smaller viruses, whilst retaining larger bacteria. This enabled the tobacco mosaic virus of plants and the foot-and-mouth virus of animals to be identified before the turn of the century. In 1901 the virus that caused yellow fever in humans was isolated, and over the next decades many more viruses were identified. By the early 1920s work at the National Institute for Medical Research in London had discovered the viral cause of canine distemper, and eventually a successful prophylactic vaccine was developed. Ferrets used in distemper research were successfully inoculated with the infected throat washings of institute staff suffering from influenza—the first, despite many attempts, successful transfer of the disease to an animal in which it could then be studied and experimentally manipulated. In 1933 a causative virus was isolated, demolishing the previously held view that a bacillus was responsible. Attempts to provide a comprehensive vaccine have been handicapped by the variety, and changeability, of the influenza-causing viruses. More successful research developed against the polio and smallpox viruses, although mishaps and accidents continued until the development of safe vaccines after the Second World War.

Major Advances in the Inter-War Period

Post First World War reconstruction included many schemes of social and medical relevance. In 1911 the National Insurance Act had been passed in the UK, which provided basic health-care provision for employed men, but not for their families or the unemployed. Those not considered by the terms of the Act had either to pay in full for treatment or apply to local medical committees. The experiences of the First World War and its immediate aftermath, especially the effects of the pandemic influenza, encouraged the belief that the health and fitness of its citizens were proper concerns of the State. The example of health-care schemes developed in the new Soviet republic inspired imitators, and detractors, around the world. In parts of Western Europe, moves were made towards more accessible health insurance, and health-education schemes were established in schools, and maternity clinics, to ensure a healthier future generation.

The Rockefeller Foundation initiated reconstruction and educational schemes to provide scholarships, fellowships, equipment, and buildings that

Diabetic girl before (left) and four months after (right) the beginning of insulin treatment.

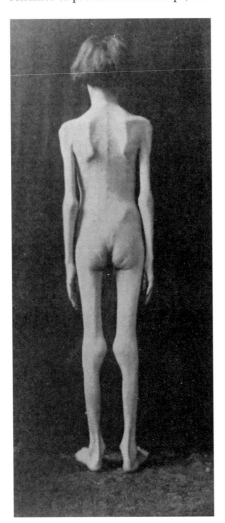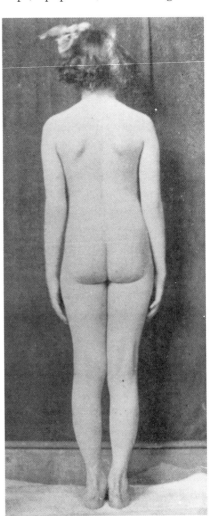

stimulated medical research centres across much of the world. In the UK, the Medical Research Council (reconstituted in 1920 from the Medical Research Committee) collaborated with the Rockefeller Foundation on a number of projects, and also, by supporting its own National Institute for Medical Research and individual scientists in universities and hospitals around the country, promoted professional biomedical research on a scale unimagined at the beginning of the century.

The first major medical scientific discovery of the inter-war period came from the University of Toronto. That the pancreas was involved in preventing diabetes had been known for several decades, and many attempts had been made to isolate an anti-diabetogenic factor, before Frederick Banting (1891–1941) and Charles Best (1899–1978) isolated the active principle, a hormone that they named insulin. An immediate problem was to determine insulin's chemical structure in order to synthesize and produce it commercially. In the event it was not until the 1950s that insulin was produced synthetically. However, chemists at Toronto University and in the Eli Lilly laboratories in the USA perfected extraction and purification methods, which they patented and licensed to reputable producers around the world to ensure judicious manufacture. In the UK, the Medical Research Council held the production patents. The idea of using animal products to replace or stimulate human functioning was not new: in the late nineteenth century the French physician and physiologist Édouard Brown Séquard (1817–94) had promoted organo-therapy, most notably of testicular extracts as rejuvenation therapy. The work of Schäfer, Bayliss, Starling, and others had established the scientific basis of modern endocrinology, from which further investigations in the inter-war period developed. These included the identification of the major sex and pituitary hormones, detailed chemical investigation of the thyroid hormones, and a growing understanding of the role of pituitary hormones in regulating other endocrine functions. The relationships of endocrine disturbances and imbalances to disease mechanisms led to the development of treatment strategies such as replacement therapies and surgical reductions.

During the same period endogenous chemical mediators were convincingly identified in the nervous system. The work of the British physiologist Henry Dale (1875–1968) and the Austrian pharmacologist Otto Loewi (1873–1961) revealed much about the role of naturally occurring substances in the normal function of the nervous system. Their work, especially that of Dale and his collaborators, suggested that the chemical acetylcholine was responsible for the transmission of nerve impulses across some kinds of synapses. Subsequent work after the Second World War on the role of adrenaline-like substances in the nervous system enhanced and developed this concept. At the time, however, these results were not of immediate therapeutic benefit, although developments from this fundamental knowledge after the Second World War subsequently initiated many major advances in pharmacological knowledge and pharmaceutical innovation.

The discovery of insulin focused concern on a pharmaceutical problem that had first been recognized during the 1890s with the advent of the antitoxins—that of standardizing, both nationally and internationally, the units by which the efficacy of such therapies was measured. Inspired by Henry Dale of London and Thorvald Madsen (1870–1957) of Copenhagen, international conferences were held in Edinburgh in 1923 and in Geneva two years later to discuss the problems and possible solutions of such biological standardization. There was general agreement that official international standards should be created, maintained, and made widely available under the auspices of the League of Nations, which established, in 1924, a Permanent Commission on Biological Standards.

An important pharmaceutical advance in the inter-war period was in chemotherapy. The success of Salvarsan before and during the First World War had demonstrated that microbes could be destroyed by synthetic drugs that did not damage the host animal, but the search for similar chemotherapeutic drugs was not particularly successful. Some promising compounds proved to be equally toxic against the host, and, although drugs were developed with some success as trypanocides, anti-malarials, and amoebicides, no major contributions to antibacterial chemotherapy emerged, despite much effort. Thus there were no successful therapeutics against the bacterial diseases and accidental infections that were common in non-tropical climates. In 1932 Gerhard Domagk (1895–1964) in the Bayer laboratories in Germany noted that a dye called Prontosil Red destroyed a haemolytic streptococcal infection in mice, without apparent ill effect on the mice. Clinical trials, most notably in the UK on puerperal (childbed) fever at the Queen Charlotte's Maternity Hospital, and concomitant chemical work in Paris substantiated the clinical claims of the drug, and also revealed that the effective moiety of the compound was a substance called sulphanilamide. This was readily synthesized, and it and various analogues, generically referred to as the sulphonamides, were rapidly manufactured by companies around the world. Particularly significant was the work on assessing the mode of action of this class of drugs. It was shown that they do not immediately kill infective bacteria, but alter bacterial metabolism such that the organisms cannot multiply and overwhelm the host's natural defence systems. Sulphonamides were immediately of vital importance in counteracting puerperal fever, pneumonia, meningitis, and other infections. Although largely superseded now by antibiotics, they still play a role in antibacterial chemotherapy, and their discovery opened up important new therapeutic vistas.

Innovative research on the role of nutritional factors also opened up new vistas on mechanisms of health and disease. The ascendancy of the germ theory, and the success of preventive strategies against infectious agents, had led to the general belief that all diseases were thus caused. In 1906 the British biochemist Frederick Gowland Hopkins (1861–1947) discovered that minute amounts of previously unknown 'accessory food factors' in certain foodstuffs were necessary for growth and development and that their absence caused deficiency diseases. Simultaneously the Danish biochemist Christiaan Eijkman (1858–1930) revealed that chickens fed on polished (husk-less) rice developed a condition similar to the human disease beriberi, which could be corrected by feeding them whole rice grains. In 1929 Eijkman and Hopkins shared the Nobel Prize in Physiology or Medicine for their discovery of what became known as 'vitamins', a word coined by the Polish-born British physiologist Casimir Funk (1884–1967), who was the first of many to link vita-

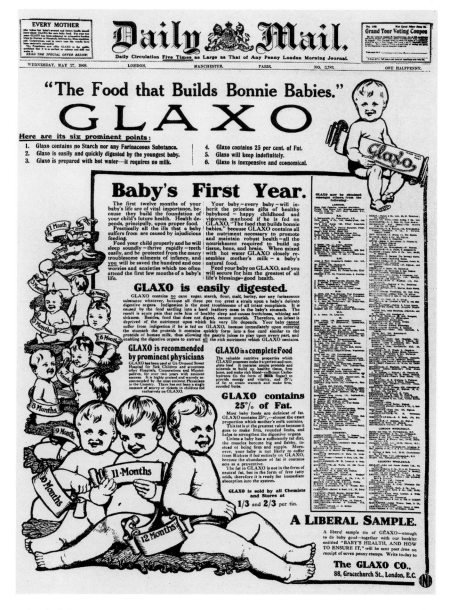

Glaxo powdered milk for babies, to which Vitamin D, the first pharmaceutical preparation of the Glaxo Department (of Nathan & Co.), was added in 1924. Nathan & Co. was one of the first companies to produce dried milk in the early twentieth century, an important contribution to infant welfare at a time when supplies of cow's milk were frequently contaminated.

min deficiencies to specific diseases, such as beriberi, pellagra, scurvy, and rickets.

Research between the two world wars established the chemical identities and physiological functions of vitamins A, C, D, E, and some of the B family, and also recognized the vital importance of certain trace elements and some 'essential' amino acids, in maintaining health and preventing disease. Rather different research approaches led to the understanding of nutritional deficits involved in the anaemias. The discovery that pernicious anaemia could be treated successfully with a raw liver extract led to the discovery of vitamin B_{12}, although it is now understood that it is not vitamin deficiency *per se* that causes the disease, but the absence of intrinsic factor in the intestinal tract, which is needed for the absorption of the vitamin.

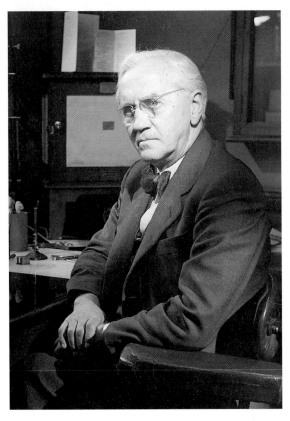

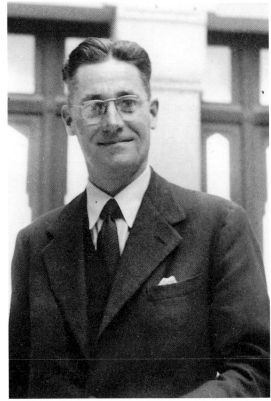

Alexander Fleming
(*left*), the discoverer
of penicillin, in his
laboratory, 1951.

Howard Florey (*right*),
the Australian-born
pathologist and
physiologist who, with
Ernst Chain, led the
Oxford team that
successfully isolated
penicillin.

The climate of knowledge about, and interest in, nutritional matters encouraged food manufacturers to market 'vitaminized' foodstuffs, one such being the dried baby food of Nathan & Co., marketed under the trade name 'Glaxo', which marked the beginning of that company's involvement with medicinal products. The concept, which matured in the later decades of the twentieth century, began to take shape, that nutritional supplements might not only correct a deficient input, but also enhance an adequate diet. Debates as to what constituted adequacy in these circumstances have raged since the late 1920s, and in 1941 the first Table of Recommended Dietary Allowances was produced by the Food and Nutrition Committee of the National Research Council of the USA.

By the end of the 1930s there had been enormous health improvements for a large proportion of the Western world's population, brought about by advances in public health, the recognition of nutritional and endocrine factors in health, diagnostic and surgical progress, and therapeutic developments in combating both infectious and deficiency diseases. Patients suffering from diabetes, pneumonia, pernicious anaemia, septicaemia, puerperal fever, or surgical sepsis could all be offered effective treatments. Twenty years earlier nothing at all could have been done for them. However, another worldwide conflagration was soon to provide new, and old, challenges to the medical systems that had developed over the past eighty years.

Advances Associated with the Second World War

On the battlefields, the Second World War created many similar problems, from a medical point of view, to those of the First World War, including the pressure of therapeutic needs which stimulated pharmacological and pharmaceutical advances. The unavailability of natural products, like the anti-malarial quinine that was produced in territories soon inaccessible to the Allies, focused British, American, and other allied scientific expertise on devising new anti-malarial compounds, and developing anti-mosquito procedures amongst vulnerable troops.

The phenomenon of antibiosis, of preventing or disrupting the growth of one type or species of micro-organism by another, was already well known to bacteriologists. Alexander Fleming (1881–1955) devised the name penicillin for the antibacterial matter he noted arising from a *Penicillium* mould that accidentally contaminated and decimated his bacterial colonies, but did not succeed in isolating the very unstable active principle. The critical chemical work in overcoming those problems was orchestrated in Oxford during the early years of the Second World War when Howard Florey (1898–1968), Ernst Chain (1906–79), and Norman Heatley (b. 1911) managed to produce, in an academic laboratory, enough crude penicillin to allow a small, successful, animal trial, which was rapidly followed by the administration of the drug to seriously ill patients. The powerful promise of the drug created immediate pressures to develop its large-scale production. Despite considerable efforts in the UK, the commercial resources of the major pharmaceutical manufacturers, cooperating as the Therapeutic Research Corporation, were unable to provide adequate quantities of penicillin. Its successful manufacture relied on important developments in US laboratories and factories, most especially the development of deep fermentation methods that increased the output. The patenting, by US industrial concerns, of some of the production techniques raised questions of the ethics of such practices that were to reoccur with increasing frequency after the Second World War. Also during the war, another fungal product, streptomycin, was developed by Selman Waksman (1888–1973) as an effective therapeutic against the tubercle bacillus. The success of the sulphonamides, penicillin, and streptomycin heralded the antibiotic era, and stimulated the search for further such therapeutic compounds after the Second World War.

The treatment of the injured resurrected many of the problems—of shock, wound control, and infection—that had presented during the First World War. Techniques in plastic surgery, developed and refined since the wave of horrific injuries emerging from the First World War, advanced especially under the scalpel of Archibald McIndoe (1900–60), a New Zealander trained in the USA who established a specialized unit in East Grinstead, Sussex. Aircraft crew were particularly vulnerable to burn injuries, and McIndoe treated personnel with reconstructive surgery that provided some restoration of damaged faces and hands. The medical officers trained in such units during the war provided the expertise on their return to civilian life to develop techniques in reconstructive surgery that could be applied to naturally occurring deformities, to post-operative and traumatic mutilations, and to disease injuries, and could even be used for elective cosmetic and aesthetic purposes.

A major new medical problem during the Second World War was that of civilian casualties; in the UK alone, air-attack victims amounted to nearly 300,000, one-fifth of whom were killed. The provision of appropriate and adequate domestic medical services became of paramount importance, and the creation of nationwide blood transfusion services had an important impact on both civilian and military casualties. Karl Landsteiner (1868–1943) had demonstrated blood groupings in 1900, which established the theoretical and technical basis for safe transfusion, although the person-to-person technique used had limited application. The discovery of anticoagulants accelerated the development of indirect transfusion, and experiences during the Spanish Civil War demonstrated that such blood could be stored and transfused safely from bottle to patient. In the USA blood banks were established at some of the major hospitals, and in the UK a tradition of on-call voluntary donors developed. In the acute conditions of wartime the Medical Research Council directed a scheme to organize blood depots, which were soon supplying blood across the country and to forces overseas. The recognition that out-of-date blood, usually about a week after donation, could be used to prepare stable cell-free plasma provided an important therapy for the treatment of shock.

Between the middle of the nineteenth century, when the cell theory and the germ theory were first propounded, and the onset of the Second World War, there had been enormous advances in physiology, pathology, surgery, therapeutics, medicine, and public health. Perhaps the most striking advance was the ability to cure or prevent a large number of infective diseases which had been the major killers of children and young people in the past. But the end of the Second World War exposed malnutrition and disease amongst displaced and ravaged communities. It also brought abhorrence and misgivings. The horrors of the concentration camps raised doubts about the power and role of the doctor—previously seen unequivocally as a member of a caring profession—in the conduct of non-therapeutic, sometimes sadistic and lethal experiments on unconsenting prisoner populations. It brought to the fore problems of medical ethics and of iatrogenic disease (disease or injury as a result of medical or surgical treatment), and growing apprehensions about the effects of industrial and environmental influences on health and illness. It also exposed inequalities of health and access to health care between social classes in Western countries, and between developed and developing nations. The benefits of previous decades of medical successes brought fresh problems. Advances in treating acute illness and injuries accentuated the problems of the chronic sick and the elderly, as typified by the creation of the new speciality of geriatrics. These and other problems were to preoccupy medicine in the second half of the twentieth century, as discussed by Stephen Lock in the next chapter.

8 | Medicine in the Second Half of the Twentieth Century

STEPHEN LOCK

EVERY age has its medical sceptics—shrewd commentators whose analysis questions or even refutes the paradigm of the totally triumphalist view of medicine. These range from Molière through George Bernard Shaw to Ivan Illich. Yet perhaps in our own day none has been so influential (certainly within medical circles) as Thomas McKeown, whose critiques of medicine in the 1970s rested not only on exceptional academic rigour, but also on an insider's knowledge, given his position as Professor of Social Medicine at the University of Birmingham.

The more controversial of McKeown's two major arguments rested on his contention that improvements in health or longevity had had little to do with developments in modern medicine. Thus in Europe the death rate from tuberculosis had started a continual decline almost 100 years before the discovery of the first curative agent, streptomycin. And again, McKeown maintained, the falls in deaths from the childhood fevers such as diphtheria, scarlet fever, and whooping cough were due more to better nutrition, sanitation, and living standards generally than to immunization with vaccines or to antibiotics.

Argument still continues over McKeown's thesis—in particular, his failure to consider the possible contribution of modern medicine to medical care as opposed to statistical evidence of cure. Less attention has been paid to his other major contention: that historically the dominant risks to life and health have occurred in three main phases: injuries and accidents, affecting humankind before it became grouped into communities; infectious diseases (many arising from animals and transmitted when man and beasts came to live in close contiguity); and (once the second phase had been largely abolished by a rise in living standards and better hygiene) the degenerative diseases of longevity.

Conceivably, then, a history of Western medicine since 1945 could be seen as comprising a mopping-up operation of McKeown's second phase and a preoccupation with the problems raised by the third. Nevertheless, there are several caveats to such a simplistic view. Firstly, even in the West, all three phases have coexisted for this period, even if the third has become dominant since, say, the turn of the century. Trauma, for example, is still the major cause of death in males between 10 and 40, even though survivors of a major car crash in the developed world are now likely to owe their recovery to highly sophisticated care. Similarly, the evolution of antibiotic-resistant strains of bacteria has led to a resurgence of professional interest in the infectious diseases.

The second caveat is that what happens elsewhere in the world has a direct effect on the West. For example, the emergence in the Second and Third Worlds of malaria that is resistant to the normally used drugs has posed a serious threat to travellers from the First World. The latter are also threatened by the breakdown in hygiene occurring in major Third World cities, with their dramatic increases in population giving rise to the formation of the megalopolis.

Thirdly, as has happened so often, hubris has been succeeded by nemesis. Just as Western societies were rejoicing in new-found freedoms, such as the sexual revolution occasioned by the development of the contraceptive pill and of antibiotics capable of wiping out the classic sexually transmitted diseases, in the last two decades of the twentieth century along came a new threat: HIV (human immunodeficiency virus) infection and AIDS (acquired immune deficiency syndrome).

Nevertheless, in at least one important regard, McKeown's thesis has been fulfilled. Western societies enjoying a high level of health care have come to realize the burden of the inexorable increase in the number of elderly people and the ever-rising costs of their care—the expense not merely of the continual new discoveries in high-tech medicine but also of long-term maintenance of life in the community. The subsequent debates about the purpose, delivery, and funding of health care, as well as the ethical dilemmas that these raised, have gradually been taken out of the hands of the professional health-care workers into the broader constituency of the community. Allied to this has been the questioning of the professional role (not only confined to medicine, but also occurring with law and education), together with a rising interest in the prevention of disease as well as in unorthodox treatments, such as acupuncture, homoeopathy, and chiropractic.

This chapter, then, will focus first on the 'triumphs' of modern Western medicine in the period from 1945 to the present, counterpointing these with the reverses. Moreover, it will not ignore the paradox that, despite widespread knowledge of the facts, much avoidable illness is produced by patients themselves—who continue to smoke, overeat, and overdrink. Not only has society been reluctant to stigmatize let alone curb this self-abuse, as by banning cigarette advertisements: it has also failed to take action against other remediable determinants of disease, such as poverty, unemployment, and homelessness. Similarly in the Third World most authorities have preferred to pursue a goal of Western-style medicine, rather than adopt proven and cost-effective methods for ensuring good health in the population: a piped water supply, simple education of mothers, childhood immunization, and simple health care delivered by indigenous aides.

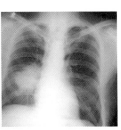

Chest X-ray film showing a cancer of the lung. Once rare, this type of cancer is now all too common, and its frequency is increasing particularly in women. The major cause, as Doll and Bradford Hill showed as long ago as 1950, is cigarette smoking—yet, despite the evidence and the publicity, people continue to smoke. This is a good illustration of how many causes of ill health are now known (unemployment, poverty, faulty diet, and lack of exercise among them), yet society does little to tackle these. Currently smoking is estimated to kill 3 million people a year prematurely (from many other causes than lung cancer), a figure that is estimated to rise to 10 million by 2025; half of all regular cigarette smokers in Britain will eventually be killed by their habit.

Triumphs

Any discussion of the principal medical 'triumphs' since the Second World War must mention at least three topics. First, the development of new drugs for major indications, not only for common disabling or even fatal illnesses such as hypertension, but also a cheap, safe, and effective contraceptive pill. Secondly, there was the evolution of surgery, including safer operative techniques; the development of prostheses, particularly the artificial hip joint; and transplantation of organs, such as the kidneys, heart, and liver. Thirdly, and linked with successful transplantation, was the elucidation of important basic structures and mechanisms, including the make-up of DNA—deoxyribonucleic acid, the building block of all living material—and its role in intricate genetic mechanisms as well as the body's response to external attack (whether infection or grafts of foreign tissues). I shall not, however, consider the last any further in this chapter, given that the first applications of this exciting subject are very recent, and are occurring explosively as I write, but their prospect for the prediction of many illnesses, as well as their prevention or amelioration, are enormous and likely to bulk large in any future history of this period.

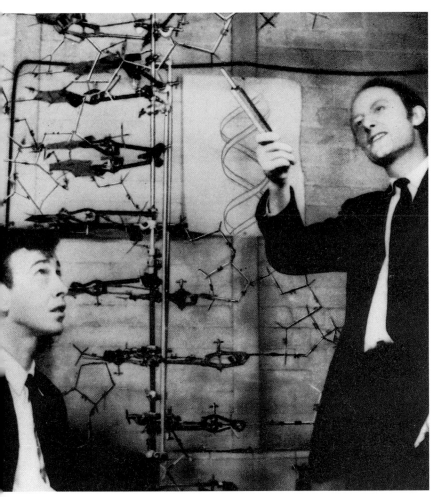

Watson and Crick with a model of the double helix. The elucidation in 1953 of the structure of DNA, the material of which genes are composed, led to a shift in the thrust of much major medical research. It enabled scientists not only to determine the basis of what was wrong in many common diseases, but also to propose ways of righting these. A further current project is to map the human genome—that is, the details of the entire sequence of genes (totalling some 50,000–100,000) on the 23 pairs of human chromosomes.

The therapeutic revolution

None of these discoveries was entirely new: as is so often the case, and even though for drug treatment they are referred to collectively as the 'therapeutic revolution', they fulfilled the tradition of evolution rather than revolution. In the 1920s, for example, the therapeutic era had been developed out of all recognition from its pre-war beginnings: the German pharmaceutical industry, in particular, went on to produce new general and local anaesthetics, the antihistamines, and hypnotics, among other drugs, while on the other side of the Atlantic the huge capacity of the US firms had been harnessed to produce the large quantities of the newly discovered insulin needed to treat diabetics all over the world. Even the first antibiotic, penicillin, had been discovered by Alexander Fleming as early as 1928, and the first group to be used in practice, the sulphonamides, was introduced into clinical practice in the late 1930s. And though the convenient form of treating pernicious anaemia by replacing the missing cobalamin by injection had to wait until after the Second World War, the discovery that eating large quantities of raw liver would cure this previously fatal disease had been made by Minot and Murphy as early as 1926. In the inter-war period also several research workers had confirmed earlier findings of the technical feasibility of organ transplantation, though they were unable to overcome the problems of graft rejection. And epidemiologists were already considering how to extend the success of immunization against typhoid fever and diphtheria to other common serious infections, such as polio and measles, as well as how to eradicate some infections altogether, such as smallpox and malaria.

Historians still argue whether war has an important role in promoting medical developments. Certainly war seems to speed these up and highlight the importance of some at the expense of others. Thus, given the hectic pace of the chemical industry in producing explosives and poison gas in the First World War, the subsequent enhanced activity in the pharmaceutical industry could have been predicted. Without the Second World War it seems unlikely that there would have been sufficient pressure to develop the therapeutic potential of penicillin so quickly and to arrange for its mass production. So much penicillin was required to treat the predicted number of battle casualties that no British manufacturer could take this on, and hence Howard Florey and his team in Oxford had to get help from US firms with sufficient manufacturing capacity.

In this way the initiation and development of new antibiotics, active initially against an ever-widening range of bacteria and later against some viruses as well, largely passed from one side of the Atlantic to the other. And this whole enterprise was counterpointed by a burgeoning programme of medical research, started in 1941 by President Franklin D. Roosevelt with the establishment of the Committee on Medical Research. This did no research itself, but placed contracts with institutions mainly into problems affecting the fighting forces: antidotes to dysentery, influenza, venereal diseases, and malaria. In 1946 this committee metamorphosed into the National Institutes of Health, developing its own large-scale units for carrying out research directly, but also continuing to give grants to others—while its research budget rose enormously (in the twenty years from 1948 to 1967 from $17 million to $803 million, respectively).

Nevertheless, though promising agents might be discovered in academic units, their evaluation and development had to be left to the pharmaceutical industry. The costs were very high, often amounting to tens of millions of dollars for a single agent, while only one of every fifty tested might end up as a drug useful in human disease. Even so, the outcome of this therapeutic revolution was impressive. The years from 1945 to 1985 saw the introduction, among others, of numerous antibiotics (meaning that cure of the then two principal sexually transmitted diseases, gonorrhoea and syphilis, could be guaranteed for the first time); anti-malarials and anti-schistosomes (against the tropical disease bilharzia); antihistamines; non-explosive anaesthetics; steroids; anti-hypertensives (reducing particularly the death rate from strokes); anti-coagulants; and agents effective against diabetes, gout, leukaemia and other types of cancer, Parkinson's disease, peptic ulcer, and serious mental illness (including depression and schizophrenia, which meant that proposals for treating psychiatric patients in the community instead of vast impersonal mental hospitals could now be implemented).

There were two new important characteristics of these developments. First, after the thalidomide disaster (discussed below), most governments set up mechanisms to test new drugs for safety, not just in pregnant women but in other patients as well. Secondly, new drugs were no longer compared with existing agents on the basis of anecdotal impressions by clinicians: instead they were subjected to a formal trial. In this development—the randomized clinical trial—roughly equal numbers of patients were assigned haphazardly to be treated with the new drug or the old one (or an inactive substance, a 'placebo'). All agents tested had to appear identical, and, until the code was broken after the study, the process was 'double-blind'—in other words, neither the patient nor the supervising doctor knew which agent had been used in the individual case. After this, statistical analysis was used to show the advantages and disadvantages of the new agent compared with the old one.

Randomized trial

The randomized trial was one of the most important developments in medicine of all time. At a stroke it began the transformation of what had been an art into a science—particularly since the method could also be applied to other medical interventions, such as surgical operations. No longer were new procedures publicized with the false enthusiasm redolent of the courtiers in Hans Christian Andersen's story *The Emperor's New Clothes*. Just as a clinical impression of anaemia was no longer enough, but needed confirmation by laboratory measurement, so increasing rigour came to be applied to many other aspects of medicine. A typical example of self-delusion even as late as the 1960s came when a new treatment for gastric ulcers was hailed as a breakthrough; this entailed freezing them by using an ice-bag passed into the stomach, but with more experience the method was abandoned as useless only a few months later.

Like other developments, the randomized trial had its roots in the past, dating back to the work in the 1920s by the great statistician Ronald Fisher on comparing different strains of wheat at the Agricultural Research Laboratory at Rothamsted. Its application to therapeutics is owed to Austin Bradford Hill, the pioneer of applying statistics to medicine, and the man who later, together with Richard Doll, was to show the connection between cigarette smoking and cancer of the lung. In 1946 the US government offered the UK, then bankrupt in the aftermath of war, sufficient streptomycin to treat 100 patients with tuberculosis. At that time in the UK 70,000 patients were dying from this every year, and over four times that number had the disease. Bradford Hill persuaded the tuberculosis committee of the Medical Research Council that the only ethical way of deciding who should be treated was a randomized trial. The results vindicated his approach, which was the start of similar trials of the new antibiotics and vaccines, which continue with increasing refinements to this day. Few claims of therapeutic efficacy would now be accepted without this approach, unless self-evidently the new agent totally cured a previously universally lethal disease.

The contraceptive pill

Possibly the most important advance on a global scale, however, was the development of a cheap, safe, and reliable contraceptive pill. For centuries women's lives had been dogged by unwanted pregnancies and their attendant risks. Even in the developed world there was widespread ignorance about contraception (particularly among the uneducated), and the methods available—the rhythm method, coitus interruptus, the condom, and the diaphragm—were both unreliable and unaesthetic. Many women resorted to illegal abortion, which carried a high risk of complications, including death. But, with the women's liberation movement given a new impetus in the Second World War as women undertook tasks normally performed by men, society's attitude towards contraception changed. This was usually irrespective of national religious attitudes, particularly once most children born were clearly going to survive to adulthood. And the introduction of a pill which was totally effective if taken regularly gave women a new freedom over their lives, and ushered in the so-called sexual revolution.

The contraceptive pill contained a combination of sex hormones, oestrogens and progestogens, and acted by suppressing ovulation (the monthly release of an egg from the ovary) without interfering with menstruation. Its discovery, development, and evaluation are a good illustration of the complexities surrounding virtually all new drugs in the modern era. Final success is almost invariably due to a team effort needing chemists, experimental pharmacologists, clinicians, statisticians, and official monitors and regulators. For the contraceptive pill, for example, the first development was the synthesis of sex hormones that could be taken by mouth, by two academic chemists, E. Russell Marker and Carl Djerassi. Thereafter, lobbied to develop a new form of contraception by a millionairess pioneer of the American birth-control movement, Margaret Sanger, an experimental biologist, Gregory Pincus, found that in animals ovulation could be suppressed by synthetic progesterone alone. Preliminary studies in women, however, conducted in Puerto Rico by two clinical doctors, John Rock and Elizabeth Rice-Wray, showed that oestrogens were also necessary for a contraceptive effect. Subsequent moni-

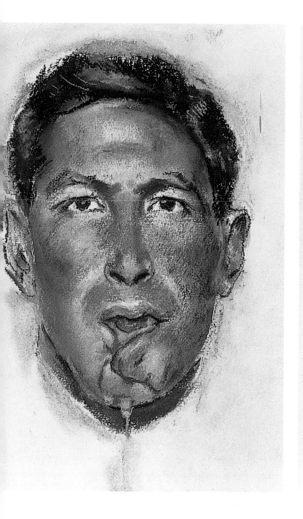
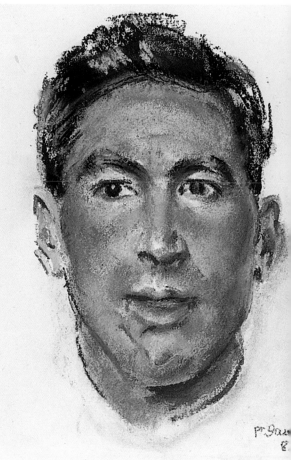

Henry Tonks was a surgeon who became an artist, returning to medical work during the First World War. These two pastel drawings by Tonks show a patient before and after plastic surgery.

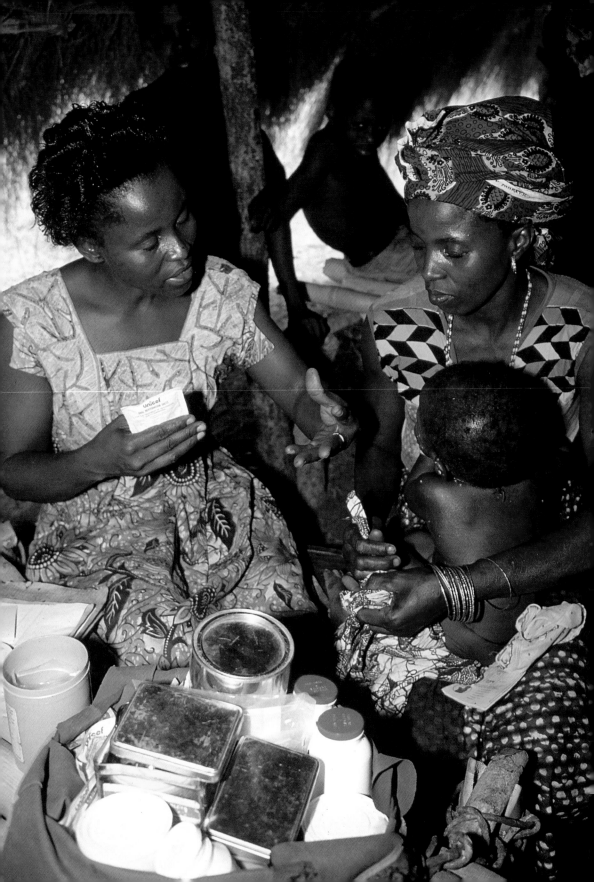

toring of the widespread field trials of the contraceptive pill by government drug safety committees showed that the largish amounts of oestrogen contained in the early preparations were associated with an increased risk of blood-clotting, diabetes, and hypertension, especially in women who were obese or who smoked or were aged over 35. These effects could largely be abolished by advising such women to adopt other forms of contraception, while for the remainder any risks were cut down by lowering the oestrogen content of the contraceptive pill to a level that did not interfere with the contraceptive effect—measures that were put into effect at the requirement of the safety committees.

Surgery

The sheer numbers and variety of battle injuries in the major twentieth-century conflicts all spelt out lessons for surgery in civilian life. New lessons (and old ones relearnt) emerged from every conflict—from the First World War, through the Spanish Civil War and Second World War, to the Vietnam War. These came as much from applying the new discoveries in basic science to problems as from clinical experience, and included the value of: delayed primary suture for battle wounds (not stitching them up for several days); anti-tetanus serum to prevent tetanus (lockjaw) arising in wounds contaminated with animal manure; measuring how much fluid, salt, and blood a severely injured person had lost, and replacing these before undertaking major surgery; effective anaesthesia and the effective control of pre- and post-operative pain; multidisciplinary specialist teams, including plastic, vascular, and neurosurgeons; and helicopters to transport the severely wounded to a well-equipped operating theatre and specialist care as quickly as possible.

Thus in this period surgeons not only became able to operate on virtually every area of the body, but they continued to improve their techniques. Often the results were spectacularly good: for example, the relatively simple technique of transurethral resection of the prostate—coring out parts of the enlarged gland by a knife passed through the urinary passage—overcame one of the commonest problems in later life in men, which had previously required a major open surgical operation carrying the additional risks of prolonged hospital stay, and subsequent urinary incontinence. Such methods were helped by adapting other techniques from science elsewhere—in particular, the miniaturization developed for the space programme and the use of computers. As a result, not only did medical apparatus become more sophisticated for treatment, but new methods were introduced for diagnosis—including better visualization with computed tomography and nuclear magnetic imaging and with small fibre-optic tubes which could be passed into many parts of the body, enabling the surgeon to view structures directly. Finally, starting in the late 1980s, a whole host of operations became possible using such telescopic control and instruments passed down a small tube inserted into the body. Such 'keyhole surgery'—for example, of hernias, the gall bladder, the kidney, and the knee joint—was liked by patients, who no longer had to stay overnight in hospitals, and by administrators, for the money it saved.

Two examples typifying heroic surgery at its most effective were operations on the heart and transplantation. Heart surgery aimed initially at repairing

Oral rehydration therapy (*facing*) first-world answer to third-world problems. Over three million children still die every year from dehydration induced by diarrhoea, but simple treatment could save many of them. In the late 1970s it was found that in cases of diarrhoea the intestines could still absorb water taken by mouth if small amounts of salt and sugar were added. This cheap and simple treatment has enabled the death rate in cholera to be reduced from 50–60% to less than 1%.

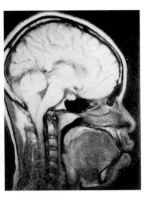

This MRI scan (magnetic resonance imaging) shows a clear picture of the brain within the skull, as well as the nose, nasal cavities, and tongue. It is not a picture of normality, however. It is a scan of a case of an uncommon disorder in which the lower part of the brain (the cerebellum, which can be seen on the left of the picture in the lower part of the back of the skull) is forced downwards into the spinal canal like a V-shaped wedge.

valves faulty at birth or damaged by subsequent rheumatic fever. A mitral valve whose leaflets had become fused by the latter was operated on successfully by Henry Souttar as early as 1925, but his example was little imitated and two important developments were necessary before the complex operations of the late twentieth century could be attempted. The first was a system whereby the anaesthetist could take over the patient's breathing, achieved by using muscle relaxant drugs to paralyse the muscles used in respiration, and simultaneously passing a tube into the windpipe through which the lungs could be inflated artificially. The second was a 'bypass' for taking over the circulation and oxygenation of the blood (particularly to the brain), allowing the heartbeat to be stopped and the surgeon time to work on an inactive heart. Developed over twenty years in the USA by John Gibbon, the heart–lung machine was first used in 1953 to repair a 'hole in the heart' and subsequently to reconstruct faulty heart valves at leisure or replace them with grafts of human or animal valves or artificial mechanical substitutes.

In the 1960s cardiac bypass was used in a surgical operation that became increasingly common (some cynics said fashionable, in the way that between the two world wars the wealthy in Western countries had had their children's tonsils and adenoids removed and their own 'slipped' organs stitched up). In this procedure—coronary artery bypass—lengths of the patient's own veins (taken usually from the legs) were sewn onto the heart muscle in order to restore the blood supply to the heart muscle, which had been threatened by arteriosclerosis. The increasing complexity of these procedures culminated in transplantation of the heart, first carried out in South Africa by Christiaan Barnard in 1967, and now used widely in various special centres, particularly for patients with serious disease of the heart muscle.

Transplantation

Nevertheless, the heart was by no means the first organ to be transplanted. In the early decades of the century surgeons had shown in animals that organs could be transplanted without excessive technical difficulty. Apart from tissues lacking a blood supply (such as the cornea of the eye and heart valves), however, the grafts were always rejected as foreign to the recipient. In human beings the first major research efforts were concentrated on transplantation of the kidney, given that renal disease often killed otherwise healthy patients who were young. Crucially, also, research in the Netherlands by Willem Kolff during the Second World War had led to the development of a successful artificial kidney for short-term use. The subsequent introduction of a permanent method for linking this to the patients' bloodstream enabled them to survive through regular dialysis in hospital or at home. Hence, if a kidney graft were to be rejected, they could always be returned to dialysis, a back-up that was not available should the transplantation of other organs, such as the heart or the liver, be unsuccessful.

For transplantation to be successful, however, two problems had to be solved. The first was to obtain organs for transplantation. In the early 1950s French surgeons had used kidneys taken from executed criminals, but, again, as in animals, though the actual operation was successful technically, the grafts were inevitably rejected by the patients. In 1969 Joseph Murray and his surgical colleagues successfully transplanted a kidney from a healthy identi-cal twin into his brother with advanced kidney disease, a procedure that won Murray the Nobel Prize for Medicine in 1990. Even so, grafts between close rel-atives were found to be as unsuccessful as between people who were totally unrelated. In work that was also recognized by a Nobel Prize, Peter Medawar, a British immunologist, and his team showed that graft rejection was due to complex immunological processes in the body. The first attempts at overcom-ing graft rejection, using X-rays, were unsuccessful, and it was not until 1970 that a drug, 6-mercaptopurine (6-MP), was found by Roy Calne, a British trans-plant surgeon, to be effective. 6-MP had originally been introduced for treating leukaemia, and to prevent graft rejection it was used together with steroids, another class of 'immunosuppressive' drugs. Subsequently, other agents, aza-thioprine and cyclosporin, were found to be even more effective, and the for-mer is now used routinely after transplant operations. Another important discovery was that tissues have different 'groups', and hence the graft can be 'matched' between donor and recipient in the same way as blood is cross-matched before transfusion.

Once the problems of graft rejection had been largely solved with continu-ous drug treatment, attention turned again to the supply of organs. Only for paired organs, such as the kidneys, could live donors be used, but most units preferred to turn to the more usual source of organs—patients proved to be 'brain-dead', whose breathing and circulation were being maintained artificially in intensive-care units, usually after a traffic accident or a brain haemorrhage. In most countries the public was closely involved in the debates about ensuring that the donors were to all intents and purposes dead and about the ethical issues of consent for removing the organs. Nevertheless, despite some disquiet and delay, by the mid-1980s many countries had estab-lished nationwide, or even continentwide, transplant programmes. Special centres kept records of potential recipients, against which the details of poten-tial donors could be matched, and new methods of cooling and preserving donor organs meant that grafts could be kept in good condition for periods varying between 4–6 hours for the heart and lungs, through 12–24 hours for the liver and pancreas, to 36–48 hours for the kidneys—and hence organs could be transported to centres where they could be used most appropriately. And the results became increasingly impressive, with functional survival of most transplants around 70–80 per cent at one year, and for well-matched kidneys 80–90 per cent at five years.

In two respects, however, heroic surgery changed. On the one hand, the increasing success of cardiovascular and transplant operations certainly encouraged surgeons to explore the possibilities ever more widely. On the other hand, however, surgeons came to realize that their strongest efforts might be ineffective and too distressing for the patient. With some types of cancer, for example, alternative approaches, such as radiotherapy or anti-cancer drugs, might be more effective. With others, controlled trials showed that often the results of simple surgery were quite as good as those of more extensive procedures.

Nowhere was this retreat better seen than for cancer of the breast, a com-mon tumour which in the UK affects 20,000 women every year and causes

13,000 deaths. From the turn of this century until the 1960s most surgeons had treated early disease with radical mastectomy, a mutilating operation which removed the entire breast and much of the surrounding tissues. The tendency had been to make the operation ever more extensive, and to use radiotherapy and treatment with hormones or anti-cancer drugs as well. Yet there was little evidence that these had improved the outlook. Moreover, controlled trials showed that simple removal of the cancer ('lumpectomy'), which had been pioneered in the 1930s by a British surgeon, Geoffrey Keynes, was as effective and usually far more acceptable to patients than the radical operation.

Patients' associations

In this evolution a new phenomenon played an important part: public opinion, in the shape of pressure groups such as patients' organizations. Coming to prominence mainly in the 1960s, these had three main objectives. First, as the proportion of a country's expenditure devoted to health care got ever larger—as it did in all Western countries, whether it came mostly from the government or from the private sector—the community needed a louder voice in how the funds were allocated, particularly as priorities changed with the ageing of the population as well as new discoveries that needed implementing. The second objective was the concern that the pace of medicine was not only getting ever faster but that it was becoming unchecked. At the lesser extreme, there was the frequent neglect of the 'hotel' aspects of health care—dirty hospitals and rude and indifferent staff. At the other extreme came the revelation of un-

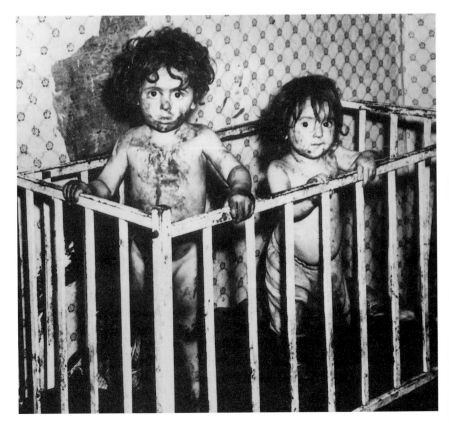

Child abuse: an old condition, recently described. In 1962 an American paediatrician, C. Henry Kempe, and his colleagues described 'the battered baby syndrome', in which there might be several serious bony fractures without obvious cause; close investigation disclosed that the cause was physical violence by an adult, most often the baby's father or the mother's partner. Clearly the condition had long gone unrecognized. Since then it has been renamed child abuse, given that it is not confined to babies nor indeed to physical violence, since not infrequently the harm may be pyschological instead, or sexual assault, or sheer neglect.

ethical research without patients having given their informed consent, with the profession doing little to prevent this.

Hence patients' organizations emerged to lobby for improvements, most noticeably the creation of local research ethics committees, with lay representation. Inevitably patients' associations pressed for more money to be spent on health in general, or on certain aspects. A particular target was mental health, always the Cinderella of medicine, whether for public esteem, visibility, or research funds. The third objective, self-help groups, arose as a natural development to tackle individual illnesses, such as multiple sclerosis or cystic fibrosis. The knowledge of patients and their carers inevitably came to be far greater than that of the professionals, and self-help groups were cheap and immensely sympathetic to individual problems in a way that orthodox institutions could never be.

By the mid-1990s, then, there were well over 800 self-help groups in the UK alone, lobbying for more money to be spent on research, campaigning for truly informed consent before patients were enrolled into trials of new treatment, and offering counselling to individual patients as well as practical advice on prostheses and implants.

Care versus cure

All this was to emphasize the return to an old concept that medicine was as much about care as about cure. However unspectacular they seemed, improved treatments for the common non-lethal disabilities benefited a large section of the population. Even if better living standards and antibiotics meant that the childhood fevers were no longer fatal, their prevention by mass immunization abolished their miseries. Replacing joints damaged by osteoarthritis (especially the hip) or rheumatoid disease (such as the knee or finger joints) with artificial substitutes, substituting plastic lenses for the natural lens removed for cataract, and sophisticated dentistry enabling people to retain their own teeth throughout their lives were three of the most prominent treatments. And the whole new specialty of geriatrics, pioneered in the late 1930s but coming into flower only after the Second World War, was to show how much care by an expert team could do for a previously neglected section of the population, the elderly infirm.

In another context, the concept of care was also revived in the hospice movement for the dying. Importantly, perhaps, its pioneer, Cicely Saunders, had come to appreciate the neglect of their medical and spiritual needs through being both a nurse and then a social worker at a university hospital before qualifying in medicine. Her new hospice, started in south London in 1967, was not only devoted to care of individuals, research, and education, but also came to include aspects such as bereavement counselling, supportive team nursing, and home care. With individual variations the movement spread rapidly, at first to the USA and Canada and then to the rest of the world. Clearly it was fulfilling an unmet need, and, as Saunders was to write later: 'The values which the hospice movement tries to establish, alongside its commitment to excellence in practice, have something akin to the earlier assurance of community, the affirmation of the individual person, and the concern for the bereaved family.'

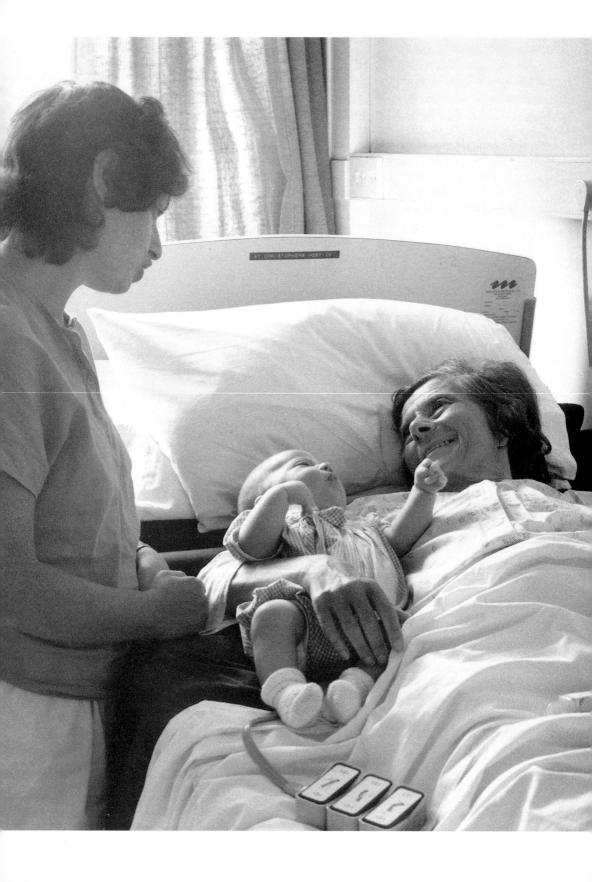

Disillusion

The onset of Western society's disillusion with modern medicine came in the 1960s. Several causes were self-evident. First were the ever-increasing costs, whether to governments or to individuals. Health care came to be funded in two major ways, neither of which fulfilled the ideal of countrywide high-quality treatment available immediately to all on demand. Countries, such as the UK and the Nordic states, where funding was largely provided by the State, had to contain costs by covert rationing: using the family doctor as a gate-keeper to the hospital, long hospital waiting lists, and even not offering certain procedures at all (such as advanced treatments for infertility). Countries, such as the USA, where care was funded by the individual, usually through insurance, might have the highest standards of medical care available immediately regardless of need. The other side was that not everybody was covered (in the USA, for instance, an estimated 15 per cent of the population had no insurance whatsoever), complex procedures such as intensive care might exhaust the insurance available and bankrupt the patient, and long-term care posed particular problems in geriatrics and psychiatry.

As the proportion of the gross national product devoted to health care continually rose (in some cases to well over 10 per cent), sceptics came to ask whether the nation was getting value for its money. How, in particular, was health to be measured? Such indicators as there were showed little correlation between expenditure and good health. For instance, one figure acknowledged as some sort of lodestone was the infant mortality rate, which consistently showed striking differences among countries: the most recent figures (1993) were as typical as any, with the rate per 1,000 births being 8.4 in the USA spending 13.5 per cent of its GDP on health care, 6.6 in Germany (spending 8.5 per cent), and 7.4 in the UK (spending a mere 6.6 per cent). And too little attention was paid to the far cheaper aspects of prevention—educating patients, for example, about the undisputed dangers of smoking, drinking alcohol to excess, and an unsuitable diet. Although some countries established official health-education agencies, mostly these were lacklustre and could do little to counter the power of large-scale industries, such as the tobacco manufacturers or the brewers. Nevertheless, sometimes prevention was pursued enthusiastically and was found to be both cheap and universally beneficial. For example, in the areas where drinking water had a low fluoride content, the load on the dental services was dramatically reduced by its fluoridation which cut down the amount of caries. In some countries, moreover, a strong anti-smoking lobby linked the concerns on health with the antisocial nature of what had become a minority habit and got stringent laws against smoking in public places enacted—a result that might have influenced many other people to abandon smoking.

The second factor in the disillusion was the feeling that health professionals were no longer interested in patients as people, but only in diseases. The Victorian physician in Luke Fildes's famous painting had been powerless; all he could do was to sit by the dying child's bedside, chin cupped in his hand—but at least he had exuded concern and compassion. In the era of safe effective surgery and the therapeutic revolution, many thought that doctors had lost

St Christopher's Hospice. Medicine is as much about comfort as cure, and nowhere is this more true than in the care of the elderly, who form an ever-increasing proportion of the population in most developed countries. In the 1930s geriatrics was pioneered as a specialty, and in 1967 Cicely Saunders, who had been both a nurse and a social worker before qualifying in medicine, established the first modern hospice devoted to the care of the dying. Here research was started into the control of intractable pain as well as into the psychological problems of the dying, with outreach and teaching programmes locally, nationally, and internationally.

135

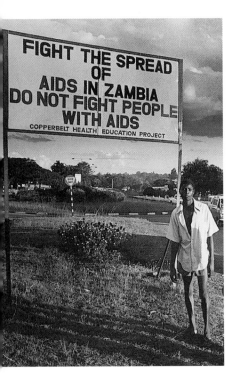

FIGHT THE SPREAD OF AIDS IN ZAMBIA DO NOT FIGHT PEOPLE WITH AIDS
COPPERBELT HEALTH EDUCATION PROJECT

Worldwide by 1996 over 30 million people were estimated to be infected with HIV (the AIDS virus), *The Economist* reported. The worst-hit region was Africa, which had 19 million people affected (63 per cent of the worldwide total) and had already had almost 8 million deaths. Health-education initiatives, such as this one in Zambia, set out to raise public awareness and change attitudes.

their humanity. The more they could do for individual patients, seemingly the less they cared about them as fellow human beings.

Intellectual attacks

Such feelings were underpinned by two influential publications: in the USA Henry Beecher's *Experimentation in Man* (1959) and in the UK Maurice Pappworth's *Human Guinea Pigs* (1961), showing how far medical research had become a vehicle for self-advancement rather than bettering the patient's condition. Another cogent intellectual attack, twenty years later, came in *The Unmasking of Medicine* (1981), delivered in the BBC's influential Reith Lectures given by Ian Kennedy, academic, lawyer, philosopher, and ethicist. Medicine, Kennedy declared, had taken the wrong path. The Cartesian theory of the body had remained central, and medicine had come to concentrate on disease to the exclusion of all else. This, in Kennedy's view, made modern medicine positively deleterious to the health and well-being of the population. 'We have all been willing participants in allowing the creation of a myth, because it serves our interests to believe that health can be achieved, illness can be vanquished and death postponed until further notice.' And Kennedy's analysis reinforced the less rigorous claims in the 1970s by the Latin American Jesuit priest Ivan Illich that health had become 'medicalized', with the individual deprived of the responsibility for his own well-being. Illich had already attacked the other professions for taking over decisions that rightfully belonged to the public, and both his and Kennedy's arguments on the state of medicine were widely discussed by an audience that had become disillusioned by experts.

Significantly, such dissent had its origins in the mid- and late 1960s, a fertile period for questioning established institutions. This was the era of protests against the Vietnam War and the atom bomb, as well as the student revolts in universities and black activism in the USA. In the UK, official censorship was relaxed. The failure of the prosecution of Penguin Books for publishing the allegedly obscene novel *Lady Chatterley's Lover* by D. H. Lawrence questioned previous orthodox values, while the vetting of all plays by the Lord Chamberlain before they were licensed for public performance was abolished at the end of the decade. Another strong indicator was the emergence of hard-hitting satirical revues and publications, including in the UK the influential fortnightly *Private Eye*.

Two important triggers

Perhaps the principal impetus in the development of modern scepticism about both science and medicine, however, came from two other important events in the 1960s: the publication of Rachel Carson's *Silent Spring* (1963) and the thalidomide tragedy. The first was a powerful depiction of a wasteland, with birds and insects dying and dead through pesticides such as DDT, trees and flowers destroyed by defoliants, and crop yields falling through pollution

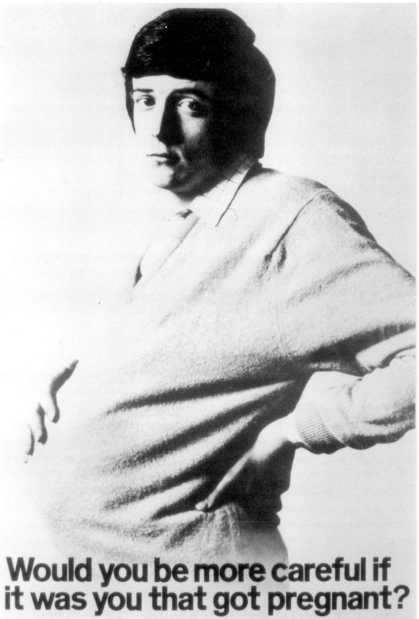

Would you be more careful if it was you that got pregnant?

Anyone married or single can get advice on contraception from the Family Planning Association. Margaret Pyke House, 27-35 Mortimer Street, London W1 N 8BQ. Tel. 01-636 9135.

It is often forgotten how relatively recently pregnancy has become almost risk-free, certainly in the developed world. Still, there is no harm in reminding men of the unique discomforts and ailments associated with the female sex. As one doctor wrote to the *BMJ*: 'men do not menstruate month after month for most of their lives; men do not have to agonise about taking the contraceptive pill every day with no-one knowing the potential risks; men do not know the discomforts of pregnancy or giving birth; they do not get post-natal depression'.

generally. No matter that subsequently many of the facts were shown to be totally wrong, or that, once DDT had been banned, many starving people must have died when insects again survived to destroy food stores. Carson wrote powerfully, her book became a best-seller, and it showed what readers at that time wanted to believe, with the added *frisson* that the author was to die from another disease perceived as modern: cancer.

Thalidomide was a hypnotic introduced in the late 1950s, with the particular attraction that it seemed safe and pleasant to take, especially since over-

137

doses did not result in coma—which were a feature of the barbiturates usually prescribed at the time. It was also apparently ideal for pregnant women, but at the beginning of the 1960s obstetricians started to see instances of a previously rare deformity in newborn children. This so-called phocomelia (seal extremities) was characterized by deformed limbs in which the long bones of the limbs were grossly shortened so that the hands and feet appeared to arise directly from the body, like the flippers of a seal; other deformed structures might include the intestines, eyes, ears, heart, and the urinary system. In Germany, where the major reports came from, between 1949 and 1959 most clinics had seen no cases at all; in 1959, however, seventeen cases were reported, in 1960, 126, and in 1961, 477. The one common factor to emerge, extensive investigations showed, was that the mothers of these infants had all taken thalidomide in early pregnancy, and such a link between the drug and the deformities was confirmed by additional reports from the UK and Australia, among other countries.

Worldwide, the estimated total of babies deformed by thalidomide was 10,000. As soon as the connection was recognized, at the end of 1961, the drug was banned by both Germany and the UK, and eventually after prolonged campaigns and legal actions many of the children received compensation for their deformities. But the episode had two important repercussions. The first was the general agreement that new medicines should no longer be introduced without full preliminary testing, including for any effects in pregnant animals. Thus many countries established committees to scrutinize the safety of medicines, and no new agent could be marketed until experts had assessed the results of extensive tests.

The second repercussion was a public perception of what doctors had recognized for some time: drugs were not harmless miracle agents, but might have predictable or unpredictable side effects, possibly worse than the disease which they were treating. And a not uncommon view then evolved: any drug-induced illness was due to somebody's lapse, whether carelessness by the prescribing doctor or inadequate supervision by the licensing authority. Such an attitude was also to develop elsewhere in medicine—particularly in the USA, where (encouraged by 'contingency litigation', whereby the lawyer took a part of any damages awarded but did not charge for an unsuccessful action) patients increasingly sued their doctors (especially surgeons and obstetricians) for any outcome that was less than ideal. So far as drugs were concerned, however, it became clear that, however rigorous the tests, not all side effects could be predicted, even though careful initial studies had suggested that a new drug was safe. It required subsequent field tests in a sizeable number of patients to confirm that rare side effects did not occur. But with the new monitoring systems as well as legal powers, the authorities hoped for an early alert, which would enable them to act swiftly (issuing warnings to doctors or even ordering the drug to be withdrawn from the market).

Complementary medicine

At a time when medicine seemed able to do more for patients than ever before, the public disillusion was signalled by a paradox: increasingly people turned away from conventional therapies to the unorthodox. Such 'alternative' ('complementary', 'fringe', or 'natural') medicine became very popular: in one survey a third of Americans had used it in the previous year, spending $13.7 billion on 425 million visits (more than those to conventional general practitioners and paediatricians); in another study in the USA 84 per cent of patients said that they would go to an alternative practitioner again or recommend such treatment to others; while in a third survey, in the UK, almost a third of adults wished some form of complementary medicine to be available within the National Health Service. And in the early 1990s the credibility of these methods was boosted by the establishment in the UK of a university department and chair in the subject and in the USA of the Office of Alternative Medicine within the National Institutes of Health.

One difficulty in all the arguments about the merits and role of complementary medicine was that it was far from homogeneous. Its spectrum ranged from methods that troubled few orthodox practitioners—such as osteopathy, homoeopathy, and even acupuncture—to those that they had difficulty in accepting as valid—such as aromatherapy and radiobionics. Nevertheless, the implications of its popularity were more far-reaching than any benefits of the actual techniques. They reflected the often-expressed disillusion with the impersonal style of orthodox medicine, the lack of empathy shown by most doctors, and the austerity of modern hospitals with their frightening arrays of machinery (not for nothing during the post-war period did the word 'clinical' come to mean stark or heartless). Most of the methods used in unorthodox medicine were much cheaper and without the serious side effects of some conventional treatments. And, crucially, with its emphasis on holism and prevention, it did what both Illich and Kennedy had been demanding: restored to individuals the responsibility for their own health.

A major impetus behind the creation of the US Office of Alternative Medicine was research into unorthodox methods for treating conditions, such as cancer and back pain, where sometimes conventional treatment was either not recommended at all or had been abandoned as having no further role. Nowhere perhaps was the demand for the rapid assessment of new therapies better seen than with AIDS. And, more than any other condition, AIDS highlights the strengths and weaknesses as well as the tensions within orthodox medicine at the latter part of the twentieth century, together with the important part well-organized patient power can play. (And, as I write, a totally new condition seems likely to be posing similar, though not identical, questions by the time this book is published. The emergence of Creutzfeldt–Jakob disease, previously a very rare condition seen only in elderly people, as an illness of young people, linked with bovine spongiform encephalopathy in cattle and possibly associated with eating contaminated beef, particularly offal, may pose major problems of all kinds in the countries where it occurs—though it is far too early to specify their nature or frequency.)

AIDS and HIV infection

Though in retrospect a few cases had possibly been seen before 1981, in this year a new and puzzling illness was first documented, occurring particularly in homosexual men in the USA. Characteristically AIDS affected the body's immune system, reducing its defences against attack so that the patients

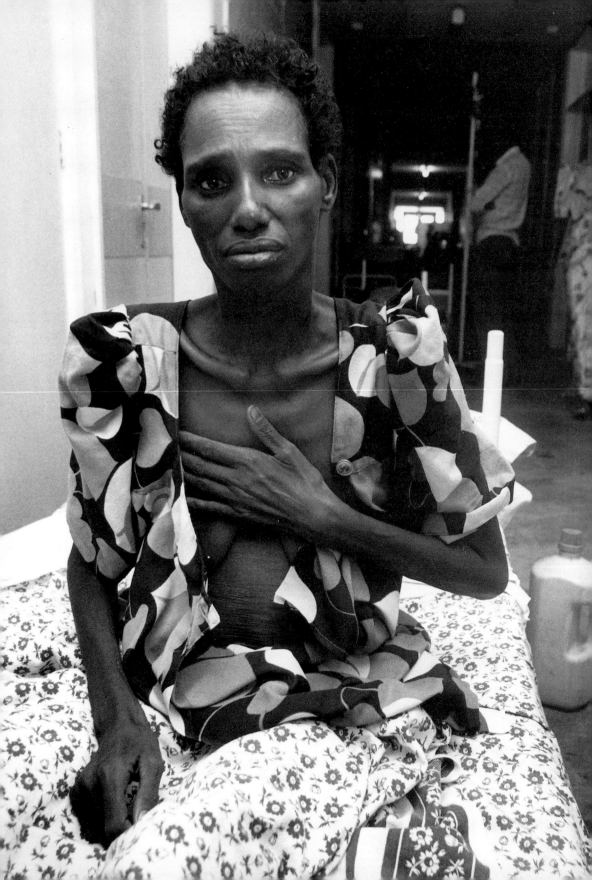

developed and often died from unusual infections or tumours. Within a few years not only had scientists isolated the responsible agent, the human immunodeficiency virus or HIV, but had also been quick to use techniques inconceivable a few years previously to determine its genetic structure and how it produced its damaging effects. Other research workers showed how HIV infection spread in the community and how treatment could prolong patients' lives; nevertheless, AIDS, which usually developed a few years after the initial infection, was uniformly fatal, the infection was spreading world-wide, and there was little prospect of a preventive vaccine.

HIV is transmitted in three main ways: sexual contact with an infected person; infected blood; and across the placenta from an infected mother to her unborn child. In the years following the first description of the disease the relative importance of the mode of transmission changed. Initially, homosexual contacts were strikingly in the majority, particularly in the developed world, and before the risks were realized many infections were also transmitted by transfusion of contaminated blood or its products, such as those used to treat haemophilia. The latter risks were overcome by special monitoring and treatment of all blood supplies, but subsequently this mode of infection came to prominence again through the contamination of needles shared by intravenous drug abusers.

In the underdeveloped world, on the other hand, infection was overwhelmingly through heterosexual intercourse, usually with prostitutes. Whatever the causes, in both the Third and the First World the scale of the problem increased rapidly to one of enormous dimensions, particularly the high cost if every individual patient was to be provided with the optimum regimen of treatment. By 1995 an estimated 17 million adults and 2.3 million children had HIV infection, and experts predicted that the burden for the developing countries would become even more overwhelming, with 21–34 million cases in sub-Saharan Africa alone by the year 2000—and even greater numbers in South-East Asia. The worst-case estimate for the whole world by the millennium was 109 million adults infected with HIV.

Given the affluence, articulateness, and influence of the group originally affected by HIV infection—homosexual men in the principal cities in the USA— the unusual pressure they exerted on society for propaganda on prevention and new methods of treatment could have been predicted, particularly during the early years of the epidemic. At first governments reacted as if they were facing a new plague. In particular in the USA the AIDS lobby accused the authorities of fanning a new holocaust, with delay in instigating preventive measures, such as closing the bathhouses where the infection was spread, or commissioning publicity campaigns about safer sexual practices, particularly the use of condoms.

The lobbyists also exerted pressure on society and government over three other aspects. First, they demanded that more money should be allocated to research. Secondly, they pressed for a reduction in the price of azathioprine (AZT), the principal drug with some effect on the infection (which included the prolongation of life). Thirdly, they lobbied the Food and Drug Administration to release drugs that might have some activity against the disease, although these had not yet been licensed for use. Hence the safety net established after

'Slim disease' (AIDS) in Africa. Infection with the human immunodeficiency virus and AIDS were described only in 1981, but aroused the public imagination to an extent comparable with previous sudden disasters, such as the plague and the cholera epidemics. Though the conditions are relatively stable in the developed world, they are currently devastating in Africa and potentially so in South and South-East Asia. With less than 10 per cent of the world's population, sub-Saharan Africa accounts for more than two-thirds of AIDS cases worldwide, with life expectancy in Uganda being the lowest in the world.

the thalidomide tragedy was breached, and the AIDS campaigners had managed to get their own way in sharp contrast to other groups—for example, some
patients with incurable cancer who had tried to get hold of an agent of
unproven value, called laetrile, and failed, thus having to obtain supplies clan-
destinely from countries such as Mexico.

Third World Problems

The worldwide current and projected figures for HIV infection/AIDS are hor-
rendously high. Nevertheless, those for the Third World have to be set against
equally stark statistics for diseases that have long been overcome in the developed world. For example, every year in the 1990s in the Third World an estimated 2 million children died from measles and a further 3 million from
diarrhoeal diseases alone. And, though this book is devoted to Western medicine, it has to be emphasized that the First World could not isolate itself from
all the problems elsewhere, which affected it in three main ways. First, the con-
science of the West was aroused by the horrendous statistics of deaths from
famine and preventable illness—and especially by the images of morbidity and
mortality flashed nightly onto its television screens. Its response was
inevitably piecemeal, from the immediate relief provided by innumerable
charitable agencies, through more sustained efforts by outsiders to instigate
policies on agriculture, pure water supplies, and family planning, to the windy
rhetoric of international jamborees, such as the 1975 conference at Alma-Ata
in the former USSR, which proclaimed the doctrine of 'Health for all by the
year 2000'.

The second interaction between the Third and First Worlds came about
because serious 'tropical' diseases were no respecters of frontiers. Some of
these were no longer the terrors they had been: for example, for well-
nourished people in the West, cholera (even that caused by new virulent
strains such as the El Tor variety) often produced only a mild illness, which in
any case could be easily treated. Some infections (yellow fever and hepatitis)
could be prevented by immunization, but where a traveller omitted to have
himself or herself immunized—and poliomyelitis is a case in point—the resulting illness and its sequels could be just as disastrous as they had been fifty years
previously, when immunization against poliomyelitis was not available. One
tropical disease, however, for which no vaccine was available, continued to be
of great concern. This was malaria, causing much illness and many deaths in
the local communities, few of which could afford the drugs for either prevention or treatment. Malaria also posed a particular problem for travellers from
the developed world. Some forgot or refused to take prophylaxis, but the major
worry was that the agent causing the lethal malignant malaria, *Plasmodium falciparum*, developed resistance to many of the drugs used for prevention or
treatment as well as to some of the newly introduced substitutes. As a result,
researchers were engaged in hectic efforts to discover yet different types of
drugs (a promising one being derived from an ancient Chinese herbal remedy),
while travellers had to return to old-fashioned means of prevention, such as
sleeping under mosquito nets impregnated with insecticide.

One early project by the World Health Organization had been the elimination of malaria from the world, using a three-pronged attack: treating all patients, eliminating all the breeding grounds for the mosquitoes, and killing the latter by extensive spraying of insecticides. Such an approach did eradicate malaria from the parts of Europe where it had persisted after the Second World War, but elsewhere the sheer logistical difficulties—as well as the emergence of strains of mosquito resistant to the insecticides—caused the campaign to be abandoned. Nevertheless, another worldwide concerted campaign by the WHO did succeed in totally abolishing another great scourge of humankind—smallpox. This was one of the two good examples of the third type of medical interaction between the developed and underdeveloped worlds: the impact of sophisticated research on large-scale problems. The other example was oral rehydration therapy (ORT).

Smallpox and ORT

Early regional attempts were made to eradicate smallpox shortly after the end of the Second World War, particularly in Latin America and China. Later, global eradication became a policy of the WHO from 1958, as a result of a proposal by Victor Zhdanov, then vice-minister for health in the USSR. The logistical difficulties in the early stages of the campaign were overcome by two important technical advances made in First World laboratories. The first was a new freeze-dried vaccine, which meant for the first time that this was stable in tropical climates for at least a month; the second a new type of needle that guaranteed satisfactory vaccination. Using the intensive methods of 'surveillance-containment', whereby any outbreaks were cut short by meticulous detection of new cases and then vaccinating all the possible contacts, the WHO campaign made impressive progress, with the last natural case being reported from Somalia in 1976. As Christopher Booth, a distinguished physician and medical historian, has remarked, the conquest of smallpox represented 'an example of what can be achieved by the unity of the human will'.

ORT was pioneered out of laboratory research by a US doctor, Norbert Hirschhorn, who found that a particular mixture of water, salt, and sugar enabled water to be absorbed from the intestines. Previously this had been considered impossible in patients with intestinal disease, and an intravenous drip was thought to be vital for overcoming the characteristic dehydration in diarrhoea, particularly in infants, and in cholera. Given together with other foods, such as starches and cereals, the special solution was found to lower the death rate from cholera from 50–60 per cent to less than 1 per cent, and was similarly effective in infantile diarrhoea. The introduction of ORT was potentially one of the most important developments since the Second World War, but, as is often the case, a major problem then arose. This was how to persuade more people who knew about the value of the treatment to use it rather than to seek the more complex and not always available alternative of an intravenous drip.

Conclusion

Self-evidently any conclusions about the role of medicine in the second half of the twentieth century are hampered by the difficulties of standing back from the events occurring in the writer's own times. But, however justified some of the scepticism may be about a Wellsian-type view of continual progress, my personal conclusions are gently optimistic. Take, for example, some statistics. Within this century for Western countries the expectation of life has increased from 45 to 75 years. In 1900 the annual death rates from diphtheria, measles, and pertussis (whooping-cough) were, respectively, 40, 13, and 12 per 100,000; by the 1960s these had fallen to 0, 2, and 1.

Adherents of Thomas McKeown might ascribe most of such reductions to improved social conditions, so a more specific indicator of improvement because of medical care is necessary. Such an example is maternal mortality. In the UK in 1900 maternal mortality was 27 per 100,000, in 1940 it was 5.4 per 100,000, and in 1987 it was 2 per million. As alternative evidence, we could play the much derided practice of historical games, seeking examples from individuals—not merely of creative artists such as Katherine Mansfield, D. H. Lawrence, and George Orwell whose premature deaths from tuberculosis would today have been averted by effective treatment, but, say, of two others who died of less common conditions. In 1911 the composer Gustav Mahler died at the age of 51 from subacute bacterial endocarditis, an illness extending over several months and due to infection of a deformed heart valve with the organism *Streptococcus viridans*. Though he had the best advice medicine could provide, at the time nothing could be done; yet today such an infection could be cured rapidly with high doses of penicillin or another antibiotic, and if the heart valve proved to be badly damaged, then it could be readily replaced by an artificial substitute.

A couple of years before Mahler died, the Irish playwright J. M. Synge had died even younger, aged 38, of Hodgkin's disease, a tumour of the lymph nodes. With modern knowledge, including new techniques of diagnosis and chemotherapy with effective anti-cancer drugs, today he would probably have been cured. And to return to general rather than specific examples, a good demonstration of the value of modern medicine is seen whenever established systems break down. In the former USSR, for example, diphtheria and polio have returned in the mid-1990s, as effective routine immunization has been abandoned—and some former Eastern bloc states stand alone in the developed world as examples of countries where the expectation of life is actually progressively falling.

Attempting to measure the contribution of medical care, in the early 1990s three US academics, John Bunker, Howard Frazier, and Frederick Mosteller, estimated that in the community medicine is currently responsible for a gain in life expectancy of about five years, with a potential for another $1^1/_2$–2 years. Nevertheless, such gains have arisen predominantly from the curative rather than the preventive health services. And their final point is one that I have tried to emphasize throughout this chapter: the importance of care versus cure.

A person who has not experienced a handicap or limitation of activity that hampers someone else may underestimate its importance to the affected person [they write]. But the miseries of depression, shortness of breath, angina, creaky and painful joints, severe pain, disabling headaches, major indigestion, urinary difficulties, toothache and sore gums, fuzzy vision, faulty hearing, paralysis and broken bones would add up to a national disaster without the relief we are able to document.

Medicine in Context

9 | The Growth of Medical Education and the Medical Profession

LISA ROSNER

WRITTEN records of the professional values governing the relationship between medical practitioners and their patients go back at least to Hippocrates, and their ongoing acceptance can be seen in the modern use of the Hippocratic Oath. Professional values governing the relationship among practitioners can also be found in the Hippocratic Oath, but those values have changed considerably over time. The modern idea of the medical profession as a unified fraternity can be traced to the emergence of the modern form of medical education.

Medical education is itself a modern term. 'Education', up to the mid-nineteenth century, meant 'moral and intellectual discipline', as an eminent London physician told a parliamentary commission in the 1830s: it had to do with imparting values and building character. Strictly medical study was more commonly known as 'medical improvement', and was the acquisition of knowledge by the already morally and intellectually disciplined adult. Education made a good man, whereas medical improvement made a knowledgeable doctor.

There were two formal, and many informal, kinds of medical improvement. The first type was university medical study leading to the Doctorate of Medicine, the hallmark of the physician, who treated internal diseases. It was based on scholarship, knowledge of medical science, including theory and treatment of disease, as conveyed in lectures and textbooks. Since medical knowledge was universal, rather than local, many students, including such famous names as Andreas Vesalius, William Harvey, and Albrecht von Haller, studied at several universities to acquire the best understanding of medical science.

The Teaching of Anatomy

From the Renaissance onwards it was recognized that medicine was an art as well as a science, and that textbooks and lectures should be supplemented by practical experience. The first practical subject to be brought within the university curriculum was anatomy: professors were expected to be experienced

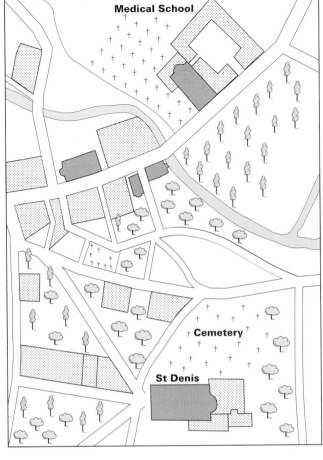

Medical School

Cemetery

St Denis

Medical schools did not
provide opporunties for
student dissection until
the nineteenth century.
Before then, the most
zealous students
supplemented their formal
training by robbing
cemeteries to obtain
cadavers. Felix Platter, for
example, went several
times to the St Denis
cemetery in Montpellier.

in dissection, and all students were required to attend anatomical demonstrations. Yet attendance at an anatomical demonstration was not a means of
defining a distinct professional identity. Felix Platter described one at the University of Montpellier in the sixteenth century, 'conducted in the old theatre
on the corpse of a boy who had died of an abscess in the stomach . . . Besides the
students, the audience contained many people of the nobility and the bour-
geoisie, and even young girls, notwithstanding that the subject was a male.
There were even some monks present.' The difficulty in obtaining and preserving cadavers made it difficult for medical students to gain hands-on experience in anatomy. For students anxious to gain that experience, robbing graves
to obtain bodies was sometimes an expedient. Platter, who made anatomy his
'principal study', described an expedition to obtain the bodies of a student and
a young boy who had been buried in the cemetery of Saint-Denis, just outside
the city walls.

When night came we left the town . . . [he wrote]. The two corpses were disinterred,
wrapped in our cloaks, and carried on poles . . . as far as the gates of the town. We did
not dare to rouse the porter . . . so one of us crawled inside through a hole that we discovered under the gate . . . We passed the cadavers through the same opening, and
they were pulled through from the inside. We followed in turn, pulling ourselves
through on our backs; I remember that I scratched my nose as I went through.

The dissections were carried out, but they were the last that Platter could complete, for 'after this the monks of Saint-Denis guarded their graveyard, and if a student came near he was received with bolts from a crossbow'.

Bedside Teaching and Apprenticeship

By the end of the seventeenth century a few universities attempted to introduce another practice subject, bedside clinical experience. The University of Leiden was one of the first medical schools to make use of a local hospital to provide clinical lectures, where actual patients substituted for the case histories presented in lectures. Hermann Boerhaave, one of the most famous medical men of the turn of the eighteenth century, gave clinical lectures on the cases in the small twelve-bed ward of the Caecilia hospital, training students, according to the course announcement, 'in the diagnosis of diseases by their signs, in a knowledge of them based on their causes, and in their cure by the remedies proper for that purpose, and thus initiate them into the practice of medicine'.

This emphasis on the theoretical, rather than the practical, side of medicine was reversed in the second type of formal medical training, apprenticeship to a surgeon, who treated external lesions or wounds, or to an apothecary, who compounded medications. Apprenticeship was a formal legal contract obliging the young man to serve his master for a set period of years, 'during which space the said apprentice [binds] and obliges himself to serve . . . faithfully and honestly by day and night, holiday and work day'. In some cities, surgeons' guilds had a monopoly on the practice of surgery in that city, and apprenticeship with a member of the guild could lead to entry into that valuable monopoly. But surgeons' guilds were comparatively rare: much more common were the surgeons or apothecaries who took apprentices to have the benefit of their labour while providing them with experience. The core of the education was the acquisition of a set of manual skills, in contrast to the science imparted to the physician by the university. Indeed, where a physician might be praised for his science, a surgeon was praised for his skill. A master might require his apprentice to read textbooks or attend lectures, but this was by no means common. More often, apprentices would carry out some of the duties of servants, only gaining access to medical tasks after a period of time, as this 1737 description of a Swedish apprenticeship implies: 'The first few years are mostly spent doing small tasks and waiting at table . . . until [the apprentice] gradually becomes accustomed to wielding the razor, opening veins, applying plasters and at most bandaging a wound or a fracture, and he may, in addition now and then be permitted to see a few operations performed by his master.'

It was also possible to combine these forms of education. A student might first serve an apprenticeship with a local surgeon, then obtain a degree at a university. Or a university student might pay an apothecary or surgeon to attend his shop for a few months, to get practical experience. Felix Platter, who lodged with a busy apothecary, wrote of the 'advantage of my master's shop', in which he 'saw something new every day'. By the end of the eighteenth century this was such a common practice that members of the Edinburgh sur-

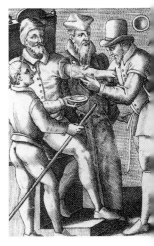

Traditional forms of medical education included apprenticeship to an apothecary or surgeon. In either case the duties required were as much those of a servant as a student: fetching medicaments in an apothecary's shop, or holding the basin during blood-letting. In part for that reason, students in the eighteenth century began to desert apprenticeship for medical lectures at universities and hospitals.

149

geons' guild complained of the practice, incidentally showing the continued division between students and apprentices, and between the cultures of physicians and surgeons: 'these gentleman students being under no sort of restraint, they take liberties, which give the very worst example to the prentices.'

In addition to these two formal types of medical improvement, there were a host of informal kinds. Young men might study with local practitioners, or, as literacy grew, study on their own. Women might do the same, for, though women were excluded from universities and guilds, they could and did practise as cuppers, bleeders, 'surgeonesses', and bonesetters. Female midwives might learn 'on the job' through their own childbirths and those of their friends and family. Hospitals run by nursing religious orders, like the Sint Jans Hospitaal in Bruges, also provided on-the-job medical instruction.

New Forms of Medical Teaching

In the eighteenth century new opportunities arose for medical improvement. One source of new opportunities came from the universities. More universities began offering more medical courses, intended, not for their graduates alone, but for guild and local practitioners' apprentices, who attended classes for a year or two with no intention of graduating. The universities at Leiden, Edinburgh, and Philadelphia are famous for developing curricula to take advantage of student demand for improvement, offering classes in all the medical sciences, as well as clinical lectures at a local hospital. But the same phenomena occurred all over Europe: in prominent universities like Göttingen, the most illustrious medical school in the German states; in Pavia, the 'best university in Italy', according to a British visitor, where 'the opportunities for dissection are superb'; in provincial schools like Ingolstadt, proud possessor of a brand-new anatomical theatre, and Stockholm, which could boast a botanical garden and chemical laboratory as well.

Even more important than the new facilities was the use that was made of them. Instead of one or two professors dividing up all the medical subjects, the ideal, at least, was that each of the courses considered essential to the study of medicine—anatomy, surgery, chemistry, botany, medical theory (physiology), medical practice (pathology), and often hygiene or dietetics as well—ought to be taught by a single professor who was an accomplished scholar in his field. This ideal could not always be realized, and it sometimes happened that a professor became a scholar of his subject only after being appointed to the chair. It is, however, the origin of the idea that each subject required its own specialized body of knowledge, and should be taught by a recognized authority in that field.

Another source of change was the transformation of surgeons' guilds. Guilds began to extend their local authority by offering certificates of competence requiring more formal study, including lectures, examinations, and dissection. This is particularly marked in France, where the surgeons of Paris were notable for enhancing their own status and that of their training: their classes attracted far more students than the Faculté de Médecine. But the same phenomenon occurred all over Europe: in Spain, where the College of Surgeons of San Carlos took the lead in redefining both the status of the surgeon and the form of education the new gentleman surgeon should have, and in Great Britain, where the Colleges of Surgeons of Edinburgh, Dublin, and London succeeded in transforming themselves from 'busy bustling mechanics', as a hostile observer called them, into eminent professional societies, consulted on questions of medical as well as surgical education.

In addition to university and guild, there were also new entrants into the area of medical education. Clinical teaching, offering far more exposure to patients than Boerhaave's twelve-patient ward, had been added to course offerings of any medical school located near a hospital. By the end of the eighteenth century it was axiomatic that university students should spend at least six months 'walking the wards' of a hospital before obtaining a degree. But if universities could borrow hospital wards for their instruction, what was to prevent hospitals from borrowing lecture halls, and developing course offerings to provide students with the medical science they needed? Indeed, hospital schools, as they were called, developed almost anywhere there were hospitals to offer opportunities for clinical experience. From the Manchester Infirmary to the Strasbourg city hospital, from the Santo Spiritù hospital in Rome to the Hospital da Mizericordia in Rio de Janeiro, physicians and surgeons offered lectures to enable students to gain clinical experience. The most famous hospital schools were in London, 'the Metropolis of the whole World for practical Medicine', according to one American student in the 1780s, and in Paris 'looked upon by the medical profession throughout the world as the one and only seat of science', according to another fifty years later. There students attended the lectures on medical subjects as far ranging as any offered by universities. In addition, they had more opportunities for the practical work universities were not well equipped to provide, in anatomical dissection, post-mortem dissection, and differential diagnosis in wards organized by disease as well as by sex.

This type of instruction especially benefited female midwifery students. By the beginning of the nineteenth century, midwives in the Habsburg territories, in some of the German states, and in France were required to be licensed by the State in order to practise; licences were given only on completion of a set course of study. The hospital schools provided the bulk of the instruction in the midwifery courses. La Maternité in Paris provided an especially impressive example. According to one attentive observer in 1818,

Besides being practically engaged in the management of natural labors, [midwifery students] attend lectures given twice a week at the hospital. . . . They also receive instruction daily from the Sage-femme en chef of the hospital, and attend the course of midwifery given exclusively to them at l'École de Médecine. They follow the Physician and Surgeon in their daily visits, and each élève makes a clinical report in writing of the patients under her care. The accuracy and minuteness of some of these reports . . . could not have been greater, if they had been made by an experienced practitioner . . . besides learning the theory and practice of midwifery, the anatomy and circulation of the foetus, and whatever is usually given in a regular course of lectures, these female students attend the dissections of les femmes enceintes ou accouchées; who die in the hospital; and they are also instructed in the practice of phlebotomy and vaccination.

There were other new institutions which arose to meet the demand for medical education. For instance, the Collegium Medico-Chirurgicum in Berlin, set

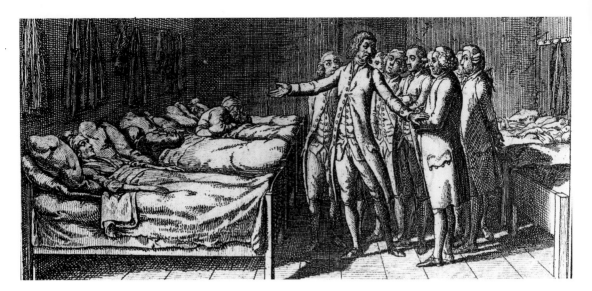

Clinical medicine was the hardest subject to incorporate into medical education, because few patients wanted to be 'practice material' for students. Hospitals for the sick poor, like the Charité hospital in Berlin, provided the main opportunities for students until the twentieth century.

up initially to train surgeons for the Prussian army, attracted more medical students in the eighteenth century than any German university. Since students could also attend clinical rounds at the Charité Hospital in Berlin, the medical school provided the same type of medical education as the best universities, though without the university degree.

The Expanding Routine of Medical Education

With all these new forms of improvement, a kind of inflation in medical education had developed by the beginning of the nineteenth century: students who might previously only have served an apprenticeship with a local practitioner now began to take courses at a university, and students who might have taken only one or two classes began to attend for many classes, for several years. In its attention to scheduling, Alexander Lesassier's daily routine at the University of Edinburgh in 1806 is the forerunner of the modern medical student's:

I rise in the morning at 8 [he wrote], finish breakfast, & get seated in Dr Gregory's class room [in Medical Practice] by 9—from 10–11 I hear Dr Hope on Chemistry From 11 to 12 Dr Barclay on Anatomy—Then from 12 till 1 I attend the Infirmary. From 1 till 2 the famous Dr Monro [on Anatomy]—from 2 to 3 I go home & take a basin of soup—from 3 till 4 . . . lectures on Midwifery—then from 4 to 5 Dinner from 5 till 1/2 past 6 Studying & reviewing what I've heard during the day—Tea over by a little past 7 & I go to the Infirmary . . . quarter past 9—Supper & to bed by 1/2 past 10.

Francis Augustus Bonney's schedule of reading and hospital attendance in Paris in the same period combined moral and medical improvement: 'Plan for the week. Monday, temperance, chemistry; Tuesday, chastity, anatomy; Wednesday, meekness, mat[eria] medica; Thursday, contentedness, pract[ice] of med[icine]; Friday, honesty, surgery; Saturday, industry, midwifery; Sunday, religion.'

With so much competition from hospital schools and other institutions, universities might have died out as places for medical education. Instead, they flourished by incorporating into their own curriculum aspects of medical study introduced by their rivals. Large anatomical demonstrations were supplemented by small dissection classes. Clinical lectures in hospitals became required courses everywhere; some hospitals were simply taken over by university medical schools and turned into a new institution, the teaching hospital. All students were required to attend surgical cases in the wards, and observe surgical operations. And, as surgeons' apprentices attended more and more university classes in medical science, and medical students were required to learn more and more anatomy and surgery, the distinction between the two professional groups blurred, as did the distinction between the 'science' of the one and the 'skill' of the other.

The unification of the two professional groups was not complete, however, until the national regulation of the medical profession, a long, slow process which took much of the nineteenth century to accomplish. There was not much dispute about the best possible course of study for a medical man: it consisted of a good liberal arts education, followed by three or four years of university medical lectures, and a year or two of hospital clinical experience. The difficulty was that this education was so expensive that to insist on it for licensing would have drastically reduced the number of physicians who could have qualified; moreover, the majority of practitioners would never have earned enough to make such an initial outlay on education a worthwhile investment. For those reasons, government and professional bodies and individuals who called for more regulation were forced to accept a compromise, the existence of two different types of practitioners, one with the best education and one which met minimal standards. France led the way in this, creating two different licences, the doctorate in medicine offered by the best medical schools, and the licence for the *Officiers de santé*, the 'médecins en deuxième classe', which required fewer years of study. Similarly, students could still obtain licences to practise as *Wundärzte*, rather than physicians, in rural parts of the German states up to the end of the 1860s, and in England practitioners could qualify under the Apothecaries' Act after serving a five-year apprenticeship and attending barely a year of classes.

Yet the two classes of practitioners proved a temporary solution. In a reversal of Gresham's law that bad currency drives out good, the second-class medical practitioners were increasingly discredited over the nineteenth century, and by the 1880s several years' study of medicine leading to a university doctorate in medicine (or in England a dual qualification by the Royal College of Physicians and the Royal College of Surgeons) was the standard qualification for medical practice. The growth of university study, and the more uniform body of knowledge it was intended to convey, led to the development of the sense of a corporate spirit among physicians, though much competition remained. The number of hours spent in study for the MD had kept pace with the growth in medical knowledge, and the following requirements, taken from the University of Vienna in the 1860s, are typical:

Zoology, 5 hours per week	1 semester
Mineralogy, 5 hours per week	1 semester
Botany, 5 hours per week	1 semester
Inorganic Chemistry, 5 hours per week	1 semester

Organic Chemistry, 5 hours per week	1 semester
Physiology, 5 hours per week	2 semesters
Anatomical dissection, 5 hours per week	2 semesters
Anatomy lectures, 5 hours per week	2 semesters
Pathology, 5 hours per week	1 semester
Pharmacognosy, 3 hours per week	1 semester
Pharmacology, 5 hours per week	1 semester
Therapy, 2 hours per week	1 semester
Bandages and instruments, 4 hours per week	2 semesters
Pathological anatomy, 5 hours per week	2 semesters
Pathological anatomy practicum, 3 hours per week	2 semesters
Clinic intern, 10 hours per week	4 semesters
Clinic extern, 10 hours per week	4 semesters
Eye diseases, 10 hours per week	1 semester
Obstetrics and gynaecology, 10 hours per week	1 semester
Forensic medicine, 5 hours per week	2 semesters
Forensic medicine practicum, 3 hours per week	2 semesters
Veterinary medicine, 3 hours per week	1 semester
Formulary, 2 hours per week	1 semester
Toxicology, 2 hours per week	1 semester
Vaccination	6 weeks

No doubt Vienna students would have agreed with John Edward Perry, who graduated from Meharry Medical School in Tennessee in the 1890s, that 'Time was all too short and often we wished the twenty-four-hour day might be stretched to thirty-six.'

Women in Medicine

The gain in professional identity and academic rigour in the preparation of medical practitioners also had its costs: it led to the exclusion from the fraternity of all those excluded from the universities. One group this affected was women, particularly the middle-class women who, in the mid-nineteenth century, began to demand the right to become physicians together with the right to vote. They were met by fierce opposition, as going outside the proper sphere of women. Elizabeth Blackwell, the first English woman to obtain a medical degree, was forced to go to a medical school in Geneva, New York State, before she was accepted. 'The whole idea is so disgusting,' said the father of one prospective woman physician, 'I could not entertain it for a moment.' Yet what was at stake was not the exposure of women to physical ailments which were, indeed, often disgusting and unpleasant, but that women should have authority over treatment of those ailments equal to that of men. Women, as nurses and midwives, had long been involved in many of the most disagreeable of medical tasks. Elizabeth Blackwell, in Paris for further study after completing her MD, complained of her 'prison life' when she attended a course of study at La Maternité in Paris, precisely because she was treated like a midwife, assigned the most menial tasks, and confined to the grounds of the hospital, with none of the freedom of the medical students. That women of the lower classes should carry out menial hospital tasks, however indelicate, under his direction was something a male physician accepted as part of the inevitable order of things, but that his sisters, daughters, and wife should join him at the hospital bedside was unthinkable. One man wrote that it was 'intolerable' that his daughters 'should go through the discipline and lead the life that I have done myself', and, as a professor of the University of Edinburgh put it, he 'could not imagine any decent woman wanting to study medicine;—as for any lady, that was out of the question'.

But ladies persisted in their study in medicine. In the nineteenth century it was Switzerland that led the way for women's admission into medical schools. The University of Zurich opened its prestigious courses and clinics to women in the 1860s, followed by other Swiss universities over the next ten years. Switzerland became the major centre for women's medical education, deciding in favour not only of co-educational lectures but also of co-educational clinical training. Women were admitted into the Écoles de Médecine in Paris in the 1870s, and to the universities in the German states from 1903 to 1908.

In the USA, where it was not difficult to obtain a charter to found new educational institutions, women founded their own medical schools when excluded from most existing ones; they also founded their own clinics when excluded from using existing hospitals for clinical teaching. In Philadelphia, the Women's Medical College of Philadelphia opened in 1850, finally acquiring facilities for hospital teaching in the 1860s. In New York, the Women's College of the New York Infirmary opened in 1865, and in Chicago the Women's Hospital Medical College opened in 1870. In the UK, too, women were excluded from existing medical schools. The London School of Medicine for Women was opened in 1874, making use of the clinical facilities of the New Hospital for Women, which had opened just two years previously. In 1876 a Bill was passed allowing women to take the licensing examination required for practice, and in 1877 they were finally admitted to the wards of the Royal Free Hospital, one of the most prominent of the London teaching hospitals.

Yet though women in the UK and the USA could study medicine, they could not attend the most prestigious of the schools of medicine. Women were not admitted to the University of Edinburgh until 1889, to many of the London medical schools until after the First World War, to the University of Pennsylvania until 1915, or to Harvard University until 1947. Legally the decision to admit women was up to each individual university and hospital, and overall those decisions were negative. The USA, first to graduate women, was slowest to admit them to full equality with men. Though many institutions opened their doors to women students and graduates during the two world wars, they kept them firmly closed otherwise. Indeed, so few women were graduated that a sociological study of the University of Kansas Medical School in the 1950s called itself Boys in White, because 'medicine is man's work ... in this country, although an increasing proportion of the people who have a part in the medical system are women, the medical profession itself remains overwhelmingly male'. The situation in the USA changed only in the 1970s, with the success of a class action suit for discrimination brought against every medical school in the country.

There were other groups excluded from universities, and thus from the medical profession. Black students in the USA suffered from the same discriminatory practices as women: they could be excluded from universities, or, even if they achieved graduation, they could be excluded from hospitals for clinical training and internships. By the 1860s only nine medical schools admitted

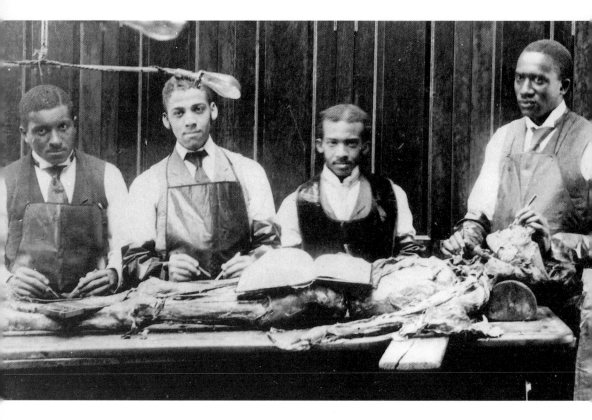

By the end of the nineteenth century, every reputable medical school required student dissection.

black students, and only in very small numbers. In the early part of the nineteenth century it was still possible for a medical practitioner to make a living without a degree, because, as a lawyer explained to James Still, a black practitioner in rural New Jersey in the 1840s, 'You can sell medicine . . . and charge for delivering, and then you can collect it just the same as for anything else. There is a fine for giving prescriptions [without a licence], but you don't give them; you sell medicine and there is nothing to stop you.' Still's practice rivalled that of the white University of Pennsylvania graduate in his township, and he eventually became a prominent landowner, but when he tried to give his children the thorough education he had lacked, the schoolteacher 'discovered eventually that he was not doing the will of God in teaching colored children . . . Consequently, my children had to quit the school.' To overcome similar prejudice, blacks, like women, created their own medical schools and hospital facilities; the two most prominent were Howard University in Washington, DC, opened in 1868, and Meharry University in Tennessee in 1875.

In the late nineteenth century, professional institutions such as the General Medical Council, the Deutscher Ärztevereinsverband, and the American Medical Association took an active role in defining the proper qualifications of the medical professional. Those qualifications increasingly focused on university-based scientific training. In the 1930s, a survey of medical schools in Europe and the USA found that the basic sciences taught in medical schools had become biology, chemistry, physics, anatomy, organic chemistry, physiology, and pharmacology. The clinical sciences included morbid anatomy, pathological histology, therapeutics, forensics, and anaesthetics. Clinical training, too, had increased, with one to two years of clinical experience within the medical school supplemented by at least a year of internship. In fact, basic medical school education began to be referred to as 'undergraduate', with postgraduate training in a speciality becoming more and more common. By the 1960s the original medical schools had grown into medical school complexes, with undergraduate clinical training divided into rotations in specific wards, such as paediatrics and obstetrics, with associated internships, and with affiliations not just at one general hospital but also at several speciality hospitals and community-based clinics. From Ghana Medical School to the University of Bologna to the Faculty of Medical Sciences at the University of Brazil, from the University of Valle in Colombia to the University of Montpellier to the All-India Institute of Medical Sciences in New Delhi, clusters of high-rise buildings, often taking up several city blocks, are physical expressions of the complexity of medical knowledge to be acquired by the twentieth-century student.

The Problems of Modern Medical Education

Though nearly all agree that medical students are now better trained than ever before, the expansion of medical knowledge has brought problems. Knowledge of the basic medical sciences seems more important than ever before, and medical schools have attempted to keep up with the new developments in pathology, histology, epidemiology by adding more and more courses: the Stanford University Medical School, for example, added 900 hours to the curriculum over the four-year medical course between 1945 and 1960. Each new course, taught by a specialist in the field in the tradition established in the eighteenth century, attempted to provide students with all a practitioner needed to know. Daily routine for medical students involved attending classes for eight hours per day five days a week, after which students spent between four and six hours studying every weekday evening with an additional five to seven hours a day over the weekend.

   Though this resulted in doctors with excellent scientific training, there were also complaints that attention paid to science took away from clinical work. This complaint about the tendency of the sciences to take over the curriculum had been noted early on: Amand Trousseau, in his clinical lectures at the Hôtel Dieu in Paris, told his students in 1803, 'You must have sufficient notion of chemistry and physics to be able to understand the application of these sciences to medicine. But I should profoundly deplore the time that you might lose in order to acquire a more extended knowledge of chemistry. ... So, gentlemen, let us have a little less science, and a little more art.' And students in the 1950s expressed their dissatisfaction with the emphasis on science more forcibly. 'All this recent research stuff is of no use to us,' complained one. 'Histology,' said another, 'that's not important. Using a microscope is something we don't have to do as doctors and looking at all those slides doesn't do any good ...' The problem, as medical school professors responded, is built into the nature of the medical profession itself. Its prestige has come in part from the scientific training involved in proper qualification for licensing, but, for many physicians, there is no direct link between the science they learn in medical school and their later practice.

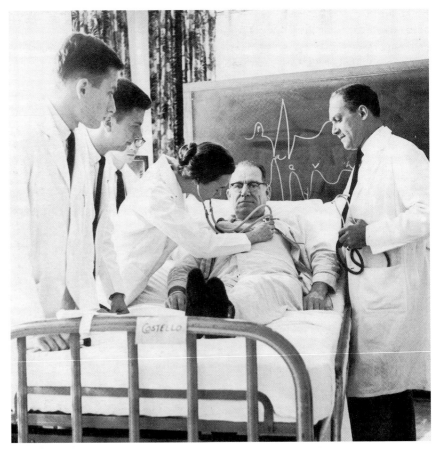

Only in the twentieth century did hands-on clinical experience become an integral part of university medical schools, due both to their association with hospitals and to the rise of hospitals as centres of medical care for the entire population.

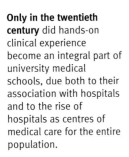

A second problem facing twentieth-century medical schools has to do with clinical training itself. Walking the wards, hailed with such enthusiasm two centuries earlier, has come under criticism for limitations both for what it does teach, and what it does not.

Because much of the teaching takes place in the hospital [wrote one commentator in the 1980s] . . . what students learn typically depends on the ailments of the patients who happen to be in the ward at that moment . . . When walking through hospital corridors, one is struck by the variable, unrehearsed quality of the teaching. Sometimes patients are seen and talked to, sometimes not. Bits and pieces of information are conveyed on the spot as problems develop and new data arrive from the laboratory or night nurse . . . Ethical issues, cost considerations and psychological problems pop up occasionally but seldom receive thorough discussion.

Even if clinical training is carried out effectively, critics argue, a university hospital does not truly prepare students for what they will experience in practice. Patients in a university medical centre are often there precisely because they have serious or unusual ailments; in treating them, students learn little about the most common ailments. Moreover, the model they acquire is of medicine carried out with sophisticated equipment for diagnosis and treatment. A complaint about this was voiced by a US state licensing board in 1930: 'A serious defect . . . is the overstressing of laboratory work . . . a student will say, when questioned, that the best way to diagnose a pneumonia is to send the patient to the hospital and have an x-ray picture taken of his chest to see if there is a consolidation of the lung, rather than to determine the clinical findings by making a personal physical examination of the patient.' In response to complaints of this type, the 1980s and 1990s have seen a new emphasis on the education of primary-care physicians, the patient's first contact with the health-care system.

The reliance on high-tech medical centres has proved to be especially problematic for developing countries, where scarce resources severely limit access for most of the population to university medical centres. In Nigeria, for example, newly certified doctors, aware of the most up-to-date research in clinical medicine, find themselves unable to diagnose and treat some of the most common health problems in the rural areas. Bayero University, Kano, has revised its curriculum to include fieldwork in a rural community; similarly, students at the Faculty of Medicine at Suez Canal University work on community health projects such as the impact on, and the treatment of, the spread of schistosomiasis following the creation of new canals. Community-based medicine, with its emphasis on primary care, has begun to supplement university hospital centres as elective, if not required, parts of many medical school curricula.

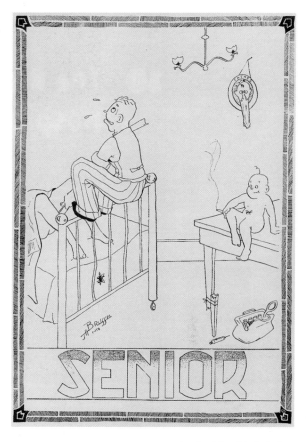

As physicians' technical competence has grown, so have concerns as to whether their medical education imparts or encourages other qualities necessary for a physician, for example compassion. In the 1920s, students had no scruples about this presentation of their care of patients.

The final problems facing medical education in the twentieth century are as old as medical education itself. Medical schools can teach basic sciences, anatomy, pathology: but can they teach compassion, responsibility, flexibility, problem-solving? They can teach the striking success of Western medicine in isolating and treating the disease—but can they teach how to understand and treat the whole patient? In other words, are they merely providing medical improvement, the opportunity to acquire medical knowledge? Or are they—and should they be—providing moral and intellectual discipline necessary for imparting values and building character, the original sense of medical education?

10 | The Rise of the Modern Hospital

ULRICH TRÖHLER AND
CAY-RÜDIGER PRÜLL

IN accounting for the rise of the hospital to the central place it now occupies in modern medicine, it is necessary to consider a number of factors—cultural, socio-political, and medical—which brought about the transformation of an earlier, medieval religious social-service system. The Enlightenment of the eighteenth century was the beginning of this process. At a pace that proceeded faster than the growth of population, new types of hospital were created and older hospices were transformed. During the French Revolution and its aftermath, through the last third of the nineteenth century, and especially after the Second World War, hospitals moved from caring for the suffering towards the provision of treatment for the sick and their diseases. The hospital has since played an ever-increasing and more influential part in the practice, teaching, and research of medicine. Accordingly, the social world within the hospital has changed, as hospital admissions have altered such that patients now come from all strata of society, as the duration of patients' stay has diminished and their age varied, and as doctoring, nursing, and hospital administration have been professionalized and specialized, and new ways of hospital funding have had to be found. The text of this chapter deals with the origin and evolution of various types of hospitals in their interplay with medicine and society.

Origins and Development of Various Types of Hospital

There were a number of reasons why in the eighteenth century new medically staffed hospitals were established particularly in Britain and the German-speaking lands. The Enlightenment, which became a vast movement of reforms touching most aspects of life, changed the previous indifference of public opinion and governments towards problems of health. Single individuals, and subsequently the State, propagated the worth of health and the value of restituting the poor sick, whose labour power was seen to be essential for the strength and wealth of the mercantilist state. These ideas also sprang from a

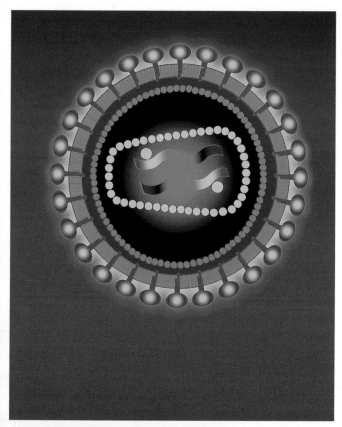

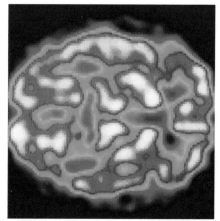

PET scan (*above*). In positron emission tomography, radioactive substances are injected into the bloodstream. The sectional images of the emissions, synthesized by computer, do not so much map the structures of the brain in the conventional manner but record areas of greater and lesser activity, designated by specially chosen colours.

Computer model of the Aids virus (*above, left*). Using data from X-ray crystallography and electron microscopy, visual models of viral and molecular structures can be created employing standard conventions of representation. Such models can be used by researchers who aspire to design drugs which might 'fit' on to the virus and neutralize its action.

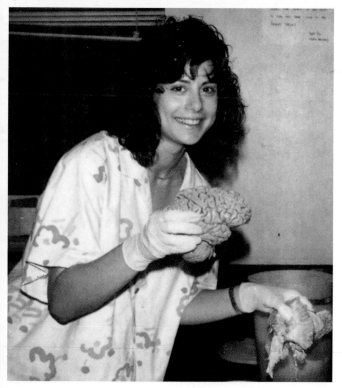

By the end of the twentieth century, preservation techniques make it possible for students to have a more intimate knowledge of anatomical structure than ever before.

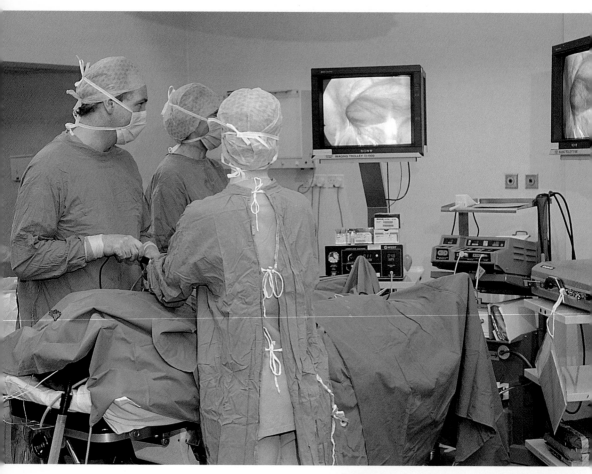

Keyhole surgery: a surgical revolution. The end of the 1980s saw the beginnings of a change in centuries-old surgical practice. Many operations could be carried out quickly, safely, and on a day-basis through small telescopes inserted into the body through tiny incisions. Thus removal of the gall bladder, the oesophagus, segments of bowel, and portions of damaged cartilage in the knee joint are all examples of this new approach, which is likely to revolutionize surgical practice within the next few decades.

A laparoscopic view of a gall bladder being removed from the liver. The telescope, with the attached television camera, is placed through the umbilicus and looks up towards the right upper side of the abdomen. The pale structure to which the instruments are attached at the top and middle is the gall bladder, with the liver on either side. In the bottom right corner, the cystic duct which carries bile out of the gall bladder is just identifiable.

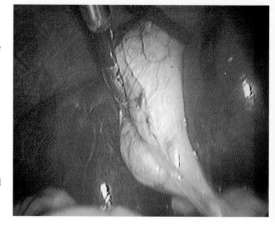

new type of socially redistributive philanthropy, itself having a root in the increasing wealth and prosperity of the middle classes. They were thus promoted from above and were certainly in the interests of the well-off, but the latter, in typical Enlightenment philanthropy, saw them as beneficial to the sufferers themselves, who became conspicuously concentrated in the bigger cities as economies expanded. Thus between 1719 and 1745 five new hospitals were opened in London (the Westminster in 1719, Guy's in 1729, St George's in 1733, the London in 1740, and the Middlesex in 1745) sponsored by groups of wealthy lay people. The similar needs of the military because of standing armies were also being met—for example, in the Berlin Charité Hospital, which was inaugurated in 1727 by government decision and provided for practical clinical and anatomical instruction for military surgeons and civilian students. The Edinburgh Royal Infirmary (opened in 1729) was planned to provide both for patients, and for students and doctors, reflecting a steady tradition of bedside teaching that could be traced back to sixteenth-century Italy. All these foundations were so-called general hospitals, which accepted 'curable' (poor) patients. The establishment of a statistically demonstrable link between poverty and morbidity and vice versa underpinned the later Enlightenment idea of State welfare. It led, for example, to the construction of the 2,000-bed Allgemeines Krankenhaus in Vienna between 1783 and 1785, which was then the world's largest hospital, providing teaching for university students as well as, in a separate department, the pupils of the military medico-surgical school (Josephinum, inaugurated in 1785). The French Revolution, which brought about radical changes in most existing social and political structures, initiated the transformation into medical hospitals of what were still medieval institutions for refuge in France and northern Italy.

In the nineteenth century the social, economic, and political drives for poor relief became more urgent and important than philanthropy as reasons for the expansion in number and size of general hospitals, particularly in urban–industrial areas. Furthermore, developments within medicine itself also enhanced this process, although they remained for some time still of secondary importance. Clinical teaching and research, consisting by 1800 at their best of immediate observations of symptoms and 'verification' by autopsy, now reached a new dimension by increasing emphasis on lesions detectable

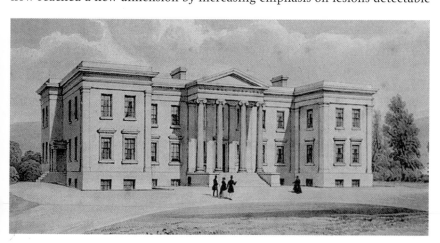

The architecture of many an eighteenth-century British voluntary hospital reflected the wealth of its benefactors and was reminiscent of contemporary country houses of the landed gentry.

only with the aid of instruments and laboratory investigations. The technical methods ranged from the stethoscope (1819), via various endoscopes (from the 1850s) and X-ray pictures (1895), to graphical recording (for example, electrocardiography from the beginning of the twentieth century). Laboratory work included bacteriology, clinical chemistry, and (microscopical) pathology, creating a scientific basis for (hospital) hygiene.

These innovations, whether or not they stemmed from hospital doctors, were certainly elaborated, tested, practised, and taught in many nineteenth-century hospitals, which were therefore involved in their development. Whether and to what extent the innovations themselves stimulated the growth of general hospitals before 1870–80 is questionable. However, medical innovations of the later nineteenth century—featuring, as they continued in the twentieth century, ever more sophisticated methods of visualization and a trend towards the increasing differentiation of microbiological, biochemical, and structural diagnostics, and the ensuing changes in hygiene and medical practice—brought with them a need for specialized hospital facilities and their continuous adaptation to new scientific insights. An early example of this new phenomenon was modern surgery, which developed during the last third of the nineteenth century based on localized pathology, anaesthesia, and antisepsis. These medical motives also fostered yet another new type of hospital: the private hospital where the privileged could receive the benefits of progress in well-furnished rooms where they could count on at least some of the privacy and freedom they were accustomed to at home.

By the beginning of the twentieth century all large and most sizeable provincial cities of the Western world possessed public and private general hospitals. Rural patients and their doctors had access to small-scale in-patient facilities,

Hospitals in cities sometimes opened specialized out-patient departments which in certain areas and times (e.g. Sweden in the twentieth century) played a fundamental role in public health care provision. Like in-patient hospitals, they offered doctors and nurses ample opportunity for acquiring clinical experience, training in practical skills, and the chance to research. The white coats worn by the staff have been a widely recognized emblem of the marriage of science and medical practice since the late nineteenth century.

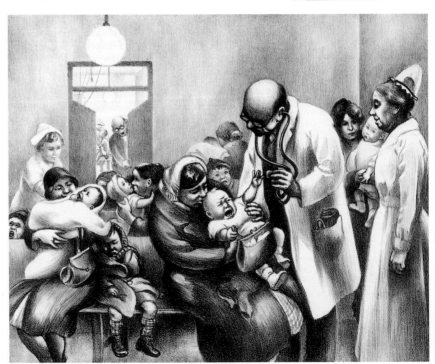

called 'cottage hospitals' in the UK and the USA and *Krankenstuben* in Switzerland. All of these institutions traditionally cared for patients with medical as
well as surgical diseases.

For a long time, patients with ailments deemed incurable, morally con-
demnable, and/or dangerous for other inmates (cancer, venereal disease,
fevers, lunacy) had been excluded from the new general hospitals. This also
held for some other groups of the population, such as children and women, for
whom special hospitals had been set up from the mid-eighteenth century,
again particularly in the UK and Germany. These specialist and general hospitals were sometimes complemented by outpatient facilities (dispensaries). By
1820 there were, in the UK alone, at least fifty-four such specialist institutions,
offering, for example, treatment for sexually transmitted diseases, fevers,
tuberculosis, eye and ear diseases, children, and lying-in women. By that date
eighteen of the twenty-two medical faculties of the German-speaking lands
had an obstetric clinic. Medical specialization was closely associated during
the nineteenth century with such specialized hospitals, or departments
within the medical faculties of the state universities, and also with private
facilities which were sometimes established by specialized medical entrepreneurs as a result of medical innovation in these fields. Special cases were
hospitals for mental diseases, the sanatorium movement for the climatic treatment of tuberculosis, which started in Switzerland in the last decades of the
nineteenth century, and the medicalization of spas on the Continent which,
after the Second World War, also became important centres for rehabilitation.

From the 1960s hospital treatment has become more and more specific, and
thus dividable into staff- and technology-intensive interventions, on the one
hand, and low-technology nursing, on the other (see Chapter 12). Hospitals
now tend to be differentiated between institutions for acute treatment and
those for long-time care. A recent development of this kind, which originated
in the 1970s in the UK in response to patient demand, was the rebirth of hospices for the incurable and dying. In fact, the underlying concept, which had
originally been a Christian one, had been modestly implemented by the end of
the nineteenth century as a consequence of the establishment of active hospital treatment for cancer, but the overwhelming commitment of the medical
world to intervention had pushed it aside.

Hospital Economics

Various models have long existed for hospital financing, the most important
distinction being between private and public funding, with many possibilities
for mixing. More than any other aspect of hospital history, funding has been
dependent on the local situation at any given time. Nevertheless a few general
features may be identified, and certainly the different forms of financing have
affected patient admissions, staff recruitment, organizational structure, technical equipment, and the spaciousness and comfort of hospitals.

Public funding goes back to late medieval times, when cities sometimes took
over the responsibility for charitable institutions. This tendency was increased
after the Reformation, particularly with the transformation of such city hospices into the modern type of hospital first seen in the eighteenth century.

Central state governments concerned with the control of the unemployed, some of whom were sick, organized and paid for their housing in so-called *hôpitaux généraux* or workhouses. From the 1720s, Prussia and Austria became involved in the care for and cure of the sick, partly because of their wish to control university education and the licensing of doctors and partly because of the perceived need to provide a military medical service. The State was ready to pay for university clinics and the hospitals attached to the military medico-surgical schools. This continued to be the means of financing teaching hospitals in the countries adopting the German 'university-type' medical education in the nineteenth century. By the beginning of the twentieth century, the functions, and consequently the financing, of university hospitals were becoming more complex, and they became dependent on the overall health-care system chosen in any given state.

Private funding was paramount for many of the other hospitals founded since the eighteenth century. In the UK they were called voluntary hospitals because they were financially dependent on voluntary contributions. After 1860 voluntary hospitals also became dominant in the USA. When, in the eighteenth century, old paternalistic alms-giving became modern philanthropy with its strict organization and definite aims, hospitals provided a popular and obvious place for satisfying the philanthropic impulse of individuals, organizations, and charities, and this is still the case in the late twentieth century. Sometimes, however, such private funding was supplemented by voluntary or compulsory contributions by patients. An example was the workers' *Kranken(haus)kassen* in nineteenth-century Germany and Switzerland.

As costs caused by the introduction of technology and the need for more and better-paid staff rose constantly in the second half of the nineteenth century, often to an extent that was not met by the original endowments, voluntary hospitals began to run into financial problems. The solutions lay in State inter-

Women's and girl's ward in a provincial hospital (Huttwil, Berne canton, Switzerland) in 1928. This staged photograph shows bedridden patients, two to a bed, with others and relatives, together with nursing staff including a doctor. The three nurses beside him are deaconesses, sisters of the Protestant order founded in Kaiserswerth, Germany, in the early nineteenth century. The other nurse (*back row, third from left*) is a novice —and Professor Tröhler's mother. The order, which owned private hospitals, also staffed public ones, as lay nurses were lacking. It was by this date quite widespread in Protestant areas of the German-speaking lands.

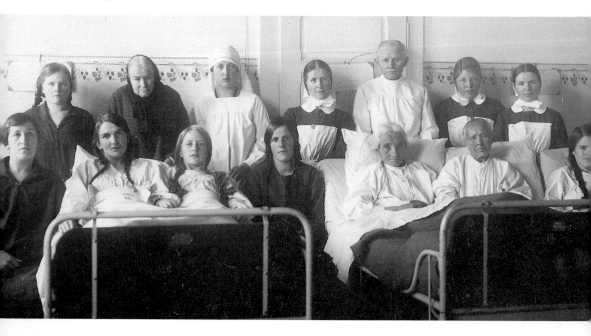

vention and/or the development of business strategies, which might involve private insurance schemes. At one end of the spectrum of responses was the nationalization of the voluntary hospitals by the National Health Service (NHS) in the UK, implemented in 1948. At the other end, hospitals in the USA became predominantly market-oriented by the 1920s. Only since the 1960s have government funding and hospitals run by government agencies become relatively more important in the USA. In between these two extremes was the financing of hospital care via public national insurance schemes, for which Imperial Germany's *Krankenversicherung* (1883) served as a model. Assuming varied forms, these schemes became crucial for funding across Europe from 1910 until the present, although there have been further modifications in the 1980s and 1990s. In summary, government has become a major source of funds for health care everywhere. It has, therefore, at all levels, steadily increased its involvement in hospital medicine.

Hospitals and People

Patients

In the centre of the whole process of the expansion of hospitals large and small, general and special, public and private, stands the patient. When, in the eighteenth century, poverty was no longer regarded as inevitable and unchangeable, hospitals were founded primarily as havens for the labouring poor, whose manpower was needed for the survival of the nation. Such an attitude was still reflected in the nineteenth century, when the German hospital population, for example, was predominantly male and of a relatively young age—below 30. According to the underlying philosophy, the criteria for admission to hospital were initially determined socially rather than medically. Socially undeserving, as well as incurables, were seen as inappropriate patients. Once admitted, patients had to comply with authoritarian discipline on pain of dismissal, regardless of their state of health. Thus hospitals functioned as a means for the social control of the lower strata of society. They maintained a certain coercive function which they shared with the prisons of the time and which developed almost simultaneously from the same common root, the early modern (that is, pre-eighteenth-century) workhouses. Such institutions also contained the multi-bed wards which both conditioned discipline and eased its enforcement. In fact, on entering a hospital, the sick were abandoning their natural milieu and habits, thus losing their autonomy to the artificial world of the institution, with its own rules demanding subordination and obedience. On the other hand, there was also demand from below, since the poor sick must have appreciated the relief offered free of charge. At any rate, the hospitals were better than their forerunners, the often prison-like workhouses euphemistically termed *hôpitaux généraux* in France and, more realistically, *Zuchthaus* (prison) in Germany. Such an interpretation helps to explain the success rate of the hospital movement throughout Europe, since in the long run patients were the ultimate judges.

The involvement of hospitals in childbirth was a totally separate issue from the treatment of medical and surgical cases. The role of the hospitals in obstetrics, and what is often called the 'birth of man-midwifery', are discussed in

165

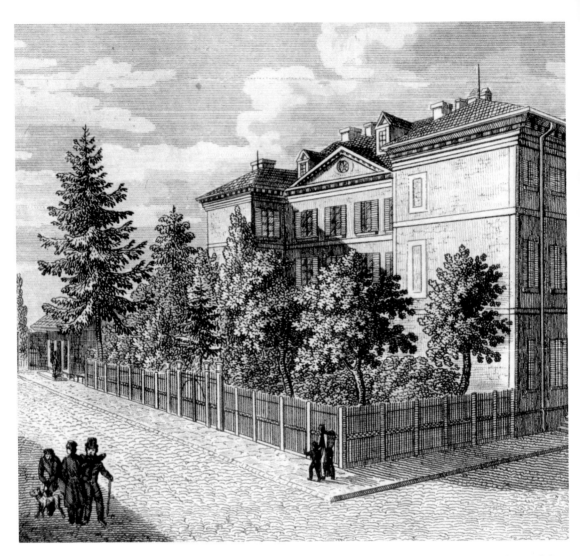

Chapter 13. By the end of the eighteenth century, however, maternity or 'lying-in' hospitals were springing up throughout Europe. The first to be opened in 1751 was the university obstetric hospital in Göttingen, where the Professor of Obstetrics, Friedrich Benjamin Osiander (1759–1822), wrote: 'The hospital is not here to serve the patients, but the patients to serve the hospital.' Until the last quarter of the nineteenth century most of the patients were unmarried women. They, in turn, were pleased, after initial hesitation, to be delivered, and sometimes even to be paid for doing so, in a relatively safe environment, although they thereby consented to be examined and treated by trainee (male) midwives. Most married and above all well-to-do women continued to be delivered at home, for, until the introduction of antiseptic Caesarian section in the 1880s, there was no apparent advantage in going to a hospital. On the contrary, in view of endemic and epidemic childbed (or puerperal) fever, it was often positively dangerous to be delivered in a hospital.

Middle- and upper-class patients, suffering from all kinds of diseases, expected doctors to see them at home, where they usually had servants to look after them privately—a service the poorer elements in society could receive only in hospitals. These domestic advantages and preferences were out-weighed only when increasingly technology-dependent diagnosis and treatment became accepted as essential by doctors and the public. This was especially true for surgical diseases which required specialized facilities and well-trained staff. Hospitals were, therefore, able to offer means of treating the sick which were sought after not only by the working classes but also by the middle and upper classes; by doing so they lost their reputation of being little more than houses of poverty and death.

Children have been considered as specific patients rather than small adults only since the Enlightenment, but paediatrics as an academic discipline did not emerge until after the First World War. Until then, with a few notable exceptions (for example, the Hôpital des Enfants Malades founded in 1802 in Paris), children were treated alongside adults in the same hospital wards.

Patients who populated the new military and naval hospitals have been little studied by historians. However, in the eighteenth century, such patients, being under military and bureaucratic orders, were used as testing-grounds for retrospective and even prospective evaluation of new treatments without concern of the ethical issues now fundamental where human experimentation is concerned.

Hospital benefactors

In the eighteenth century most of the new civilian hospitals, with the exception of the German-type university clinics, were initiated by private donors. They had rights in proportion to their financial contributions for the admittance of those patients they favoured; moreover, upon request, they were empowered to give a ticket for free treatment. A selected group of donors, the governors, decided on all administrative matters, including the appointment of medical staff. This private and lay dominance played an important role in spreading the idea of modern hospital foundations in European societies. It was most pronounced in Britain, where it formally persisted until the establishment of the National Health Service after the Second World War. Medicalization of hospitals—that is, a reversal of the power relationship between benefactors and doctors as a consequence of medical progress—was a gradual development of the nineteenth century: while doctors typically were not admitted to boards of governors in the eighteenth century, they became the decisive members of such boards in the nineteenth, a position they still hold in many private hospitals in the late twentieth century, although a new profession, the hospital administrators, has also become more and more influential.

Doctors

Although doctors were at first excluded from governorships, an appointment to a hospital was a symbol of success much sought after by ambitious doctors. In addition to their symbolic value, hospital appointments provided ample opportunity for gaining practical experience and allowed contacts with wealthy and influential donors, opening the door to private practice in the highest social circles. In short, from the eighteenth century, a consultancy at a

The Neues Accouchierhaus (facing), the first purpose-built university lying-in hospital, was opened in the German university town of Göttingen in 1791. Since no model existed, its style followed that of eighteenth-century aristocratic domestic architecture. However, it was specifically designed to provide sufficient light and ventilation in all rooms, in accordance with Enlightenment precepts for the prevention of childbed fevers. It also featured a dissection-room, and had its own chapel where the mostly unmarried clients could carry out the penance required for their misdemeanour in private rather than publicly in church.

charitable institution became a public label of professional success which also increased the consultant's income. The high reputation of hospitals, especially teaching hospitals, meant that, during the course of the nineteenth century, senior hospital physicians all over Europe were regarded as the leading exponents of their disciplines. Hospital appointments were granted only to regular practitioners, usually those with university qualifications, to the detriment of all kinds of lay healers and quacks, who had played a large part in providing care in the medical market place up to the early nineteenth century. Thus the growth of the hospitals played a central role in the rise of medicine as a profession during the nineteenth century, accompanied by a rise in the number of medical societies and scientific hospital periodicals.

Not all of the exponents of academic medicine were able to obtain posts at general hospitals. Some of the more entrepreneurially inclined set up their own private institutions and practised in a specialized field. Such special hospitals were 'medicalized' earlier than the general ones, in the sense that admission was necessarily determined by medical rather than social criteria—that is, primarily by the doctors. From the late nineteenth century, hospitals provided an environment which encouraged specialization amongst the medical staff, a process which has accelerated through the second half of the twentieth century, leading to an ever-increasing number of 'super-specialists'.

Nurses

Another important factor in the rise of Western hospital medicine has been the development of professional nursing, which paralleled the expansion of treatment possibilities and the widening and intensifying use of technology (see Chapter 12). Traditionally, religious orders had been at the forefront of patient care in Catholic hospitals, as long as very few specific skills were necessary and nurses mainly had to do household-like work. In Protestant countries, the situation was both more complex and on the whole less satisfactory, as uneducated lay nurses, not necessarily with Christian ethical underpinning, prevailed. Therefore, reform movements came in the 1830s from Germany and the 1860s from Britain, changing the social origins and transforming the image of the nurse. While previously nurses had often been recruited among the convalescent or former patients, who were necessarily from the labouring or poorer classes, from the late nineteenth century they increasingly came from middle-class backgrounds. Better organization of the wards, the design of uniforms, provision of accommodation, progress in education, and the advance of medical knowledge with its demands for cleanliness and order made nursing socially attractive even if not well paid in comparison to the doctors. The terms of employment improved over the next 100 years, reflecting the growing importance of nursing as medical interventions increased. Further changes as the nurse-to-patient ratio increased and nursing became more specialized are discussed in Chapter 12.

Administrators

Until the end of the nineteenth century, hospitals were administered by laymen who were often benefactors or retired civil servants or officers. As health-care facilities became larger and more complex, and ideas and practices designed to increase efficiency became dominant, increasing claims were made on hospital administrators. This began in the USA in the early twentieth century and led to the professionalization of hospital administrators, whose power increased enormously in subsequent decades. Like doctors and nurses, hospital administrators now have their own professional associations, meetings, and publications. In Europe this change was slower, as hospitals continued to be run as charities or institutions of state welfare rather than as businesses. Furthermore, doctors retained their exclusive power in the process of decision-making, acquired in the nineteenth century, and this relegated administrators to subordinate roles for a longer time than in the USA. However, the growing quest for efficiency has by now also had a marked influence upon hospitals in Europe.

The Role of Hospitals

The role of all types of hospital can be approached from different viewpoints: social policy, medical practice, medical education, midwifery, nursing, and research. Although formal teaching and research have been confined to a few hospitals, all hospitals reflect changes in social policies and medical practice.

Social welfare

Hospitals were clearly planned for the poor sick rather than the sick poor. Yet in practice they could not help simultaneously fulfilling the traditional custodial and even coercive functions of the old hospices that served the elderly, blind, lame, invalid soldiers, and lunatics. Despite their enormous internal and external modernization throughout the nineteenth century, most hospitals—albeit decreasingly so, in the case of university clinics—remained important tools for the social provision of poor relief. Until about 1870 the primary attraction of the hospitals to the sick poor was 'care' in the sense of food, warmth, a clean bed, and a roof over their head. After 1870, patients began to look for specific therapeutic treatment as well—in other words, they looked to hospitals to provide cure (or at least alleviation) as well as traditional nursing care.

Medical practice

Active medical intervention was for long uncommon in hospitals, but the increasing number of poor people in cities had somehow to be cared for, particularly when they had ailments treatable by minor surgery—such as fistulae, haemorrhoids, abscesses, or general signs of fatigue, scabies, and rheumatoid pains, and so on. For such patients the general hospitals fulfilled the important social and medical function for which they had been conceived in the eighteenth century. According to contemporary opinion, specialized institutions, underpinned by their own possibly biased statistics, showed high rates of cure for fevers, venereal disease, and children's diseases. 'Cure', however, must not be understood in our sense of *restitutio ad integrum*; it often meant alleviation of pain or the provision of comfort. From this perspective, eighteenth-century hospitals, for all their limitations, were not the 'gateways to death' their critics have claimed.

Certainly, from time to time, and in various places through the nineteenth and twentieth centuries, criticism and even crises of confidence in hospitals were produced by opponents of medicine based on the natural sciences, as it was taught first in the German universities. These critics included a few doctors who claimed that university hospital patients were (ab)used for experimentation. A widely publicized incident thereof was the inoculation of syphilitic pus into women and children in order to test an 'anti-syphilitic serum' for which Professor Albert Neisser (1855–1916) was actually sentenced in 1900. In the same year, the Prussian Ministry of Public Health and Education issued the world's first directives for clinical professors concerning the conducting of research on human beings.

Further general criticism, increasingly advanced by doctors and insurance agents, related to both the unhygienic and the over-regulated living conditions of hospital patients. Of particular concern were the infections which seemed to have become endemic, particularly in surgical and obstetric wards (hospitalism). They continued to be combated by various traditional measures such as whitewashing and disinfecting the premises, burning the clothes, and improving ventilation. Then hospital hygiene found a new scientific basis through the advances of bacteriology in the last quarter of the nineteenth century. An extraordinary case was the actual boycott of the Berlin Charité by left-wing doctors and health insurers in 1893, resulting finally in a thorough reconstruction of many departments. The same group also requested that the military-style discipline to which patients were subjected should be abolished, that patients should give their consent before becoming the object of demonstration to students, and that there should be a free choice of reading materials; in short, they asked for some autonomy and privacy.

Such liberalization was introduced only very slowly, probably following similar developments in society at large. There were also structural changes in hospital design—such as smaller wards. These modernizations, together with the glamour surrounding technology in such fields as surgery and diagnostic imaging, provided the catalyst for a more general acceptance of scientific medicine in the hospitals. By 1960 standards were set for optimal treatment and nursing in all fields to which both doctors and patients of all ages and classes aspired. Later in the century, with the arrival, for instance, of minimally invasive or 'keyhole' surgery, short-term hospital treatment for acute diseases became easier, and a number of what were formerly hospital-based diagnostic and therapeutic methods can now be performed as outpatient procedures. These phenomena have significantly reduced the duration of in-patient hospital care, and the resulting rise in turnover rate has also changed the nature of the work and the relations of hospital staff to their patients and vice versa. On the other hand, chronically ill and geriatric patients with little diagnostic or therapeutic problems need in-house nursing care above all, for which high-tech hospitals are over-equipped and their staff often inappropriate.

Teaching

From the beginning, one of the purposes of the hospital as we know it today was the teaching of medicine. The system of bedside teaching, which was slowly introduced throughout Europe in the eighteenth century, was estab-

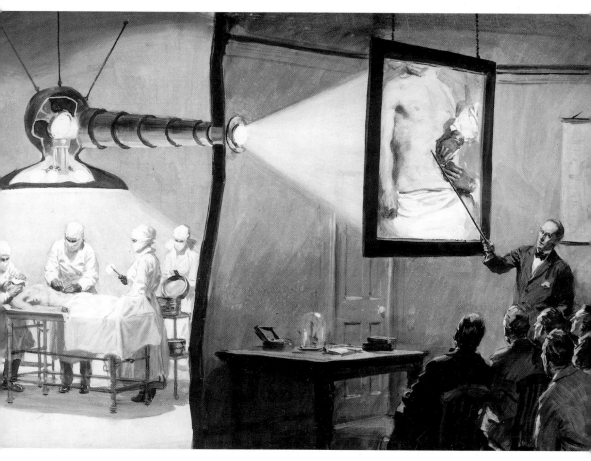

lished by Hermann Boerhaave (1668–1738) in Leiden. He took about a dozen 'interesting cases' from the inmates of the St Caecilia Gasthuis and admitted them to separate 'clinical' wards. Although this model was not a general feature of continental universities, it caught on in cities such as Halle (1717), Edinburgh (1729), Vienna (1753), Freiburg (1768), Würzburg (1769), Pavia (1773), and Göttingen (1780). Thereafter, the term 'clinic' (from the Greek *kline*, meaning a bed) was used for bedside observation combined with teaching, and the small numbers of selected patients suggest that the primary purpose was to impart orthodox knowledge rather than shed light on new scientific perspectives.

It was, however, a model of learning medicine which opened the way for the study of hospital patients by students acting on their own initiative, as happened in the Royal Infirmary at Edinburgh (a hospital with 150–200 beds) after 1741. Students could buy a ticket which allowed them to walk the wards and gave them access to the ward journals—a practice later introduced in the London teaching hospitals. Teaching in midwifery, as practised in most of the eighteenth-century lying-in hospitals, was more practical in so far as students delivered patients, practised obstetrical operations, and used new instruments such as forceps and pelvimeters.

The large metropolitan areas such as London, Paris, and Vienna offered students the chance of practical training based on a wide variety of diseases. Whether teachers and students grasped these opportunities for questioning

Technological development offered early possibilities of combining delicate surgical treatment with teaching, by optical transmission from the operating theatre to a lecture room. Note features of modern surgery such as inhalation anaesthesia, rubber gloves and, to the right, an aseptic instrument-case. The operating table, however, still looks rather domestic. Operating theatres acquired the marble-glass-and-steel look customary today only in the twentieth century.

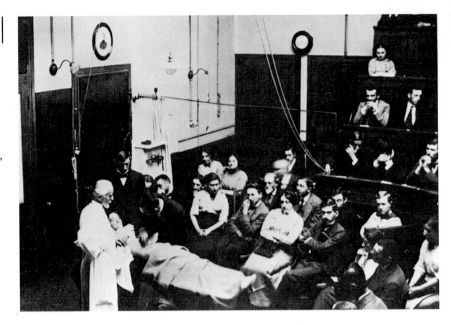

Professor Theodor Kocher,
(1841–1917) the first
surgeon to be awarded a
Nobel prize (1909)
teaching students using a
patient in the University
Hospital, Bern, 1914. A
considerable number of
(foreign) female students
is present, which was
quite common in Swiss
medical faculties of the
period.

existing knowledge depended on their intellectual vigour, and on local political, professional, and cultural factors. In Paris these opportunities were
grasped at the time of the Revolution, and medical education was completely
reorganized on the principles of 'peu lire, beaucoup voir, beaucoup faire' (read
little, see much, do much). Teaching at Parisian hospitals, which reflected
political and ideological changes associated with the Revolution, was essentially practical and focused on common diseases. As such it provided an ideal
basis for the introduction of new methods of physical examination such as percussion (1751) and auscultation (1819).

German professors, however, remained to a certain extent wedded to the
Boerhaavian tradition. While they were quick to grasp new technical methods
of physical examination, in the university clinics the teaching continued to be
centred on classroom demonstrations of rare and interesting cases rather than
bedside instruction. Even when university hospitals in Germany were providing a service function for whole regions, the habit remained of professors
selecting patients for special 'clinical' wards for teaching purposes. Teaching
in Germany was therefore oriented rather more towards research than care.
Furthermore, laboratory training played an increasingly important part in
medical education. But now it was necessary for young doctors to complement
their training by compulsory postgraduate internships, where they worked at
general hospitals without links with the university clinics. These differences
in hospital-based medical education between the French 'school-type' and the
German 'university-type' persisted throughout the nineteenth century and
have, to a certain, if limited extent, persisted until the late twentieth century.

The UK, which had long adhered to the French school-type, integrated elements of the German laboratory education after the Franco-German War of
1870–1. Japanese and US medical education was completely reformed according to the German model around the turn of the twentieth century. In all these
systems, hospitals were seen as indispensable, albeit with varying emphasis.

The lying-in (maternity) hospitals, first established in the eighteenth century, were used for teaching midwives—a process which brought midwives (or at least those who worked in lying-in hospitals) under the control of doctors, who then insisted that they and not the midwives should make use of new instruments such as the obstetric forceps. The same holds true, although with a century of delay, for the training of nurses. The first German and British training schools, of Theodor Fliedner (1800–64) in Kaiserswerth (1836) and Florence Nightingale (1820–1910) in St Thomas's Hospital (1860) respectively, both had hospital attachments. These reforms greatly improved the hospital image and contributed to its acceptance by the middle classes.

Research

In eighteenth-century Britain, partly as a result of the greater number of patients, and partly because of certain administrative requirements imposed by the new hospitals and policlinics, surgeons and physicians, mostly Edinburgh-trained, began to examine new methods of classifying diseases (nosology), and also the evaluation of therapies by simple statistical methods. Numerical methods complemented by autopsy became, by the early nineteenth century, the essence of the clinico-pathological method. This was also elaborated in Parisian hospitals and exported to many other countries. The use of statistics to evaluate therapies was known as 'the numerical method of Louis', after Pierre-Charles-Alexandre Louis (1787–1872), the Parisian founder of medical statistics as opposed to vital statistics (the statistics of mortality). These methods, based on the 'objective' classification of disease entities, led to an increased understanding of clinical and pathological–anatomical problems throughout the Western world.

By contrast, research—and teaching—in the German clinics had hitherto concentrated more on the individual subject. Yet from about 1850, both gained another face through a focus on the application of the methodology of natural sciences, and on technology as described above. The teaching hospitals, because they were so conspicuous, played an indispensable role in creating and propagating the acceptance of this new approach by both the medical profession and the general public. An immense volume of experimental research *in vitro*, on corpses, on animals, and on patients has underpinned modern medicine ever since it was taught, learned, and practised, albeit with national idiosyncrasies, in universities throughout the world.

The growth of aetiologic and technological knowledge has brought with it a continuous development of new methods of diagnosis and treatment. Since the Second World War, however, before a new treatment can be introduced in general practice, it is subjected to testing, usually by a randomized controlled trial, and sometimes to ethical scrutiny by ethical committees. Such concerns have given further impetus to increasing numbers of human experiments, for which hospital patients and facilities are indispensable.

Conclusion

The quantitative and qualitative role of hospitals in shaping both social policy and modern medical practice, teaching, and research, and vice versa, leads to

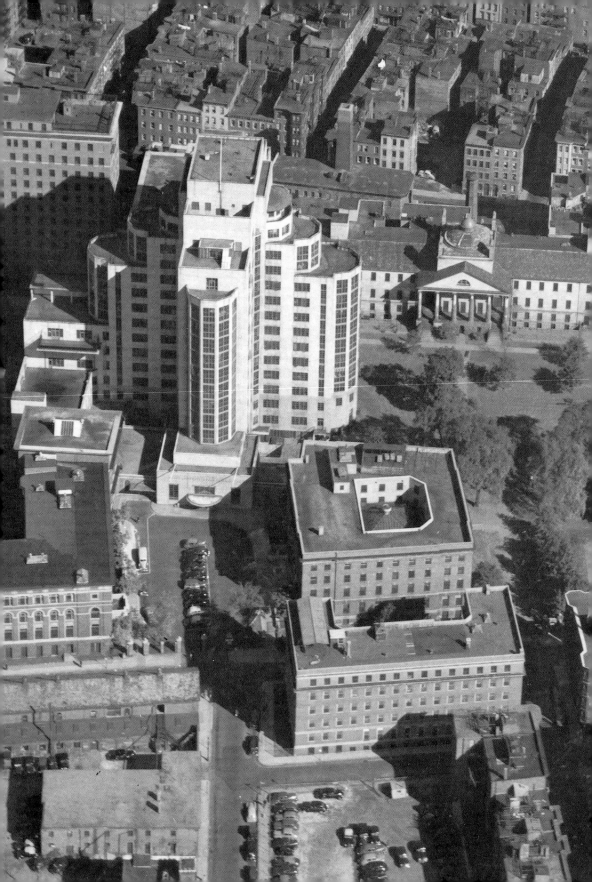

considerations of their significance, on a more general level, for public health and society. The stabilization of overall mortality at a high rate after 1800 and its decline from the last third of the nineteenth century are well-known features of the recent demographic history of developed countries. However, the role of medicine, and therefore also that of hospitals, in these phenomena, and the concomitant epidemiological transition, are still being debated among epidemiologists, historians, and clinicians. There are doubts as to whether hospital treatment has contributed positively to the massive rises in life expectancy. For example, there has been a marked decline in maternal mortality (or 'death in childbirth') in all developed countries since the end of the Second World War. This seems easily attributable to increased antenatal observation and management of birth in hospitals. But, contrary to expectations, comparative evidence, based on critical observation and experimental evaluation, indicates that interventive obstetrics in hospitals has not been the decisive factor in rendering childbirth safer. As a counter-reaction to what some have termed 'over-medicalization' of birth-assistance, new kinds of ambulatory facilities for 'natural' deliveries directed by midwives have become popular.

This example shows that hospital treatment is at the crossroads of competing interests. Today these interests involve medically trained staff, suppliers of technical equipment, hospital administrators, (state) insurers, and, not least, patients. This is why any hospital system can be criticized from one perspective or another. In fact, this has always been the case.

From their beginnings, for instance, innovative hospitals encompassed practice and/or teaching and/or research. In daily practice they stood first for the medical care of the poor sick, then for the medical treatment of ill people, and finally for the medico-technical assistance for almost everybody at birth and death, and at times of disease. Such focusing has not met with universal approval. The hospice movement and the outpatient midwifery institutions, for example, are responses to the preoccupation of today's autonomous lay population with the medicalized management of the three anthropological constants of birth, life crises, and death. In the late twentieth century, routine hospital treatment for acute diseases is not the social issue it was only a few decades previously, nor is it a matter of social control.

For chronic cases, however, such as psychiatric, geriatric, drug/alcohol dependent, and AIDS patients, specific hospitals are objects of social policy and retain custodial functions. These latter functions have always contained elements of constraint and therefore the dangers of abuse and stigmatization of the patients concerned. Admission to a given type of hospital is a question of therapeutic perspective and prognosis, just as it was in the eighteenth century. From this perspective, developments have gone full circle. The overall authority for enforcing innovations rested after the eighteenth century with medically unconcerned lay benefactors and the State, and after the nineteenth century with expert doctors; since the 1970s it has lain with concerned lay groups and the State. These developments, too, have gone full circle. Hospitals thus have been shaped by, and in turn have mirrored, the varying cultural, socio-political, and medical needs, wishes, obligations, and responses of their times and places.

Conclusion

A bird's-eye view of the Massachusetts General Hospital, Boston, in the 1950s which reveals its physical growth and architectural development. Its oldest building, at the back on the right, dates from 1821, in the centre of which is the cupola of the operating theatre, nicknamed 'ether-dome' following the pioneering 1846 operating under inhalation anaesthesia there.

11 | Epidemics and the Geography of Disease

MARY DOBSON

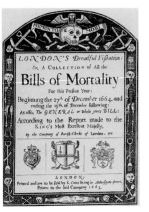

The Great Plague of London, 1665–6, was the last 'dreadful' visitation of plague in Britain. Bills of Mortality were compiled from the early sixteenth century to record the deaths of Londoners and document the impact of plague. A searcher, often an elderly woman, was responsible for identifying the victim and the cause of death. The Bills of Mortality were not always accurate but they provide an important source for historians studying epidemics of the past.

THROUGHOUT human history, successive epidemics and devastating pestilences have punctuated and scarred the populations of the world. Of the four horsemen of the Apocalypse, Pestilence has struck humankind with the severest blows. The Black Death of the mid-fourteenth century, one of the most dramatic episodes of all times, killed in a few years at least one-quarter or one-third of the population of the known world. During the Great Plague of 1665–6, over 100,000 Londoners died, and, at the height of the epidemic, there were as many as 6,000 deaths per week. Between the fourteenth and the eighteenth centuries, some 50 million Europeans are believed to have died as a direct result of plague, as the epidemic periodically tracked its way across the world from east to west.

On the other side of the Atlantic, the impact of epidemic diseases was also, at times, catastrophic. Following European contact with the New World, wave after wave of smallpox, malaria, and other epidemic diseases struck the indigenous peoples of the Caribbean and the Americas, drastically reducing their populations by as much as 90 per cent in some places. The opening-up of the African continent further set in motion not only the shipment of thousands of slaves across the Atlantic but the exchange of millions of lethal microbes over the seas.

Even in the twentieth century, statistics on death, disease, and epidemic mortality make chilling reading. In the aftermath of the First World War, a pandemic of influenza pervaded the entire globe killing in a single sweep some 20 to 30 million people. Fatalities as a result of battle and combat, religious and political wars, pale by comparison with the far-reaching global and historical impact of epidemic diseases like plague, smallpox, malaria, and influenza.

Today, we are faced with a new and escalating global epidemic—AIDS (acquired immune deficiency syndrome). With a projected 40 million infected with the AIDS virus by the year 2000, the current tragedy continues to remind us of the ever-present threat of epidemic disease to humanity.

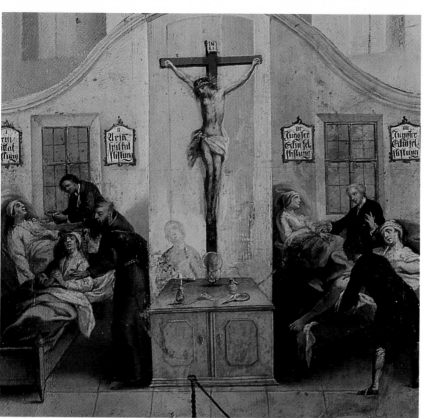

Two hospital scenes in late eighteenth-century Freiburg im Breisgau (Germany). The painting seems to illustrate the characteristic shift of emphasis from the hospice for the sick poor to the hospital for the poor sick. While the inmates of the lefthand side are cared for by lay and religious staff in the hospice tradition (*Armspittalstiftung*), those in the ward on the right, recently opened by a private benefactor, are attended by medical personnel. As in the Freiburg institution for which these scenes were painted, the needs of both groups long continued to be met in modern hospitals.

By the eighteenth century, the well-equipped medical school had a library open to both students and professors, as well as an anatomical theatre, botanical garden, and a room for chemical demonstrations.

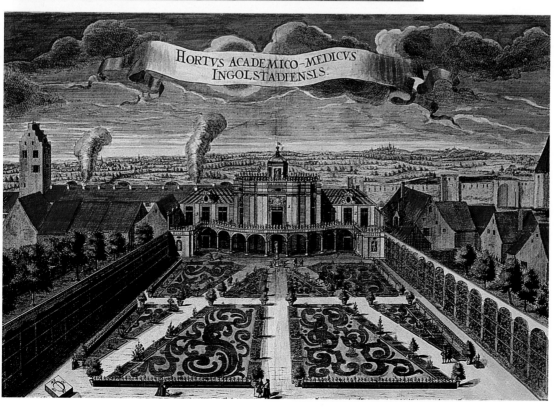

HORTVS ACADEMICO-MEDICVS INGOLSTADIENSIS.

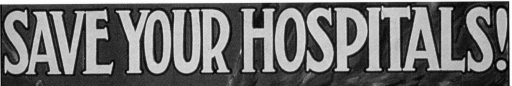

SAVE YOUR HOSPITALS!

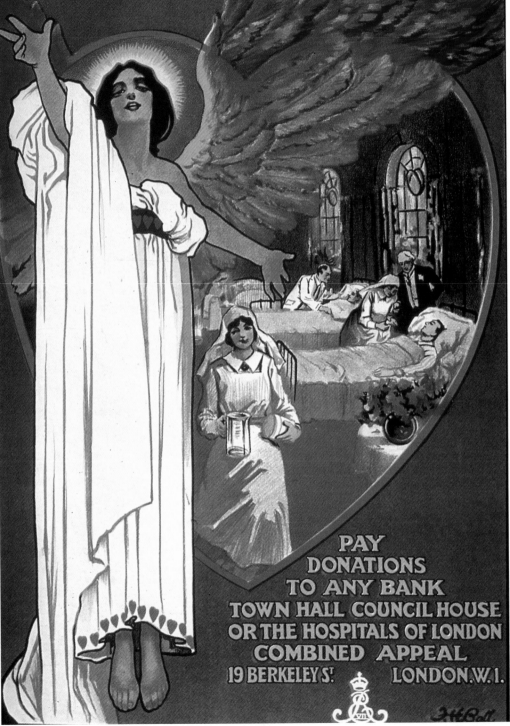

PAY
DONATIONS
TO ANY BANK
TOWN HALL COUNCIL HOUSE
OR THE HOSPITALS OF LONDON
COMBINED APPEAL
19 BERKELEY S⫶.   LONDON. W.1.

The Global Impact of Disease

The influence of epidemic disease on societies, past and present, cannot be underestimated. Countless lives have been lost, civilizations destroyed, nations disrupted, armies defeated, and economic development affected as a direct or indirect consequence of disease. Some historians have argued that malaria was one of the vital forces behind the decline of the classical world. William McNeil in his *Plagues and Peoples* and Alfred Crosby in *The Columbian Exchange: Biological and Cultural Consequences of 1492* have forcefully drawn attention to the holocaust of the American Indians and the extent to which smallpox, measles, and other epidemics contributed to the collapse of the Inca and Aztec civilizations. Military historians have also accorded disease a prime role in the history of global and civil wars. Indeed, until the twentieth century, more people died on the battlefield as a result of disease than as a consequence of war wounds. Typhus plagued Napoleon's catastrophic expedition to Russia in 1812 and an epidemic of typhus accounted for two to three million deaths in the First World War. Economic and social historians have, likewise, reminded us of the devastating effects of epidemic disease on world development and trade. Malaria—that million-murdering death—yellow fever, sleeping sickness, leprosy, river blindness, cholera, and a host of other diseases which have plagued tropical lands unremittingly for centuries, are recognized as prime stumbling blocks in the path to economic progress in many Third World countries.

The forces of history are clearly endlessly complex, and disease is only one factor among many to have affected the tides of change. Some historians have criticized the McNeilian view that plagues and pathogens have changed the course of history and others have recently downplayed the impact of epidemics on the native American populations. But, while recognizing all the

As the nineteenth century progressed, hospitals had to cope with increasing financial burdens. Fund-raising campaigns became quite common in the voluntary sector. Orderly nursing staff, their white coats representing outer—and inner, i.e. moral—cleanliness, often featured prominently.

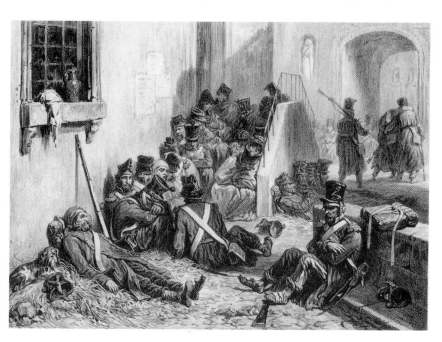

Epidemic typhus is transmitted by the human body louse. In the past, major epidemics of typhus have been associated with wars, famines, and conditions of filth and poverty. Typhus has been variously known as jail fever, ship fever, camp fever, and famine fever. The military connection is illustrated in this nineteenth-century lithograph by E. Leroux, showing soldiers suffering from typhus, lying in the streets.

complexities of historical events and situations, there nevertheless seems no doubt that tiny microbes have, in sometimes quite powerful and subtle ways, made an important impact on the human history of the world.

Behind the grim mortality statistics of pestilence and death, moreover, have always lain the fear, the anguish, the shock, and the panic generated by an epidemic. The very whisper of an epidemic disease has set up all sorts of ramifications—people fleeing in the wake of plague, often carrying with them and spreading further the seeds of contagion; religious groups, Jews, and social outcasts blamed, stigmatized, and punished for bringing pestilence on the world; pesthouses and lazarettos set up to contain the afflicted and banish the infected. During the Black Death, Jews were tortured and murdered in some European cities, accused by their violent attackers of poisoning Christian wells and spreading plague. Flagellants, groups of frenzied men, went from town to town whipping themselves or each other with knotted leather

London 1665: List of diseases and casualties

Plague was the most fatal disease in London in 1665. Bills of Mortality recorded the cause of death of London citizens—the lists contain both familiar and strange diseases and casualties of past times.

Disease or casualty	Deaths	Disease or casualty	Deaths
Plague	68,596	Drowned	50
Ague and Feaver	5,257	Grief	46
Consumption and Tissick	4,808	Kild by several accidents	46
Teeth and Worms	2,614	Overlaid and Starved	45
Convulsion and Mother	2,036	Quinsie	35
Spotted Feaver and Purples	1,929	Rupture	34
Aged	1,545	Palsie	30
Dropsie and Timpany	1,478	Gout and Sciatica	27
Griping in the Guts	1,288	Frighted	23
Chrisomes and Infants	1,258	Executed	21
Surfet	1,251	Found dead in streets, fields, &c.	20
Flox and Smalpox	655	Livergrowne	20
Childbed	625	Bleeding	16
Abortive and Stilborne	617	Plurisie	15
Rickets	557	Headmouldshot & Mouldfallen	14
Rising of the Lights	397	Lethargy	14
Stopping of the Stomack	332	Spleen	14
Impostume	227	Meagrom and Headach	12
Bloudy Flux, Scowring & Flux	185	Bedrid	10
Collick and Winde	134	Murthered, and Shot	9
Appoplex and Suddenly	116	Burnt and Scalded	8
Canker, and Thrush	111	Hangd & made away themselves	7
Jaundies	110	Measles	7
Scurvy	105	Plannet	6
Stone and Strangury	98	Blasted	5
French Pox	86	Distracted	5
Kings Evill	86	Calenture	3
Sores, Ulcers, broken and bruised		Leprosie	2
Limbes	82	Shingles and Swine pox	2
Cold and Cough	68	Poysoned	1
Cancer, Gangrene and Fistula	56	Wenn	1
Vomiting	51		

Source: A. H. Gale, *Epidemic Diseases* (1959), Appendix, p. 151.

and iron spikes to expatiate the sins of humanity. Lepers, from biblical times, have been cast out of communities as unclean and uncleansable. In medieval Western Europe, they were identifiable at a distance by a yellow cross sewn to their cape and a clapper or bell rung to warn people of their presence. A long pole was sometimes carried in order to point to items they wished to purchase, but, in many places, they were denied access to public areas and had to resort to begging or alms.

There have been times in the past when there were not enough able-bodied to care for the sick and the dying, when large numbers of infants have been abandoned and orphaned, and cohorts of young adults have been severely depleted for generations to come. The well-known story of the 1665–6 plague visitation to Eyam, Derbyshire, reminds us of the power of a single epidemic to deplete nearly an entire village. The Rector, William Mompesson, having advised his community to cordon off the village with a circle of stones, quickly had to bury many of his flock. Over 250 inhabitants succumbed to the agonizing torment of the plague in Eyam. As one medical chronicler described it: 'shut up in their narrow valley, the villagers perished helplessly like a stricken flock of sheep.' Social and medical historians are only now beginning to unfold the traumatic experiences of individuals and families whose lives have been shattered by disease—the infinite number of human tragedies embedded between the layers and dramas of global epidemics.

Epidemics and Disease Ecologies in a Changing World

The classic, and often most dreaded, epidemic diseases have been those that have appeared unexpectedly and killed quickly, like plague, yellow fever, smallpox, and cholera. These epidemics have periodically spread from their geographical heartlands to reach distant parts of the world. The term *epidemic* itself derives from the Greek 'upon the people', while *pandemic* is applied to a disease extending across the globe within a limited span of time. The Black Death of 1346 to 1353 and the influenza pandemic of 1918–19 were both widespread in their ravages—the former taking seven years to move along its westerly, northerly, and easterly trajectories, and the latter, for reasons still not fully understood, erupting simultaneously in many parts of the world within a dramatically short space of time. Some diseases have entered new terrain as virgin-soil epidemics, causing havoc on populations with no prior experience of the disease. Following their initial onslaught, such diseases have established themselves on a permanent basis, settling down as endemic diseases or rising up from time to time, within their local setting, in epidemic cycles and waves. Smallpox has existed in a range of epidemic and endemic forms in different parts of the world and across different epochs of time, until its final eradication from the globe in the 1970s.

Different ages and different parts of the world have had their own characteristic diseases and epidemics. Hunter-gatherers and early agricultural societies of the Old World are generally believed to have been free of epidemic diseases, their lives more often shortened by brute violence and physical attacks. Pre-Columbian America and the Caribbean were infested with diverse intestinal and parasitic diseases, and some forms of treponemal infections or syphilis, but the native Indian populations appear to have been isolated from the major epidemics of the Old World.

Ancient South Asia was one of the first regions to develop civilizations of a sufficient population density to support many epidemic diseases. From this cradle of the globe, epidemics like bubonic plague, smallpox, and cholera spread along trade routes to engulf other parts of the world. The Justinian plague, probably bubonic plague, originated in the Himalayas and reached Europe in AD 547. For the next 800 or so years plague smouldered in China but did not reach the Western world. The arrival of the Black Death from the East in the 1340s heralded the beginning of a new epidemiological era, and, for the next five centuries, successive waves of epidemics followed the paths of sailors, traders, armies, merchants, and missionaries from Asia to Europe.

Africa was another ancient locus of a range of diseases, its vast and varied ecological settings giving rise to a complex biological and epidemiological flora. The antiquity of malaria on the African continent is evident from the widespread prevalence of a number of genetic traits refractory to malaria, including sickle-cell anaemia, a genetic trait that protects against falciparum malaria (though sickle-cell anaemia itself can be potentially fatal), and the Duffy negative factor, which appears to give 95 per cent of black Africans and their descendants resistance to vivax malaria. Malaria spread from Africa to the Mediterranean world, and here, too, genetic defences, including a variety of thalassaemia traits, have evolved, carrying forward certain deleterious consequences for future generations in these ancient cradles of disease. The treponemal disease yaws, an infection related to venereal syphilis, also has an ancient history in the African world, as do smallpox, yellow fever, and a host of insect-, water-, food-, and air-borne infections.

The Black Death of the mid-fourteenth century was one of the most dramatic epidemics of all times, killing in a few years perhaps one-quarter or one-third of the population of the known world. The plague moved along a westward trajectory from its ancient heartland in the east.

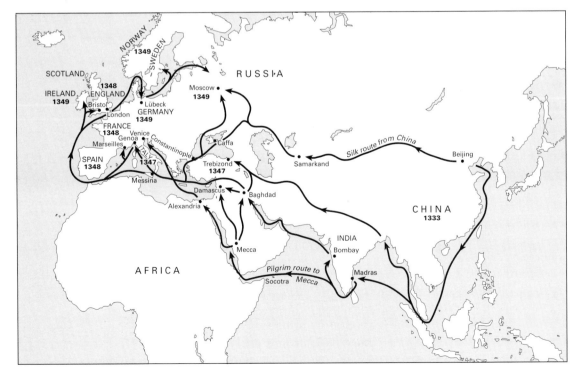

An explosion in the rate and scale of disease exchange began around the six-teenth century with the fusing of the Old and the New Worlds—an epoch that the French historian Emmanuel Le Roy Ladurie has aptly called 'l'unification microbienne du monde'. As Africa entered the biological exchange, it unwit-tingly released its multifarious pathogens to distant horizons. At the same time, its own rich disease pool had a tremendous impact on non-immune Europeans. Soldiers and sailors often died at the rate of 500 to 700 per 1,000 per annum when stationed in the tropics, earning equatorial Africa the label 'White Man's Grave'. The opening-up of the New Worlds—from the Americas and Caribbean to the Pacific lands of Australasia and Hawaii—provided 'new' seedbeds for the ancient epidemics of the Old World. The devastating effects of these epidemics on virgin-soil populations, isolated and without immunity, have been the subject of much research and discussion in historical epidemi-ology. Some historians have suggested that the demise of the native American Indian labour force, following epidemics of smallpox, measles, and other infectious diseases, led to the subsequent acceleration of the African slave

The opening-up of the Americas and the fusing of the Old and New Worlds gave rise to an explosion in the rate and scale of disease exchange. Europeans introduced many diseases to America with severe consequences for native populations. The transfer of slaves from Africa to America added a new element to the Columbian exchange.

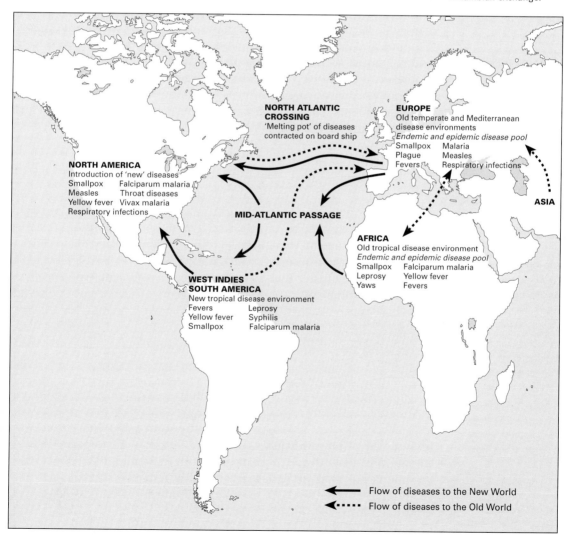

NORTH ATLANTIC CROSSING
'Melting pot' of diseases contracted on board ship

EUROPE
Old temperate and Mediterranean disease environments
Endemic and epidemic disease pool
Smallpox   Malaria
Plague   Measles
Fevers   Respiratory infections

NORTH AMERICA
Introduction of 'new' diseases
Smallpox   Falciparum malaria
Measles   Throat diseases
Yellow fever Vivax malaria
Respiratory infections

ASIA

MID-ATLANTIC PASSAGE

AFRICA
Old tropical disease environment
Endemic and epidemic disease pool
Smallpox   Falciparum malaria
Leprosy   Yellow fever
Yaws   Fevers

WEST INDIES
SOUTH AMERICA
New tropical disease environment
Fevers   Leprosy
Yellow fever Syphilis
Smallpox   Falciparum malaria

Flow of diseases to the New World
Flow of diseases to the Old World

trade to the American colonies, which, in turn, carried forward its own twist of epidemiological fate. Europeans, in the subtropical climates of the southern colonies of America, succumbed all too readily to malaria and yellow fever imported from Africa. The black slaves, on the other hand, seemed immune to both. With slave labour justified for all sorts of reasons, including their ability to withstand these lethal diseases, thousands of African slaves were shipped across the ocean to work on the plantations. The enduring consequences of the Columbian exchange, the rise of large-scale tobacco plantations, as well as the embittered struggles generated by racial tension, are still with us in the late twentieth century.

The mysteries that surround the route taken by syphilis—whether it came from pre-Columbian Indians in America and thence to Europe or whether the Europeans and/or Africans shipped it across the Atlantic—are fascinating questions still unresolved. There seems no doubt that there was a devastating epidemic of syphilis which swept through Europe in the late fifteenth century, when it behaved in many ways as a virgin-soil disease characterized by high fever, rashes, and skin sores and a high fatality rate. The epidemic is said to have begun in France (hence its initial name *morbus gallicus*) and spread rapidly to Spain and Italy and thence to the rest of Europe. No country wanted to be held responsible for such a vile disease, so the French called it the Spanish, or Neapolitan, pox and everyone else the French pox! The author of a famous treatise in 1503 said it was 'so disgusting, so appalling, that until now nothing so horrifying, nothing more terrible or disgusting, has ever been known on this earth'. It was so dreadful that smallpox paled in comparison; hence the disease was the 'great pox' and in contrast variola became the 'smallpox'. It was named syphilis in 1530 by an Italian physician Fracastorius of Verona, who wrote a light-hearted poem, called 'A Poetical History of the French Disease', about a shepherd called Syphilus who cursed the sun during a burning-hot summer and drought. In revenge the Sun-God inflicted the French pox on poor Syphilus. Whether syphilis was, in fact, a totally new disease in fifteenth-century Europe remains a tantalizing question. A number of historians believe that it was present in antiquity in a quiet non-sexual form, possibly as a mild disease spread by direct skin contact and common in children, who thus acquired early immunity. The visitation of acute epidemic syphilis in the 1490s may have been a new virulent strain imported from America. The two worlds, the Old and the New, when isolated, may both have experienced their own treponemal infection, which then came together in the 'unification microbienne' as venereal syphilis, a notorious disease which ravaged large parts of the world for several centuries.

Countless other diseases, less explosive in their eruption, more familiar to their victims, and often more divisive in their social impact, have also gnawed at the fabric of society. Tuberculosis, sometimes called the White Plague, was for hundreds of years endemic within many countries of Europe and Asia. A chronic infectious disease, tuberculosis destroys its victims more slowly than bubonic plague, smallpox, influenza, or cholera. Yet it, too, ranks amongst the greatest killers of the world. In the rapidly urbanizing and industrial centres of nineteenth-century Europe, millions of young children and adults succumbed to this lingering disease. Indeed, it is likely that in some of the poorest

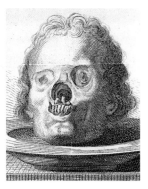

This preserved skull of a woman who died in 1796 from venereal syphilis reminds us of the horrors and disfiguring condition of syphilis, also known as *morbus gallicus* or the French Pox. The geographical origins of this disease and the role of Columbus in transferring it from the New World to the Old World in the 1490s still remain in dispute. Skeletal evidence from all over the world is being examined, using modern techniques, and may throw new light on the historical epidemiology of this notorious disease.

parts of cities like London and Paris and amongst certain occupational groups, such as textile workers, almost everybody developed tuberculosis at some point in their lives, and, even if they died of some other cause, countless numbers suffered from the debilitating consequences of tuberculosis.

The great scourges of the Western world underwent a marked decline in the mid-twentieth century and an age of optimism was reached in the post-Second World War decades. The level of incidence and mortality of many of the world's major contagious diseases was, at last, on the wane. Bubonic plague had seemingly disappeared from Europe. Smallpox, cholera, and malaria were now of minor significance in temperate regions. The death rate from tuberculosis in the UK, Europe, and the USA had fallen sharply. Infant mortality (the number of infant deaths under one year per 1,000 live births), one of the most frequently used measures of the health of a nation, had dropped dramatically from around 150 in mid-nineteenth-century UK to 22 a century later. In many Western countries today, infant mortality is now less than 10 per 1,000. Life expectancy at birth (the number of years lived, on the average, by a given population) correspondingly improved from around forty years in the mid-nineteenth century to over seventy years in the 1970s. The life expectancy of the Japanese now exceeds eighty years. The pace of improvement was considerably slower in the world's poorer countries, but by the 1950s the World Health Organization had already begun to anticipate that many of the most persistent tropical diseases, like malaria, would in due course be eradicated.

Historians are still uncertain of the causes of the changing epidemiological and mortality spectrum. Preventive measures, such as public health, quarantine, sanitation, improved nutrition, infant and maternal welfare, better living conditions, personal hygiene, and changing patterns of behaviour, along with a range of curative therapies and drugs, antibiotics, immunizations, and increasingly sophisticated medical care and technologies, have each, in some way and at different times, played a significant role in the secular decline of mortality. Medical historians, such as Thomas McKeown, have argued force-

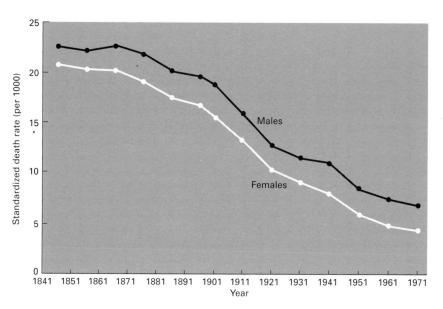

Death-rates in the Western world have fallen substantially since the mid-nineteenth century. The cause of this mortality decline remains a subject of debate amongst historians. It has been argued that immunization, medical therapies, and other scientific advances made little contribution to the mortability decline, except possibly in the case of smallpox and vaccination.

fully that the downward curve of mortality and the declining incidence of many infectious diseases was already in play well before the introduction of miracle drugs and magic bullets, but precisely how and why the great pandemics and epidemics of the Western world receded remains an area of intense historical debate.

At the end of the twentieth century, non-infectious diseases, like cancers and cardiovascular diseases, have soared into prominence on the lists of causes of death. A wide array of chronic and degenerative diseases, some related to problems of ageing, others to environmental toxins, cigarette smoking, and patterns of behaviour, and some to hereditary or genetic conditions, are posing enormous problems for the health services of many countries in the late twentieth century. These are the epidemics of the modern Western world. These, too, are inflicting their toll 'upon the people' of the earth.

Such diseases have not, however, entirely replaced the pestilences and plagues of the past, as we have seen from the recent comeback of tuberculosis in the West, the recurrent epidemics of plague, malaria, meningitis, and cholera in Asia, Africa, South America, and elsewhere, and the increasing number of diseases which are currently proving resistant to drugs and antibiotics. Nor has the present epidemiological era reached a climax in its experience of new epidemic visitations. Mysterious invasions of new strains of disease, mutations of old infections, and the recent introduction of a host of hitherto unknown human diseases, including Lassa fever, Marburg and Ebola viruses, Lyme disease, Legionnaires' disease, and, most significantly, HIV (human immunodeficiency virus), continue to overshadow the world of the late twentieth century. The scale and novelty of the AIDS epidemic, caused by HIV, has, above all, drastically changed our perception of the epidemiological future of our globe. In an age of continuous uncertainty and in an era of vast intercontinental networks across land and air, the recent threat of new diseases and the reminder of past pestilences remain as disturbing as ever.

The Search to Understand and Control Epidemic Disease

Contemporary descriptions of the worst mortalities of past times remind us of the confusion and mystery shrouding each epidemic visitation. Some epidemics of the past were so widespread and so sudden in their impact that they appeared as if from 'a blast of stars' sent from some heavenly influence, as the Italians believed when they coined the word 'influenza'. Others, like leprosy and syphilis, were earthly loathsome diseases associated with filth, human contagion, and moral sin. Plagues were invariably seen as the arrows of divine wrath for the evils of mankind which were spread through the air by way of vapours, stenches, and putrid breath. Malaria was so closely associated with the noxious miasmas of stagnant marshes and coastal swamps that the disease was literally understood to be caused by 'bad air' or *mal'aria*. This miasmic view of disease continued to hold sway into the nineteenth century. The foul water and stinking sewers of European cities were seen by many as an obvious haunt for fever and cholera epidemics. Today, with the sudden appearance of several new epidemics, the stubbornness of many old infections, and the uncertainties surrounding the geographical clustering of diseases such as leukaemia

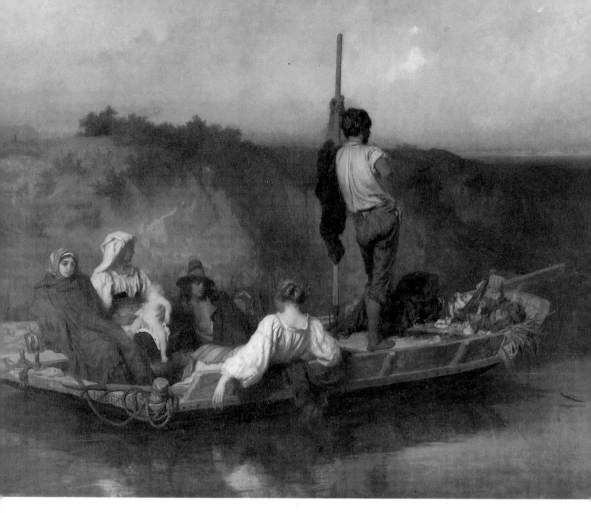

and meningitis, we continue to search for explanations of the epidemiological mysteries of the modern world.

The range of ideas surrounding disease causation has over the centuries, inevitably, led to a plethora of different reactions and measures of control. Prayers, preventives, and preservatives of all kinds have been adopted, tried, and tested during the epidemics of the past. Patients and physicians, public-health authorities, and governments have taken whatever steps have seemed appropriate and necessary to prevent the spread of an epidemic. Citizens and communities have adapted, survived, and fought back in the aftermath of an epidemic.

Flocking to church to pray both for forgiveness and for protection was often an immediate response to the first signs of an epidemic threat. Fumigating the air with strong-smelling essences was an important way of dispelling the poisons of plague and pestilence. Cleaning up the environment, removing rubbish and dung heaps, killing rats and wild dogs, separating the sick and healthy, and burning infected clothing were amongst the many local sanitary measures adopted, with varying degrees of legislation and success over time, to counter the spread of epidemic disease. Imposing *cordons sanitaires* around towns and cities or putting under quarantine for forty days potential carriers

Malaria, a disease transmitted by mosquitoes and still widespread in many tropical areas of the world, was once endemic in temperate latitudes. *La Mal'aria*, by A. Hebert, which hangs in the Musée d'Orsay, Paris, shows a group of people adrift in a boat in the Pontine marshes as a result of malaria. Prior to the late nineteenth century it was assumed that the disease emanated directly from evil-smelling marshes— hence the name 'mal'aria', literally meaning 'bad air'.

Cholera has long been a major disease of the Ganges Delta of India and Bangladesh, whence it has spread to other parts of the world in periodic epidemics. Asiatic cholera first reached western Europe and North America in 1831/2. At the time, its cause was unknown and, as this 1832 satire of a London Board of Health searching the city for cholera suggests, a bad smell was a popular sign of the disease.

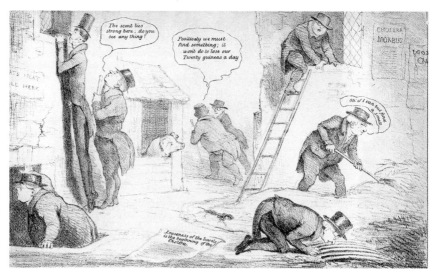

of infection were restrictions that were more strictly enforced in some states, especially in Italy and the Mediterranean in the early modern period, where ideas of contagion and isolation influenced the policies of official public-health boards. Migrating from the countryside to the town to fill the empty spaces left by victims of the plague was an effective way of rebuilding the social, economic, and demographic fabric of a city in the wake of a major epidemic. Preserving native customs and adopting a range of survival strategies have, in turn, demonstrated the resilience of many small groups of survivors whose worlds were once shattered by devastating virgin-soil epidemics.

John Snow drew a mark or bar on the houses where deaths from cholera took place in Soho during a period of eleven days in 1854. He noted that the people who had drunk water from the Broad Street pump fell ill, and when the pump handle was removed the epidemic ceased.

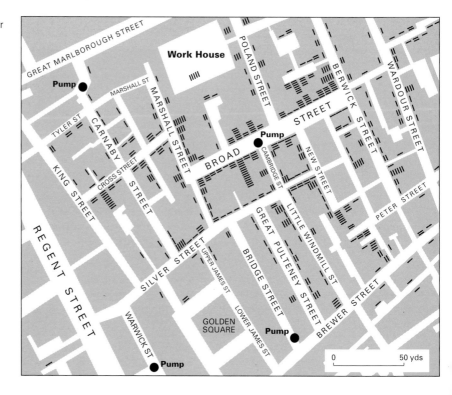

Before the discovery of the germ theory, endless arguments were waged over the role of miasmas or contagion in the origin and aetiology of epidemic disease, and numerous disputes were fought over the relative effectiveness of sanitary measures or isolation controls in preventing successive incursions of epidemic disease. Observation, not of the germs or microbes that transmit disease, but of the paths and chains along which epidemics have appeared to spread, has, at times, led to rational methods of prevention and control. Avoiding the stagnant marshes was seen as one of the best ways of avoiding the marsh fevers or malaria. Cleaning up the polluted watercourses of London was a sensible precaution during the cholera years, and the well-known demonstration of the water-borne nature of cholera by John Snow was conducted three decades before the identification of the cholera microbes in the 1880s. The recognition that smallpox was passed on by human contact and could be prevented by inoculating the pus of one sufferer into the body of a healthy individual was one of the most remarkable feats of empirical medicine. Vaccination using the cowpox (the word vaccination being derived from the Latin for cow, *vacca*) extended this idea in the early nineteenth century and, 180 years after Jenner's famous discovery, vaccination finally enabled the eradication of smallpox in the 1970s.

This outstanding victory in the ancient battle to fight epidemics, however, stands alone. In the late twentieth century, in spite of our impressive scientific understanding of the nature of viruses, parasites, and bacteria that invade the human system, in spite of our intimate knowledge of the genetic make-up of the human body, of the dynamics of DNA, and of the role of cells, antibodies, proteins, and enzymes in the process of human disease, with all the powerful drugs at our disposal and the mass of immunizations ready to eradicate diseases, the great killers—plague, cholera, malaria, sleeping sickness, meningitis, tuberculosis, cancers, and now AIDS—continue to haunt us.

Exploring the Mysteries in the Epidemiological Landscapes of the Past

Epidemic diseases can be as mysterious and as perplexing today as they were in the past. The complex chains and mechanisms that link together the human host, the agents, and the paths of disease—the animal and insect vectors, the human carriers, the invisible pathogens that steal along the watercourses, pass through the bite of an insect, or emanate from the breath of an infectious patient—have been delicately arranged in a fragile balance of equilibrium. Over time that balance has tipped and spilled in many different directions with diverse results; it has varied according to an array of conditions and often poorly understood sets of circumstances; it has manifested itself in a range of ways in different epochs and in different parts of the world.

In order to re-create the epidemiological landscapes of the past and track the routes and pathways of the world's major epidemics, we need to understand these dynamics in an ever-changing natural and human world. The ecological and biological chains of disease transmission—where and how each epidemic is spread; the environmental parameters and constraints—geographical and seasonal variations in the natural and physical world; the demographic vari-

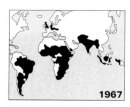

1967

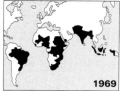

1969

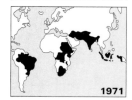

1971

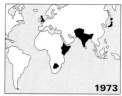

1973

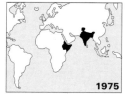

1975

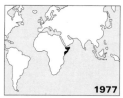

1977

■ Areas affected by smallpox

In 1967 the World Health Organization embarked upon a ten-year global smallpox eradication programme, with mass vaccination and selective control.

187

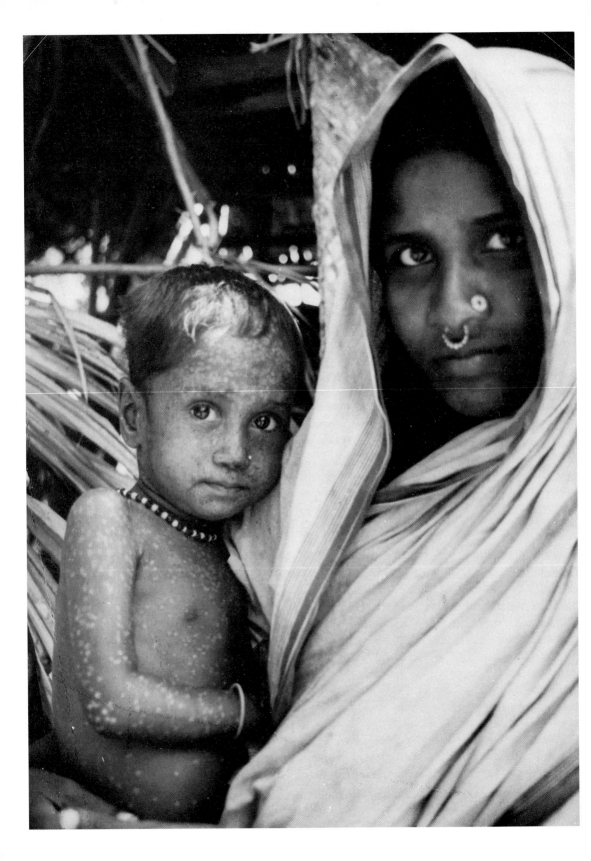

ables—the density and age structure of a population needed to support an epidemic disease, levels of contact and crowding, and the prior immunological experience of a community; the multifactorial social, economic, domestic, and personal factors that enter into the equation—standards of living, the nutritional status of a host population, its level of domestic and public hygiene, patterns of residence, occupation, and migration—have each combined with a multitude of elusive factors, from disease mutations to animal–human disease transfers, to govern and determine the spread of each epidemic disease and its global impact.

The interplay of factors that give rise to an outbreak or epidemic, moreover, varies for every single disease. Even within a single disease complex these can vary over time and space. Bubonic plague, for instance, is a rodent disease transmitted to humans by the bite of an infected flea. Historically the most important rodent is the black rat, *Rattus rattus*, which lives in close proximity to humans. Human plague occurs when the rat population itself experiences a high mortality from an *epizootic* (animal epidemic) of plague. Infected rat fleas, deprived of rat hosts, seek their blood meal from humans and, in so doing, disgorge the plague organism, *Yersinia pestis*, into the human bloodstream and infect a new population. At times in the past, other hosts besides rats have been implicated in the chain of bubonic plague, as happened in San Francisco in the 1960s. Human fleas, as well as rat fleas, may also have been responsible for spreading the plague, perhaps explaining some of the seemingly puzzling geographical manifestations of European plagues in the past.

The Black Death has, furthermore, appeared at various times and places in its pneumonic and septicaemic forms, spreading through airborne particles from person to person—a pathway evoked in the children's nursery rhyme:

> Ring-a-ring o' roses,
> A pocket full of posies,
> Atishoo, atishoo
> We all fall down.

One of the greatest puzzles of our epidemiological past remains the reason for the disappearance of bubonic plague from Britain after 1665–6 (with the exception of one brief outbreak in twentieth-century Suffolk). Traditional ideas, such as the displacing of the black rat by the less friendly brown rat, *Rattus norvegicus*, or the cleansing of the urban environment by the Great Fire of London, have long been dismissed by historians as inadequate explanations. A plethora of alternative hypotheses have been presented in the literature but the sudden shift in Britain's epidemiological cycle of events still retains its place as the mystery of history.

Malaria is another example of a disease with a complex and multi-faceted past. Once believed to be caused by the bad air of the marshes, we now know that this parasitic disease (of which there are four malaria types, *Plasmodium falciparum, P. vivax, P. ovale,* and *P. malariae*) is transmitted from person to person by an anopheline mosquito. There are, nevertheless, several hundred species of *Anopheles*, of which at least sixty are important malaria vectors. Each mosquito species has its own unique set of ecological and environmental requirements: some, like the English malaria vector, *Anopheles atroparvus*, do breed in

The last person in the world to catch smallpox (*variola major*) was a three-year-old Bangladeshi girl called Rahima Banu (*facing*). Rahima survived and in 1979 the World Health Organization declared that smallpox had been eradicated from the globe.

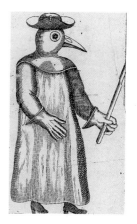

A traditional protective costume worn by physicians attending plague patients. The long beak-like nose piece was filled with aromatic substances to combat the stench associated with plague epidemics as seen in this picture:

In Rome the doctors do appear,
When to their patients they are called,
In places by the plague appalled,
Their hats and cloaks, of fashion new,
Are made of oilcloth, dark of hue,
Their caps with glasses are designed,
Their bills with antidotes all lined,
That foulsome air may do no harm,
Nor cause the doctor man alarm,
The staff in hand must serve to show
Their noble trade where'er they go.

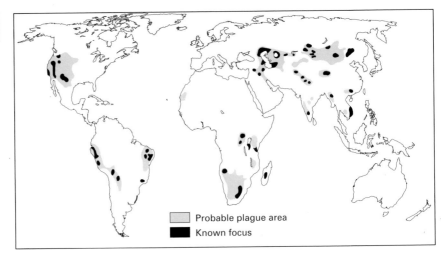

Plague was a notorious
disease of past times. Foci
of plague still exist in
many parts of the world
today, as this map shows.

Probable plague area
Known focus

swampy, stagnant, and foul-smelling waters, but other mosquito species pre-
fer holes in trees, some like freshwater sites, and yet others are found in standing water in paddy fields or in artificial water containers. Malaria transmission
in any one locality depends upon the complex interaction of mosquito vectors,
parasites, and human hosts, which, in turn, is critically affected by physical,
environmental, and socio-economic factors, human biology, demography,
and behaviour. As one malariologist has described it: 'Everything about
malaria is so moulded and altered by local conditions that it becomes a thousand different diseases and epidemiological puzzles. Like chess, it is played
with a few pieces, but is capable of an infinite variety of situations.'

Understanding that infinite variety of situations poses numerous complexities to historians exploring the epidemiological landscapes of malaria in the

The global distribution of
malaria has been very
extensive in the past. In
the 1920s, parts of north-
west Europe and other
temperate areas, including
south-east England and
the Fens, were still subject
to malaria.

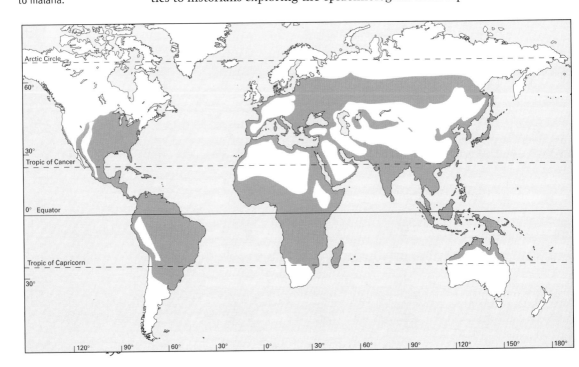

Arctic Circle

60°

30°

Tropic of Cancer

0° Equator

Tropic of Capricorn

30°

| 120° | 90° | 60° | 30° | 0° | 30° | 60° | 90° | 120° | 150° | 180°

past, when the disease extended and manifested itself in a thousand different ways across wide parts of the tropical and temperate world, including the fenny and marshy areas of England. It presents enormous challenges, too, to scientists and sufferers today, who are battling to break the connections between the few pieces of the disease, but are experiencing a host of new problems in many parts of the tropical and subtropical world, where drug resistance, vector resistance to insecticides, and changing mosquito behaviour are creating their own infinite variety of local idiosyncrasies and confounding attempts to eradicate, or even control, this devastating death.

Conclusion

Historians of medicine, epidemiologists, and medical scientists cannot always explain or understand the ebb and flow of epidemic disease in time and space. The questions surrounding the origin and recent epidemic of AIDS in far-reaching parts of the world in the late twentieth century have proved as tantalizing as the sudden disappearance of bubonic plague from the Western world in the late seventeenth and early eighteenth centuries or the persistence of malaria in late twentieth-century Africa, Asia, and South America. The future epidemiological map of the world remains uncertain: mortality rates *should* continue to fall in many parts of the globe; epidemics of infectious diseases *should*, at some point in the future, be within the control of medical science and public health; new cures for epidemics, like AIDS, *should* be found; explanations and interventions for cancers, heart disease, and many genetic conditions *should* be within reach—but, against this background of progress and optimism, we can also anticipate unexpected changes and new scenarios. The mysterious and elusive cycles of epidemic disease will continue to outwit human understanding and control into the twenty-first century and beyond.

12 | Nurses and Ancillaries in the Christian Era

ANNE SUMMERS

THE nurse in the historical context frequently eludes discovery or definition. The term nursing is susceptible to multiple meanings, including suckling and childminding; the nurse's contemporary role is easily confused with that of the doctor or paramedic. Nevertheless, there is widespread understanding of the meaning of nursing care in sickness. At its best it involves attending to all the needs of a permanently or temporarily disabled patient: administering food and drink as well as medicaments; keeping the sick person's body at a comfortable temperature by attention to clothing, bedding, and ventilation. It involves keeping the patient and everything around him or her clean: bodily evacuations must be seen to, laundry taken care of, floors, walls, and furniture scrubbed as necessary. The patient must be treated as the subject as well as the object of the treatment, and helped to keep quiet, calm, and as cheerful as possible. Accurate medical observations, by eye or by instrument, of physical or behavioural reactions to diet and therapy, must be made and reported. The patient must be nursed for as long as the illness continues, regardless of outcome.

This spectrum of tasks, as necessary to the success of scientific diagnostic medicine as to what may be called the self-healing process, has been practised with varying emphases and priorities throughout the period under discussion. While it has frequently been acknowledged that nursing requires the application of learned skills as well as particular qualities of character, and that it is a paid, and latterly professional, occupation, it is nevertheless inseparable from the ideas of service and self-abnegation. It is, therefore, unsurprising that it should have been promoted as a religious exercise; unsurprising, also, that it should have been associated with women. The care of small children, and to a lesser extent the care of other family members in sickness, has traditionally fallen to mothers; selflessness is a conventional attribute of maternity, and subordination associated with the female gender in societies in which males are dominant. This stereotype of the nurse as female has often obscured the important role played by men in religious, military, naval, mental, and private nursing.

For much of the Christian era nursing was a function which could be practised with little or no reference to licensed medical practitioners. As long as medical science was poorly equipped to predict the outcome of disease, the concept of cure could easily be subsumed within that of care. The relative importance of cure and care began to shift in the eighteenth century. Doctors and their historians were swift to bury the record of a period when the possibility of cure was remote and contingent, and they were so successful that many nursing reformers and historians have followed suit and disowned their autonomous history. Since the nineteenth century, nursing has sought respectability and modernity by linking its fortunes firmly with mainstream medicine, and by seeking a secular model for the profession to distance it definitively from its religious, unscientific, and often unremunerated past. So far, this professional model has tended to lead nursing into a position of educational and occupational dependence on doctors—an unstable coexistence marked by shifting and disputed boundaries. The survival or revival in the next century of what is distinctive to nursing may depend upon clinical developments which alter once again the balance between care and cure.

The Religious Model

The Early Christian Era and the Middle Ages

The personal service of the sick and helpless is embedded in a number of precepts dating from the earliest years of the Christian tradition. The seven corporal works of mercy derived from Matthew 25, the parable of the Good Samaritan, the teaching 'inasmuch as you have done it to the least of these, you have done it to me', and the reiterated commandment to 'love thy neighbour as thyself' placed the activity of nursing on a different moral and spiritual plane from the practice of diagnostic medicine as a profession. When Christianity was adopted as the official religion of the Roman Empire, nursing acquired a public dimension. From the fourth century individual and civic acts of piety led to the endowment of hospitals for the sick as well as shelters for the poor, the foundling, and the traveller. Nurses and nursing may date from time immemorial, but it is only with the Christian era that they enter the historical record as a distinct social group.

While in principle the works of mercy were enjoined on all pious individuals, in practice a spiritual division of labour was effected whereby the institutional nursing of the sick poor became the preserve of those gathered in separate religious communities. Some nursing was carried out in the domiciliary sphere: deaconesses of the first-century Church are said to have gone into the homes of the poor to offer care and religious instruction, and this tradition was from time to time revived. Most domiciliary nursing seems, however, to have been undertaken by lay attendants. The care provided by the first hospitals was supposed to be supplemented by that of large monasteries and convents, which constructed infirmaries for their own members and maintained at least hospice accommodation for the neighbouring or vagrant poor. Disparities between infirmaries and hospices were open to criticism, and the establishment of religious orders dedicated exclusively to nursing was an important feature in the life of the Church of the eleventh and twelfth centuries. Communities of *conversi*—lay brothers or sisters under Augustinian rule—were placed in charge of hospitals and hospices throughout Europe; in many cases these foundations were inspired by the example, and adapted the regulations, of the Knights Hospitallers of the order of St John of Jerusalem. In the thirteenth century the nursing vocation was promoted further, particularly by the male order of St Francis and the female Franciscans known as the Poor Clares.

The pattern of unpaid religious and charitable nursing in institutions, alongside paid nursing care in the domestic setting, was a feature of nursing during the whole period before the sixteenth century. Motivations for founding and joining nursing orders and for maintaining hospitals will have waxed and waned with responses to specific crises and challenges such as the spread of leprosy, the needs of soldiers during the Crusades, and sudden increases in the numbers of the poor. What remained constant was the religious model for provision. A permanent body of resident staff, without distracting family ties, with a capacity for living according to discipline, and imbued with *esprit de corps* and a sense of heavenly justification, was hard to better for the task of imposing routine and social order on a mixed population in varying states of debility, and of ministering to their basic and often repellent physical needs. Such a corps could be trained as to when to consult medical practitioners, but could function without their continuous supervision; could employ non-religious workers and co-opt religious voluntary helpers; could manage autonomous institutions, and transfer between sister houses.

Until recently, nursing historiography has equated the religious orders with ignorance, superstition, and hostility to medical progress. This is partly because they have been associated with an indiscriminate mission to care, which might or might not have been conducive to cure. Of their many unhygienic procedures, the practice of cramming more than one patient to a bed was notorious. All the orders, however, set themselves goals of cleanliness, with elaborate procedures laid down for washing and delousing the bodies and heads, and changing, cleaning, and where necessary burning the clothing and bedlinen of their patients. If they were falling short of their goals, they were, nevertheless, often reaching higher sanitary standards than those previously known to the sick poor. Pictorial and other evidence that wealthy patrons of the orders were nursed by the sisters in their own homes suggests that their services were considered the best available. Multi-occupancy of beds arose from unwillingness to turn away anyone in need; we may compare and contrast such measures with decisions in our own day to deny life-saving treatment to certain categories of patient where this is not considered 'cost-effective'. Many orders functioned with minimal recourse to licensed physicians and surgeons; but there was no necessary antithesis between care and cure, spiritual salvation and bodily healing. The influential regulations of the Knights Hospitallers of St John paid great attention to the separation of clinical from surgical cases, and fever patients from those suffering from mental afflictions; religious nursing orders showed themselves able to adapt to new developments in medical perceptions and techniques in fourteenth- and fifteenth-century Florentine hospitals.

The Reformation: change and continuity

In the sixteenth century the hegemony of the Catholic Church in Western Europe was broken by the Reformation. In many countries Protestant regimes dissolved monastic and conventual orders, and with them lost, very often, both infirmaries for the sick and their nursing personnel. Even before these upheavals—and in countries which did not make the ultimate break with Catholic tradition—there had been attempts to impose lay municipal authority on ecclesiastical hospitals whose prosperous incumbents had increasingly delegated their active charitable functions to non-religious staff, or had abandoned them altogether. Moreover, outbreaks of plague from the fifteenth century onwards had compelled municipalities to set up their own machinery for preventing and containing the spread of infection. Measures taken included the payment of lay women nurses to 'search' corpses to identify the cause of death, and to attend the sick in their own homes or in pesthouses. The plague further stimulated the employment of lay nurses in private families, and there were also private initiatives to house and nurse plague victims in return for cash. Despite these apparently secularizing tendencies, however, the religious model was restored wherever the Counter-Reformation triumphed and indeed, as we shall see, entered a dynamic new era.

It is, therefore, only within Protestant societies that a secular model for nursing provision can be looked for, and evidence suggests that it was in England that the abandonment of the religious model was the most wholehearted. The evidence is, however, piecemeal and elusive, often because of the domiciliary character of the work; and also because it has been overlaid with prejudice and hearsay. What the documentary record shows is that the new system of poor relief inaugurated in Britain by Elizabeth I's Poor Law Acts of 1598 and 1601 empowered parish officials to pay nurses and midwives, as well as surgeons and apothecaries, to attend the sick poor. Nursing care was provided mainly in the patient's home; it should not be forgotten that this was a position of trust, exercised within communities whose members were well known to one another; it is unlikely that a nurse would have been allowed across a threshold if that position had ever been abused. In some parishes infirmary wards were constructed, particularly for the elderly, and here, too, patients were nursed without scandal.

Until the early eighteenth century, the Poor Law system seems to have provided adequately for the nursing needs of the poor in Britain. The capital had always had special needs: the dissolution of St Thomas's, St Bartholomew's, and St Mary's Bethlem hospitals after 1536 had been followed in 1538 by a petition of the City of London for their refoundation, which was effected within the decade. Other cities appear to have been less anxious to construct hospital accommodation, perhaps because they suffered lower levels of crowding and distress. In the eighteenth century this picture began to change, both because rapid urban growth prompted demands for innovations in institutional care, and because changes in the discipline of medicine were to alter the educational formation and public status of practitioners. Until this period the independent lay nurse, attendant, 'tender', or 'keeper' was a representative of a valued occupation.

He or she was able at the very least to relieve family members of the strain of watching, and enable them to continue earning their livelihoods, or caring for their children. At a time when much Poor Law medical relief consisted in the supply of extra rations, the careful feeding of a patient was as visibly useful as the prescription and administration of medicines. Moreover, while unlicensed medicine was practised by family teams of wives as well as husbands, daughters as well as sons, it was not automatically assumed that, if a nursing attendant were female, she would also be ignorant and incompetent. She might, indeed, have many specialist skills, in addition to midwifery and a repertoire of herbal remedies; she might be capable of bleeding a patient, applying leeches, or giving rheumatic, arthritic, or otherwise immobile limbs intense 'rubbing' or massage. Medical recollections and hospital records of the late eighteenth and early nineteenth centuries indicate that a number of such women were both engaging in independent practice and working on contract to the new voluntary hospitals in these capacities; it is a plausible assumption that such nurse practitioners had an established 'pre-hospital' history and lineage.

Across the Channel, religious models of nursing continued to flourish. In France, St Vincent de Paul and St Louise de Marillac were responsible for a major new initiative, creating the 'Filles de la Charité' in 1633. Going against the grain of the Counter-Reformation ruling on enclosing all female religious orders, this new order's members engaged in work amongst the poor, did not take perpetual vows, and moved easily between their own and kindred institutions. Their services were speedily requisitioned by older-established nursing houses such as the Hôtels-Dieu of Paris and Angers. They influenced the foundation of similar orders throughout France, and the term 'sister of charity' became synonymous with a respected, and increasingly feminized nursing vocation. A number of older religious nursing orders, despite their formal enclosure, also expanded their sphere of action in this period, opening hospitals in Quebec and Montreal under the sponsorship of female philanthropists, notably Jeanne Mance and the Duchesse d'Aiguillon. Their example was followed in the eighteenth century by Marguerite d'Youville, founder of the Grey Nuns in Montreal.

Studies of the Filles de la Charité in individual hospitals show that they undertook much diagnostic, pharmaceutical, and surgical practice (including venesection), together with the care of the insane and the normal round of housekeeping tasks. Their regulations formally precluded attendance at childbirth, but did not prohibit their presence in, and overall responsibility for, hospitals with labour wards. After a very brief hiatus during the French Revolution, they returned to serve the hospitals of France and its Empire, including many secular foundations, throughout the nineteenth century. Possibly in direct emulation of the successful Catholic systems of their close neighbours, a number of communities in the Protestant states within Germany and the Netherlands established orders of deaconesses to run schools and asylums for the poor, or to make domiciliary visits. Members in no case took vows for life: they sometimes continued to reside in their own homes. Deaconesses were appointed for the city of Amsterdam from 1566, and the Mennonite sect established them throughout Holland from this period

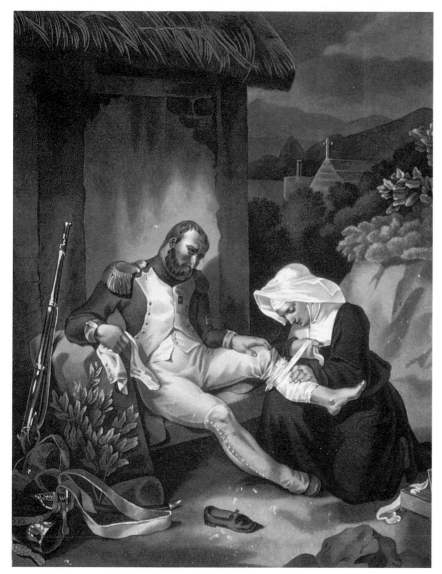

The nursing carried out by female religious orders in France was essential to the functioning of French hospitals. Far from being superstitious and hostile to advances in medical science, it succeeded in surviving the ideological challenges of the French Revolution, and was responsible for important developments in the care of the sick in Canada and other French colonial territories; it was also an important influence on Florence Nightingale and other nursing reformers in the Protestant world.

onwards. The example of the Béguines, a religious order active in the Catholic Netherlands and northern Europe from the twelfth century, who nursed the sick poor in their own homes and were not under perpetual vows, may have been important here. Deaconesses were consecrated by the Hussite Moravian sect from the mid-eighteenth century, and shortly after the Napoleonic Wars this form of organization for social and religious work was being actively promoted within both the French and German Protestant communities.

Modernization and Professionalization: A Secularizing Trend?

The nineteenth-century movement to reform and professionalize nursing (by no means identical ambitions) is usually associated with the rise of hospitals as teaching institutions in France and England from the eighteenth century,

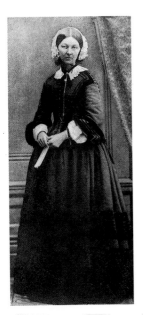

Considered the founder of the modern secular school of nursing, Nightingale was profoundly imbued with the ideas of public health 'sanitarians', and endowed with something close to genius in framing and pushing reforms through the national legislature. Although she was also deeply religious, her character was far removed from the sentimental Victorian imagery of the 'Lady with the Lamp' and the 'angel of mercy'.

and with an increasing clinical focus on diagnosis and more adventurous surgical intervention. It has been assumed that a more scientific approach required the hospital nursing staff to undergo more formal training in order to ensure a greater continuum of treatment. The nurse became as much part of the curing as of the caring process; his or her (but increasingly her) work was more closely linked and more clearly subordinate to that of the doctor, and the religious element in treatment became subsumed within a secular, scientific, and professional model. This by now conventional narrative centres particularly on the person of Florence Nightingale (1820–1910), the outstanding Englishwoman who rose to fame during the Crimean War of 1854–6 and who dedicated her life to the cause of public health and the role of the trained nurse in promoting it. Her own Training School for Nurses was opened at St Thomas's Hospital in London in 1860.

There are many important caveats to be made to this broad interpretation of the modernization of nursing. Over the same historical period the growth of scientific medicine in France was accomplished with the nursing aid of a flourishing religious sector. The first calls for a more systematic approach to the home and hospital nursing of the poor in the UK came from those who had observed the successes of religious organizations on the Continent. In the 1820s, as a result of her work with female prisoners, appeals were made to the Quaker Elizabeth Fry to create an English order of Sisters of Charity. She finally did so in 1840 after a visit to Pastor Theodore Fliedner's Deaconess Institute at Kaiserswerth on the Rhine. (Fry's non-denominational Protestant organization for home, hospital, and mental nursing was later renamed the Institution for Nursing Sisters so as not to offend British anti-Catholic sensibilities.) Her initiative was followed by the formation of a strictly Anglican order, St John's House Training Institution for Nurses, in 1848. This sisterhood took over the nursing of King's College Hospital, London, in 1856, and of Charing Cross Hospital, London, in 1866, and supplied nurses and superintendents to other provincial and metropolitan hospitals; it should be noted that the Nightingale Training School was able to turn out few reliable 'graduates' before 1870.

These and similar movements to replace what seemed a haphazard system of recruiting attendants from the general female working population were informed by a genuine desire to give the sick poor the benefit of the highest levels of nursing expertise. However, though they often found sympathetic professional support, they were most actively promoted by non-medical persons: the impulse behind them was principally social and pastoral. Britain's rapid urbanization had removed many of the poor beyond the effective reach of parish clergy, and breached many of the informal links between social classes. The wish to create goodwill between rich and poor—and the anxiety that no deathbed opportunity for salvation should be neglected—were as strong as any clinical imperatives. Where clinical considerations were at work in giving nursing a higher public profile, they may well have related less to developments in hospitals than to events outside them, most particularly the cholera outbreaks of 1831–2, 1848–9, and 1854. For most patients the only remedies seemed to lie in being nursed: in the maintenance of warmth and hydration, and the prevention of physical rigidity and spiritual terror. Possibly uniquely in the annals of nineteenth-century medicine, one physician wrote of the

1849 outbreak that 'the nurse was then of more use to the patient than the doctor'.

A nursing development apparently more closely related to scientific advances in hospital medicine in this period was the increasing emphasis on hygiene. However, the wish of hospital governors to impress subscribers with shining wards and smartly turned out attendants could have had more to do with the new middle-class vogue for uniformed domestic servants than with any interest in antisepsis. The introduction of new nursing regimes rarely coincided with the recognition and application of Listerian principles; and it should be noted that nurses were not always admitted to the operating theatre, and that medical students or 'dressers' were often assigned to post-operative care. Nightingale herself did not believe in the possibility of contagion by micro-organisms, and her commitment to 'sanitarian' principles in fact placed her in lifelong opposition to the major development in modern medical science.

Now that some of the non-clinical and traditional factors involved in the so-called 'modernization' of nineteenth-century nursing have been considered, it is necessary to stress the distinctive features contributed by Nightingale to the innovations of her period. Her Training School, while requiring evidence of impeccable character and broadly Protestant church membership of its pro-bationers, did not impose any further tokens of religious affiliation. This made it an uncontroversial model for the Protestant non-denominational nursing reformers of the USA and Canada as well as the rest of the British Empire. The model was adapted in parts of Scandinavia and Germany (where two of Queen Victoria's daughters, married into the royal houses of Baden and Prussia, were devoted Nightingale disciples), recommended itself to westernizing elements in Japan, and also to the founders of the international Red Cross movement.

Nightingale's decision to locate a training school within a general hospital, where she was eventually able to enlist the teaching services of its physicians and surgeons, linked the training of nursing firmly to the professionalism of established medical practice: nursing skills were no longer to be acquired piecemeal and 'on the job' according to the occasional needs of employers. Her system was followed in many general hospitals worldwide. Nightingale herself felt ambivalent about professionalization on the medical model—in which a system of examinations led to a qualification which was nationally registered and recognized in law; but it is significant that many of her own disciples pressed for such developments.

Moreover, while Nightingale's overwhelming concentration on the layout, hygiene, and ventilation of the sick ward may have turned much nursing train-ing into a higher branch of domestic service, her insistence that effective nurs-ing depended on the totality of the clinical environment enabled nurses to claim a great share of responsibility for the management of a patient's recov-ery. Despite her vocal deference to doctors and her rejection of the formal model of professionalization, Nightingale's very large claims for nursing's place in the prevention and cure of ill health gave succeeding generations enormous confidence in expanding the social, clinical, and academic aspects of their work. This confidence was nourished by the growth of feminist move-ments, particularly in the UK and the USA. The International Council of Nurses

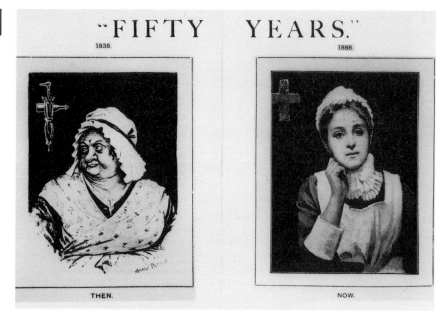

"FIFTY YEARS."

1838   1888

THEN.   NOW.

Sarah Gamp, Dickens's fictional character, was used by the growing nursing profession of the nineteenth century to blacken the reputation of the working nurse who had provided a service in home and hospital without benefit of 'modern' training.

was founded in London in 1899 as an offshoot of the International Women's Congress first held in Washington in 1881. Most of the leading figures in the campaign for the professional registration of nurses were also suffragists. Nurses in New Zealand, where women were enfranchised in 1893, achieved the goal of registration in 1901; registration came for nurses in most US states between 1903 and 1915, and the female suffrage in 1920; in the UK registration was granted in 1919, and the female suffrage in 1918 and 1928.

Nursing and the State

While Nightingale was adamant that the laws of hygiene were the laws of God, hers was, nevertheless, a more secular vision of the role of the nurse than that embodied by sisterhoods and deaconesses; and by situating nursing prominently within the broader context of public health she commended the Nightingale model to governments and social reformers engaged in the negative struggle to contain the spread of infection in cities and the positive battle to foster the growth of a healthy population. From the outset, her career was associated with the health of soldiers in peace and war, and her concerns coincided with those of civilian and military leaders on at least three points: the need to reduce the mortality among soldiers from secondary infections contracted away from the battlefield; the fear that urban living was weakening the physique of future generations of military recruits; and the need to train a reserve of ambulance and nursing personnel for wartime emergencies. Nightingale's sanitary preoccupations and campaigns to improve the status of the Army Medical Service played a key role in the first area. She contributed indirectly to the development of mother-and-infant welfare schemes to prevent national 'physical deterioration' through providing trained nurses for clinics and home-visiting schemes. And, although she did not design a blueprint for national ambulance reserves, Henri Dunant, promoter of the Geneva Convention, was inspired in 1859 to found the Red Cross movement and claimed Nightingale's Crimean work as his inspiration.

The second half of the nineteenth century was an era of European and American wars involving larger and larger numbers of troops and a corresponding increase in casualties. All nations, whether belligerents or observers, realized that these large-scale engagements drew heavily on the resources, both moral and material, of the entire citizenry. The needs of governments and the desires of soldiers' families converged with the formation of voluntary medical, nursing, and sanitary corps: these required training in a purely military discipline. It is sometimes forgotten that the Red Cross, so widely associated in our own day with international humanitarian relief, had its nineteenth-century origins in the need for national armies to coordinate the work of their own volunteers in caring for their own sick and wounded. In many countries which had only a meagre secular nursing tradition in this period, it was the Red Cross which provided training for many men and women in both military and domestic nursing skills, and which planned and funded the staff and equipment needed at the various staging posts of a wounded soldier's journey from front to rear of battle. The example of Japan's well-drilled Red Cross volunteers in the Russo-Japanese war of 1904–5 strongly influenced the formation of the UK Voluntary Aid Detachment scheme in 1909, through which the Red Cross and the Order of St John recruited and trained many thousands of the Empire's First World War nursing volunteers.

War has given nursing its principal public aspect other than the Christian religious vocation. At the beginning of the twentieth century, those nurses struggling for professional registration insisted that the demands of war service required national standards and a national register, and their war service certainly contributed to securing this goal. However, women's war nursing has been exploited by authority in ways unrelated to their professionalism. Although stretcher-bearers and field hospital staff remained predominantly male through both world wars, it was the female nurse whose image was blazoned on propaganda in every medium: she represented an idealized version of motherhood, the prime civilian value, transposed to the military bedside; she also represented the pretty young womanhood which was the sexual reward for the demonstration of the ultimate masculine virtues. For the nurses who wished to carry their part of the patriotic burden, and to be taken seriously as medical professionals, these images were, and still are, unhelpful.

Despite these stereotypes, there is no doubt that, especially where the middle classes were concerned, military nursing in the age of total war

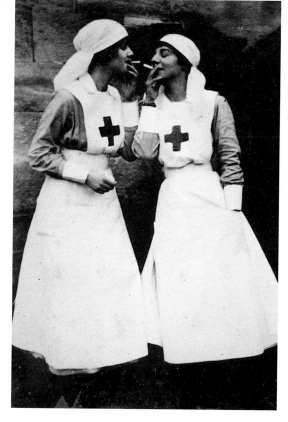

For many girls, war nursing offered an opportunity for freedom and excitement as well as caring for the sick and wounded.

The nurse is depicted as androgynous and as a soldier. Technology has modified the structuring of emotional, sentimental, and gendered roles in the hospital.

broke down many of the social barriers between young men and women; and, despite the cross worn on so many uniforms, for the first time it placed the nursing profession outside the context of either other-worldly self-denial or the social subordination involved in domestic service. This opened up the possibility of putting the secular ideals of meritocracy and gender equality into practice. The combat fatigues of the US nurses serving in the Korean and Vietnam wars are, perhaps, the visible emblem and final demonstration that military service, in fact if not always in fancy, has emancipated the female nurse from the persona of nun, maid, or mother so pervasive elsewhere; and has perhaps also presaged the entry of women into both the combat and medical wings of the armed services on equal terms with men.

The status of the nurse associated with the purely civilian state is less clear than her role in a society at war. There is normally more political consensus surrounding military objectives than there is concerning public-health policy in modern nation states. Public-health employment has in many ways enhanced the prestige of nurses: the district or visiting or school nurse has been accepted as an independent practitioner with educational functions and legal powers. This status is, however, insecure. Public-health budgets are always contested; the function of the nurse as instructor in parenthood, regulator of infant and school-age development, and sometimes dispenser of welfare benefits is seen in some ideological perspectives to threaten the independence and liberty of the individual citizen. All state health measures, from vaccination onwards, have aroused controversy, and nurses as well as doctors have been tainted by connection with extreme practices such as those associated with racist and eugenicist theories. It may be in the so-called developing countries, where the average level of access to medical resources is extremely low, that the public-health nurse will be most valued in the twenty-first century.

The Academic Model: An Uncertain Future

The logical extension of the movement to professional registration was to follow the medical model, and to make nursing an academic discipline taught within higher education as well as learned through practical experience. The pioneers of this development were the nurses of the USA and Canada. The first university-based hospital training school for nurses was established at Johns Hopkins, where Isabel Adams Hampton Robb was the first Superintendent in 1890. The school had its first Professor of Nursing in 1907. This example was not followed outside North America until well into the post-Second World War period, possibly reflecting other societies' lesser commitment to the goal of mass higher education. From the late 1920s US nurses were, indeed, proceeding to the next logical step of promoting nursing as a research-based discipline generating doctoral degrees and scholarly journals.

Nurses can very properly argue that many developments in modern medicine, particularly in acute conditions and intensive care, have increased the scientific and technological content of their work and training. The modern nurse measures blood pressure, administers oxygen, injects medicines, and cares for patients undergoing open-heart surgery, laser surgery, cardiac

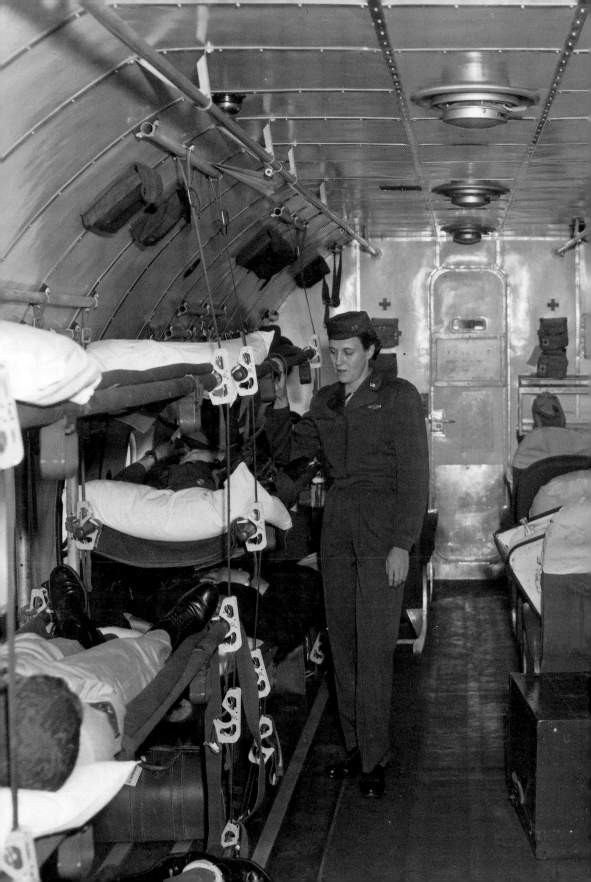

catheterization, or renal dialysis. Frequent changes in technology, constant additions to the pharmacopoeia, and extensions to the range of monitoring devices have to be mastered. A succession of official commissions and academic analyses of the 'nursing process' have broken down the practice of care into components requiring varying degrees of intellectual rigour and preparation, and different titles have been attached to different roles. Historically, institutional—but not domiciliary—nursing has usually been a graded occupation. A woman of greater experience, or higher social class, or both, supervised a number of nurses and domestics in a ward; with the advent of formal training schools, tasks requiring lesser skills and experience were performed by probationers. Professional bodies have been anxious to distance nursing from its less academic functions; the drive to replace an apprenticeship model of training with university-based nursing education is linked with the attempt to strip ancillary and less qualified staff of any claim to the title of nurse, and to create clinical specialists and consultants at the top of nursing's own hierarchies.

There are many stubborn obstacles in the way of this development, such as have indeed hampered professionalizers at every stage. In the first place, there

A British 'district nurse' visits an elderly patient. Modern domiciliary nursing, with its absence of 'high-tech' procedures, and resemblance to social work, often carries less professional prestige than institutional practice; at the same time it offers the potential for a high degree of nursing autonomy. The term 'district' derives from the nineteenth century Church of England tradition of dividing parishes into 'districts' for pastoral and charitable home visiting.

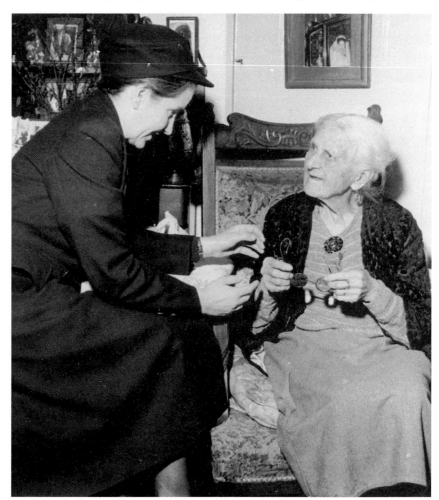

is the distrust or at least apprehension of medical practitioners that nurses will exchange subordinate for rival roles. In the second place, there are employers' objections on grounds of cost: higher qualifications mean higher salaries. A third factor is the growth of management as a profession with almost autonomous concerns, invested with increasing power in hospital and health-care systems, and conceding progressively less influence over staffing issues to medical and nursing personnel. Underlying, and in addition to, all these undermining forces is the factor of gender. In societies where the male sex is still dominant, nursing's overwhelming association with a female labour force drastically reduces its political and economic leverage.

Proponents of the academic model feel that the personal-service elements of the 'nursing process' militate against its being given equal weight with other forms of medical practice. And yet common-sense definitions of nursing care are likely to resist hijacking. The patient may be able to come to terms with computer diagnosis of symptoms, with remote consultation of a physician, even with remotely controlled surgical operations. But he or she will not easily come to terms with a remote care programme, or one broken down into a multitude of tasks performed by a bewildering variety of individuals. We are certainly living in an age of mental stress; the populations of the West are ageing; we may well be entering an era of increasing vulnerability to incurable or chronic diseases. The technology of modern hospitals may become irrelevant to most of these conditions. Though the market value of their labour may remain shamefully and counter-productively low, good cancer, psychiatric, or geriatric nurses, male or female, who are able to relate to every aspect of a patient's experience, are irreplaceable. The academic model of nursing may be thwarted for many negative and ignoble reasons; but in the home or the hospice the personal-service model, wholly compatible with a high level of nursing education, is likely to be the one most sorely needed.

13 | Childbirth

IRVINE LOUDON

To a historian of childbirth, the illustration of the grandmother, mother, and newborn baby of a sharecropper's family in the Mississippi Delta in 1937 raises a series of questions. Where was the baby delivered? Who was the birth attendant? What kind of maternal care was available to such a family and how did it compare with maternal care in other parts of the world and other periods? From what is known of the history of childbirth in the USA, the baby was probably delivered at home, either by a midwife or general practitioner, or possibly a neighbour, and the risk of such a mother dying in childbirth was about twice as high in Mississippi as it was in New England, and about three times as high as it was in Scandinavia in the 1930s. This illustration serves as an introduction to this chapter, which will be concerned as much with systems of maternal care in various countries as the traditional landmarks and great names in the history of obstetrics.

Childbirth before Man-Midwifery

Today, when most Western women are delivered in hospital maternity departments, it is not always appreciated that in historical terms childbirth is a recent addition to the medical curriculum. Until the late seventeenth century on the Continent and the early eighteenth in Britain, childbirth was not so much a medical as a social occasion, like weddings and funerals. At births, deaths, and marriages there was usually an 'official' or 'expert' (priest, undertaker, midwife), but the event centred around the immediate community of family and friends. Childbirth, however, differed in one important respect. It was exclusively female. The mother chose a midwife and a group of friends (the 'gossips') to attend her delivery. Men were rigorously excluded, unless some complication arose which left no alternative but to call in a surgeon to use the crude instruments available at the time to deal with an obstructed labour. It follows that before the eighteenth century medical practitioners knew very little about the nature or management of normal and abnormal labour. Only a handful of men such as François Mauriceau (1637–1709) in Paris and Hendrik van Deventer (1651–1724) in Holland had made a special study of childbirth and its complications and could therefore be thought of as the obstetricians of

Grandmother, mother, and newborn baby of a sharecropper. A memorable photograph raising the questions: Who delivered the baby? Where was it delivered, at home or in hospital? What maternity facilities were available for the poor in the Mississippi Delta in 1937?

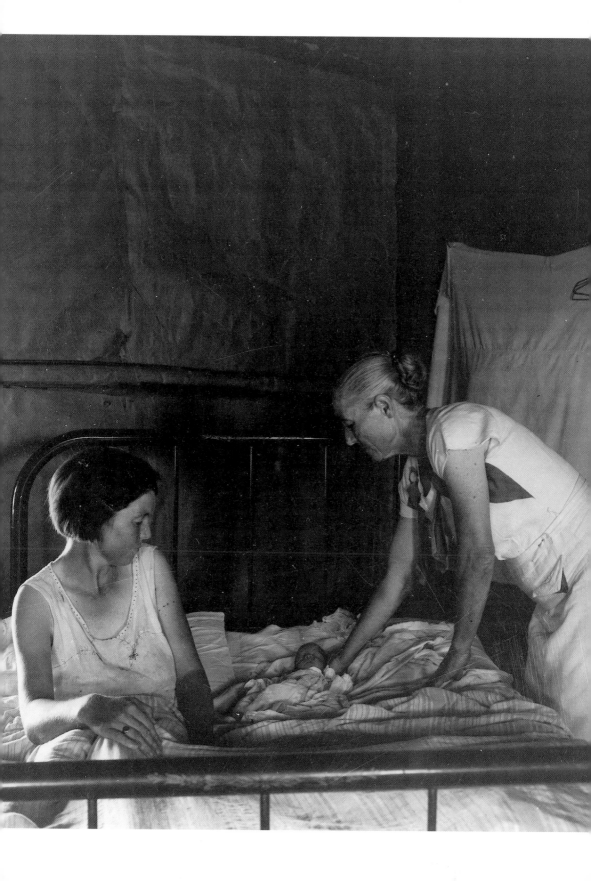

A detail from Brueghel's *Triumph of Death* (c.1562). The Black Death of 1347, which killed between a quarter and a third of the population of Europe, was seen at the time as a manifestation of the powers of evil and darkness.

their day. But only a tiny and negligible proportion of women were attended in labour by a doctor.

In short, midwifery was in the hands of women, and until recently we knew very little about the history of midwives. Everyone has heard of Sarah Gamp, and it is sometimes imagined that, if she was typical of the nineteenth century, midwives in earlier periods were probably worse. While there is no doubt that there were always ignorant and illiterate midwives, the more we learn about early midwives the more impressive they seem. By the mid-fifteenth century municipal councils in Germany were overseeing and licensing midwives. In seventeenth-century Holland it is clear that the midwife was recognized as an important and respected member of the community on whom the welfare of mothers and babies and the future of the population of a prosperous country depended. By 1656 the surgeons' guild and the town council in Delft were responsible for ensuring that midwives were educated women and members of a respectable craft or profession, and by the eighteenth century Dutch midwives who applied for a licence had to be women of good name and reputation, legally married or a widow, with children of their own. Moreover, they had to be strong and healthy, able to read and write, and they served a long apprenticeship. That should not surprise us if we look at the portraits of rich seventeenth-century Dutch burghers and their families, with their clothes, furniture, and immaculate houses. Would they have entrusted their wives and children to Sarah Gamps? Of course not.

And so it was in most of Europe, especially in Sweden and Germany, where

This Dutch woodcut which shows a series of events surrounding childbirth in the sixteenth century, illustrates the fact that childbirth was a social rather than a medical occasion: not only childbirth but the upbringing of children were affairs conducted by women. Left centre, a woman is being delivered by a midwife; right centre, she is lying-in after childbirth; and in the foreground there are children playing and coming to the table for food.

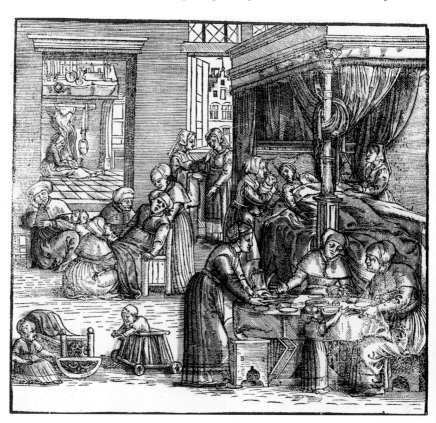

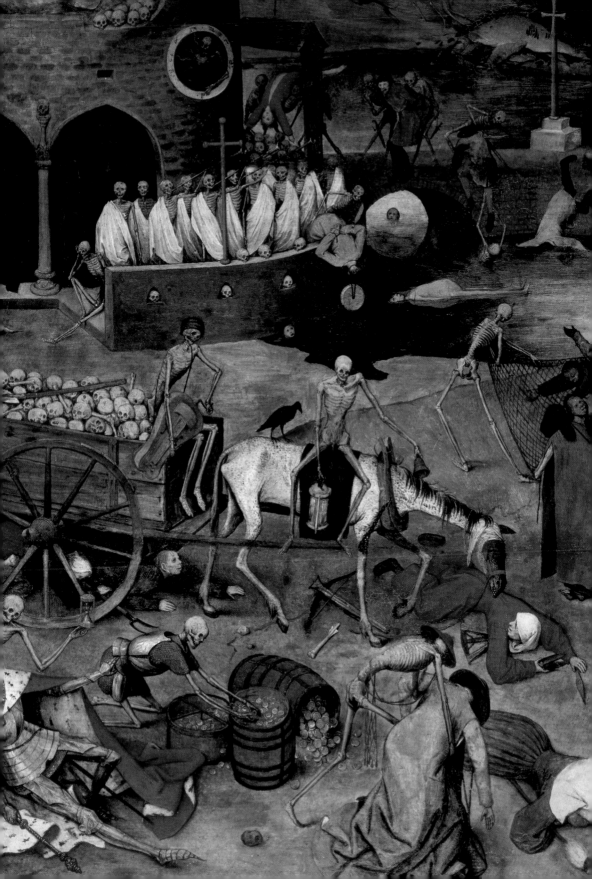

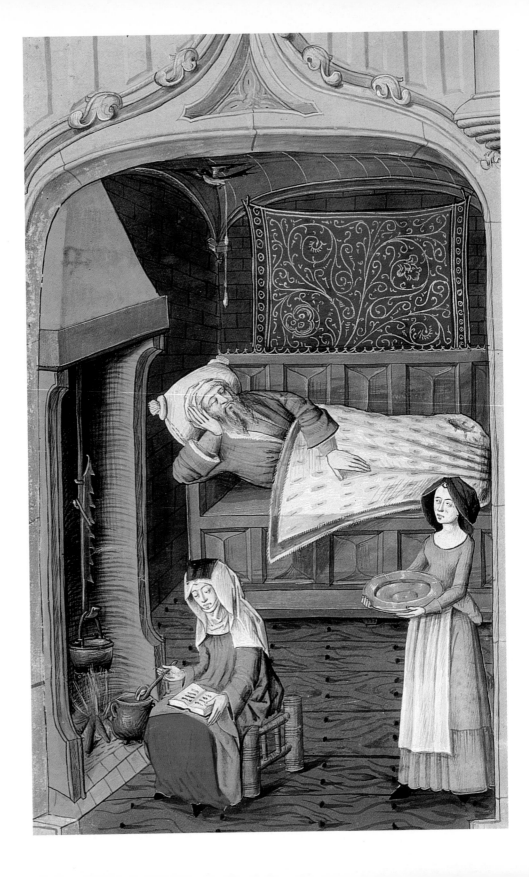

the regulation of midwives by the State probably began earlier than anywhere else. From France we have the memorable story of the midwife Mme du Coudray, a woman of impressive charisma, talent, and literacy with a profound knowledge of the management of childbirth. During the second half of the eighteenth century, King Louis XV, fearing that the population was shrinking, placed the future of midwifery in France in her hands. Armed with a royal warrant, a model of the female pelvis and infant (her own invention), and a remarkable *entourage* of assistants and servants, she toured almost the whole of France teaching hundreds of students in each region of the country.

Compared with the Continent, England was backward. In most continental countries it was the State or municipalities who were responsible for midwives, and later the same bodies were also responsible for establishing and maintaining lying-in (maternity) hospitals. In England, however, apart from occasional licensing of midwives by bishops (a process in no way comparable to what happened on the Continent), it was not until 1902 that the first Midwives' Act was introduced to regulate the training and practice of midwives. Likewise, in contrast with the Continent, lying-in hospitals in England were 'voluntary hospitals', dependent on charitable contributions. Although recent research has shown that eighteenth-century midwives in England were much more literate and capable than had been generally supposed, continental midwives played a much larger part in the provision of maternal care than the midwives of England before the twentieth century.

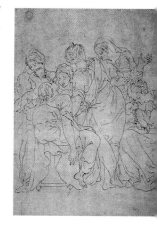

Before the eighteenth century women were delivered by women in the presence of women with never a man in sight, least of all a doctor.

The Rise of Obstetrics and the Obstetrician

At the beginning of the eighteenth century, the employment of medical men in the conduct of normal as well as abnormal labours was rare. By the end of the century, however, many women of all social classes engaged a medical practitioner rather than a midwife to attend them in their labours and virtually all the surgeon-apothecaries (the predecessors of the general practitioner) were also 'men-midwives' or 'accoucheurs'. Naturally, this development was deeply resented by the midwives. Sarah Stone, an experienced and literate midwife of firm views, tells us in her book *A Complete Practice of Midwifery* (1737) that when she began practice in Somerset, men-midwives were unknown. But when she moved to Bristol in 1730 she found that 'every young MAN who hath served his apprenticeship to a Barber-Surgeon, immediately sets up for a man-midwife, although as ignorant, or indeed much ignoranter than the meanest women of the Profession'.

At a rough guess, by the 1790s something between a third and a half of all deliveries in England were attended by medical practitioners. This change in the pattern of maternal care was only one aspect of the astonishing rate at which midwifery/obstetrics in the modern sense was created. Between about 1730 and the end of the century, the essentials of the anatomy, physiology, and pathology of parturition as we know them today had been established. The management of the three stages of normal labour, especially the dangerous third stage, was described so clearly by Thomas Denman in his treatise *An Essay on Natural Labours* (1786) that, with a few minor alterations, it could serve as a text for students today. Before the eighteenth century so little was known of

A skilled woman under religious discipline ministers to a male patient without the supervision of a male physician. There is no clear distinction visible between her responsibilities and those of the physician or apothecary.

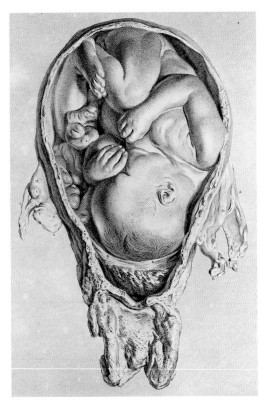

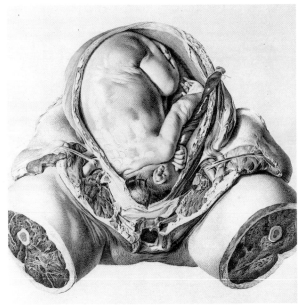

The pathology of the condition known as *placenta praevia* (*above*). The placenta lies across the mouth of the uterus preventing the birth of the baby until the placenta has come away, usually with profuse bleeding. Hunter noted that in this case haemorrhage caused the death of the mother.

From William Hunter's huge and magnificent *Anatomy of the Gravid Uterus* (*above right*), this is one of the early accurate illustrations of the lie of the normal full-term baby in the uterus.

the lie of the baby in the womb that William Hunter's famous illustrations of the gravid uterus represented new knowledge. Malpresentations and most other causes of obstetric complications were also described in detail. Puerperal fever, which we come to later, was recognized for the first time. From about 1740, lying-in (maternity) hospitals were established in Britain and on the Continent, as well as outpatient maternity charities from which midwives trained by the charity sallied out to deliver the poor in their own homes, knowing they could call on the charity's accoucheurs to deal with complications. This explosion of knowledge and new forms of maternal care in the latter two-thirds of the eighteenth century was accompanied by a flood of treatises and papers, with Paris as the centre of publications on midwifery before 1750, and London and Edinburgh afterwards.

In England almost all of this activity was due to a surprisingly small number of London accoucheurs such as William Smellie (1697–1763), William Hunter (1718–83), Thomas Denman (1733–1815), and William Osborn (1763–1808), all of whom held appointments at lying-in hospitals, taught large numbers of pupils, and were prolific authors. In Britain, the élite accoucheurs were to be found in Dublin, Edinburgh, Glasgow, and most of all London. Young apprentices and surgeon-apothecaries, eager for instruction in this new subject, flocked to these cities, just as their contemporaries on the Continent flocked to Paris, Amsterdam, Copenhagen, Berlin, and Vienna.

Why did man-midwifery/obstetrics appear so suddenly in this period? Historians have sometimes suggested it was due to the publication of the design of the obstetric forceps (a secret which had been held by the Chamberlen family for nearly a century); but there are strong reasons for believing that this was not the case. It was probably a combination of two factors: first, a new spirit of medical enquiry, especially in the fields of anatomy and physiology; secondly, the sudden rise of the surgeon-apothecary as the family doctor—the practitioner who, from now on, was trusted to deliver your babies, attend your children's complaints, treat your fevers and indigestion, set your fractures, dress your wounds and ulcers, and draw your teeth. One thing is sure: the rapid adoption by the surgeon-apothecary of the role of man-midwife could have taken place only if it was actively sought by women and their husbands.

Indeed, midwifery came to play a central role in general medical practice, for it became an article of faith that delivering babies created a bond between the patient and the family doctor. Although midwifery was the key to family practice, it had its disadvantages. It was not a well-paid aspect of general practice, and a maternal death could destroy a practitioner's reputation more rapidly than anything else. As the Bristol surgeon Richard Smith junior (1772–1843) commented, the surgeon-apothecary as man-midwife 'cannot be compensated at all by the mere lying-in fee, unless it leads to other business. I know of no surgeon who would not willingly have given up attending midwifery cases provided he could retain the family in other respects—but that is unprofitable as every accoucheur knows . . . midwifery destroys those who practise it.' 'Destroys' may be an exaggeration, but many found it exhausting. Matthew Flinders (1755–1802), a surgeon-apothecary in Lincolnshire, attended forty-three deliveries in 1775 and on one occasion complained he had 'not been in bed or my boots off for forty hours'. All through the long first stages of labour he sat at the bedside fretting at the thought of lost fees from his other patients who could not get hold of him. But he fretted even more at the prospect of losing a midwifery case to a midwife, or worse still, to another practitioner. Likewise, in 1892 a general practitioner wrote: 'I have no hesitation in saying . . . that midwifery is the most anxious and trying of all medical work, and to be successfully practised calls for more skill, care and presence of mind on the part of a medical man than any other branch of medicine.' Midwifery may have been the linchpin of general practice, but it was often the most wearying and worrying part of the job.

Who Delivered the Babies?

Let us start with England. The élite obstetricians who held appointments at maternity hospitals and private practices amongst the well-to-do were almost entirely confined to London; and even there they were greatly outnumbered by consultant physicians and surgeons. As late as the end of the nineteenth century, an observer who travelled from London to Penzance, passing circuitously through Reading, Portsmouth, Winchester, Oxford, Bath, Bristol, Exeter, and Plymouth, would have been hard put to it to find a single practitioner who was in any sense a consultant obstetrician. But he would have found hundreds of midwives and general practitioners busily delivering babies. What, then, was the role of the lying-in hospitals? There were two kinds: the prestigious voluntary lying-in hospitals and maternity departments in general hospitals, first established in the eighteenth century, and the workhouse hospitals dating from the mid-nineteenth. There were also many outpatient lying-in charities. Altogether these lying-in institutions—which catered only for the poor and never for the middle classes—accounted for a very small proportion of total births in a few cities in England. In Scotland the proportion was even smaller. Even at the end of the nineteenth century in the UK, over 90 per cent of deliveries were home deliveries by midwives and general practitioners. This can be seen in Figure 13.1, which is a reminder of the extraordinary extent of change in maternal care over the last century.

The major lying-in hospitals were both symbols of charitable care and centres for teaching. In the UK the teaching of midwifery in the nineteenth and twentieth centuries was often disgraceful, although (and this was often remarked by obstetricians at the time) general practitioners could save more lives by skill in midwifery than in any other branch of medicine. The trouble was that midwifery was regarded as the Cinderella of the medical curriculum, despised by physicians as an unsuitable occupation for gentlemen with a university education, and spurned by the surgeons precisely because midwifery

The Dublin Lying-In Hospital or 'Rotunda'—so called because of the circular building which was added some years after it was established—was by far the largest in the British Isles and was famous for its teaching. It suffered a horrific level of deaths from puerperal fever.

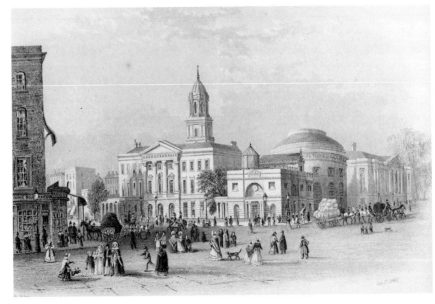

La Maternité, the famous lying-in hospital in Paris. Specially designed and built in the early nineteenth century on healthy high open ground to avoid infection, it nevertheless had an appalling high rate of deaths from puerperal fever—higher than in any of the lying-in hospitals in London.

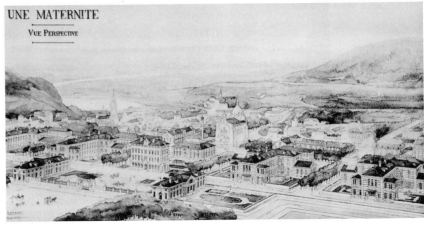

UNE MATERNITE

VUE PERSPECTIVE

was one of the hallmarks of general practice. Elizabeth Garrett Anderson, one of the first women in the UK to qualify in medicine, wrote in 1898:

It is unfortunately true that the puerperal mortality all over England is higher than it ought to be ... The responsibility for this rests in great measure with the examining bodies. When they recognise that a sound and extensive knowledge of practical mid-wifery is infinitely more important to a practitioner than a minute acquaintance with organic chemistry and with the refinements of physiology there will be a chance of improvement but not till then ...

Her recommendation that every student should spend six months in 'acquiring skill in midwifery' was still a far cry from reality in the 1930s. Obstetric training was still crammed into a few weeks. Students were told to 'get their "midder" out of the way' as quickly as possible so that they could get down to the real subjects of medicine, surgery, and pathology. Training consisted to a great extent of being sent out to deliver poor women 'on the district' with minimal instruction or supervision. On the Continent, however (and especially in the Netherlands and Scandinavia), obstetrics was treated with as much respect as medicine and surgery. In general it is a self-evident truth that the attitudes of teachers affect the standard of medical education, and in turn the standard of medical care. The blame for the generally low standard of obstetric care in the UK (and the USA) until the mid-twentieth century lies fairly and squarely on the teaching hospitals. Now, however, we must change direction and consider the major changes in obstetric knowledge and the means by which standards of maternal care can be measured and compared.

Anaesthesia, Antisepsis, and Puerperal Fever

There were many minor advances in nineteenth-century obstetrics, but the two major ones were anaesthesia and antisepsis. Anaesthesia in childbirth was introduced by James Young Simpson (1811–70) of Edinburgh in 1847. He began by using ether, but soon changed to the more pleasant but potentially more dangerous agent, chloroform. His technique was rapidly adopted throughout Scotland and on the Continent, but it was opposed in England. It is often said that the opposition was based on the biblical injunction: 'in sorrow thou shalt bring forth children' (Gen. 3: 16), to which Simpson replied in anger (and correctly) that in the first place the original meaning of sorrow was 'labour' or 'work', not 'pain and sorrow', and in the second that it was little short of blasphemy to assert that a loving God would oppose the relief of pain in childbirth. But the real opposition came from London obstetricians, who, without any evidence, argued that chloroform might cause delayed side effects such as convulsions. It was only when Queen Victoria had chloroform in 1853 for her eighth delivery that opposition collapsed. Simpson's method was generally adopted and became known as chloroform à la reine.

The other major change in obstetrics was the introduction of antisepsis. To appreciate the importance of antisepsis it is necessary to understand that the most common cause of death in childbirth was puerperal or 'childbed' fever, an infection of the genital tract of women following childbirth due in a large majority of cases to one micro-organism, *Streptococcus pyogenes*. Puerperal fever was first recognized as a specific disease of childbearing women, as opposed to

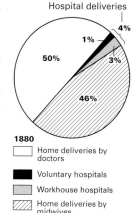

Hospital deliveries

50% · 1% · 4% · 3% · 46%

1880

- ☐ Home deliveries by doctors
- ■ Voluntary hospitals
- ▨ Workhouse hospitals
- ▨ Home deliveries by midwives

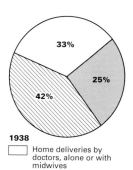

33% · 25% · 42%

1938

- ☐ Home deliveries by doctors, alone or with midwives
- ▨ Hospital deliveries
- ▨ Home deliveries by midwives alone

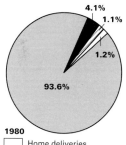

4.1% · 1.1% · 1.2% · 93.6%

1980

- ☐ Home deliveries
- ▨ Deliveries in other hospitals
- ■ Deliveries in GP obstetric unit
- ▨ Deliveries in an NHS hospital with consultant obstetric unit

The distribution of deliveries in terms of deliveries by midwives or doctors, and deliveries in home or in hospital. England and Wales, 1880, 1938, and 1980.

a common fever, in the mid-eighteenth century, when lying-in hospitals were first established and began to experience recurrent epidemics of the disease. Sometimes whole wards of lying-in women were 'swept away' by the disease. Epidemics also occurred in towns. An epidemic in Aberdeen which lasted from 1789 to 1792 was studied by Alexander Gordon (1752–99), who showed that puerperal fever was contagious in the sense that it was transmitted from one lying-in woman to another by the birth attendant.

Many others confirmed Gordon's finding, and one who is often quoted was Oliver Wendell Holmes (1809–94), the poet-physician who was Parkman Professor of Anatomy and Physiology at Harvard University. In 1843 he published a paper on the contagiousness of puerperal fever (it is one of the finest essays in the history of obstetrics) which was republished in 1855 as a pamphlet entitled *Puerperal Fever as a Private Pestilence*.

Holmes's work was soon followed by the work of the famous Hungarian-born obstetrician Ignaz Phillip Semmelweis (1818–65), who is often believed (incorrectly) to have been the first to show that puerperal fever was contagious. In 1847 he was appointed assistant physician to the Vienna Maternity Hospital, the largest maternity hospital in the world. The hospital was divided into two clinics. The first clinic (in which Semmelweis worked) was reserved for medical students, the second for student midwives. To the dismay of the authorities, the mortality from puerperal fever in the first clinic was very much higher than it was in the second. Many suggestions were made and alterations introduced, but in vain until Semmelweis made the key observation that the medical students at Vienna began their day by carrying out post-mortem dissections of women and then went straight to the wards to carry out vaginal examinations on women in labour. It occurred to him that the soiled hands of the students conveyed something to the genital tract of lying-in women which caused the disease. At first he was sure that the 'something' was 'morbid matter' from the dissected corpses, but later he concluded that the infective agent was 'decomposing animal organic matter'. He therefore insisted that before entering the wards every student had to wash his hands in a chlorine disinfectant. The mortality in the first clinic instantly declined to the level of that in the second clinic.

Although in retrospect the work of Gordon in 1795, Holmes in 1843, and Semmelweis in 1861 is seen as critical for the understanding and prevention of puerperal fever, they made almost no impact in their lifetime. In theory, Semmelweis's discoveries should have led to a fall in deaths from puerperal fever, and many historians have assumed there was such a fall. In fact national levels of mortality from puerperal fever increased. The reasons why Semmelweis's work was almost totally ignored are complex. Until the advent of bacteriology, it was almost universally believed that fevers in general, and puerperal fever in particular, were due to many different causes. Few were disposed to accept a unitary explanation, and Semmelweis insisted that all cases of puerperal fever whatsoever were due to the single cause—the transfer of decomposing animal organic matter. Also, he made few converts because of his extreme dogmatism, egocentricity, and intolerance of even the mildest criticism. These characteristics were exaggerated by the onset in the mid-1850s of mental illness, the nature of which is uncertain. At all events he died miserably in a common lunatic asylum in 1865, possibly from a septic hand, possibly from a head injury inflicted by brutal asylum attendants.

Antisepsis was finally introduced into obstetrics because of the work of two men—Pasteur and Lister. In the 1860s, Louis Pasteur (1822–95) and others began to study the role of micro-organisms and to frame the germ theory of disease. By 1880 Pasteur and a number of others had identified the organism which was later named *Streptococcus pyogenes* as the cause of the large majority of fatal cases of puerperal fever. In 1865 (the year of Semmelweis's death) a Glasgow surgeon, Joseph (Lord) Lister (1827–1912), who was profoundly influenced by Pasteur but totally unaware of Semmelweis's work, developed the principles and practice of antiseptic surgery.

While this was going on, in spite of numerous sanitary measures, deaths from puerperal fever in the lying-in hospitals had risen throughout the nineteenth century in the UK, the United States, and on the Continent. To the utter despair of obstetricians, even the newest hospitals, carefully designed on the latest sanitary principles, were not immune. Indeed, the London obstetrician Robert Barnes noted in 1865 that: 'It is in a model hospital (Beaujon) that there rules a mortality so enormous that if it were the type for the whole country, out of the 900,000 to 950,000 labours taking place yearly, there would be 80,000 deaths, and France would be a desert in less than fifty years.' By 1870 it had come to the point that mass closure of these hospitals was seriously considered. Then a dramatic change occurred. In the late 1870s Listerian antisepsis, which had been so successful in surgery, began to be used in obstetrics. The results exceeded all expectations. Puerperal fever in hospitals was almost completely abolished. As one London obstetrician put it in 1887:

From being hotbeds of death and disease in which no woman could be confined without serious risk . . . in the majority of well-managed lying-in hospitals a woman is now as safe, if not safer, than if she was confined in a large and luxurious private house, with nurse, physician, and all that money can now procure. This is no exaggerated statement.

Unfortunately, for many years the antiseptic revolution was confined to the hospitals and had little effect on home deliveries.

Childbirth in the Twentieth Century and the Continuing Problem of Maternal Mortality

From the eighteenth century obstetricians had been deeply interested in mortality statistics, largely because of the appalling mortality rates of the lying-in hospitals compared with the mortality of home deliveries. The maternal mortality rate came to be defined as the number of maternal deaths in a given number of births; until the second half of the twentieth century it was usual to express the maternal mortality rate as the number of maternal deaths per 1,000 or per 10,000 births. Now that maternal deaths have become rare, it is customary to use 100,000 births as the denominator. In effect the maternal mortality rate is the cost in terms of mothers' lives of producing a given number of live births. By the 1870s there was growing concern over the number of maternal deaths in home as well as hospital deliveries. Further, in spite of

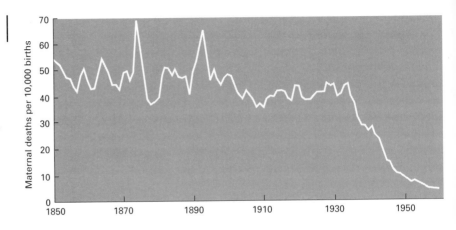

England and Wales,
1850–1960. Maternal
mortality rate shown as
number of maternal
deaths per 10,000 births.

what were seen as advances in obstetrics, national rates of maternal mortality showed no signs of declining. Figure 13.2, which shows the annual maternal mortality rates in England and Wales from 1850 to 1960, demonstrates that maternal mortality remained on a high plateau from 1850 to the mid-1930s, and that the plateau was very 'spiky' from 1850 to 1900 but less so afterwards. From the mid-1930s, however, there was a steep and continuous fall in maternal deaths which has continued to the end of the century, and we shall come back to that. This striking graph shows that the risk of a mother dying in childbirth was as high in 1934 as it was in the 1860s. In contrast, the risk of dying in childbirth in the 1980s was *forty* times less than it had been only fifty years before. It is easier to grasp if one puts it this way. In the 1890s there were on average thirteen maternal deaths a *day* in England and Wales. In the 1990s there is less than one maternal death a *week*, even though the population of women of childbearing age has doubled.

Maternal Care and Maternal Mortality, 1900–1940

From the end of the nineteenth century there was a steady decline in mortality in general, in infant mortality, and in mortality from most infectious diseases. The causes of this decline are still debated by historians, but very little of this improvement was due to clinical care 'at the bedside'. Maternal mortality was the great exception. Yet there were many features of maternal care which, it seemed at the time, should have led to an ever steeper decline in maternal mortality. Deaths from puerperal fever should have disappeared because of the introduction of antisepsis and asepsis. Caesarean section, which, before the 1890s, was so dangerous that it was scarcely ever performed, rapidly became a safe operation after 1900. By the 1920s one saw the widespread introduction of maternal welfare clinics and antenatal care. At the same time there were more obstetric specialists, maternity beds, and supposedly better medical education. Furthermore, in England and Wales the Midwives' Act of 1902 produced a rapidly increasing number of trained and supervised midwives. Yet, in spite of all these supposed advances, instead of declining, the maternal mortality rate actually rose from the beginning of the century to the mid-1930s. This pointed to a massive and scandalous failure in maternal care which was not confined to the UK but occurred in many Western countries. It was a situation crying out for analysis and action.

One of the striking features of the early years of the twentieth century was the substantial international variation in the levels of maternal mortality, reflecting wide differences in systems of maternal care and standards of training. In the Netherlands and Scandinavia, home delivery by a trained midwife was the central form of maternal care. In the USA there was a deliberate and largely successful policy of banning midwives and delivering all women (apart from those in remote rural areas) in hospital by specialist obstetricians. In the UK, the midwife and the general practitioner provided the backbone of maternal care, with hospitals reserved for high-risk cases, women whose homes were judged unsuitable ('social admissions'), and emergency admissions. The USA had by far the highest rate of maternal mortality in the Western world, the Netherlands and Scandinavia the lowest. England and Wales, France, Germany, Australia, and New Zealand came in between.

It might be argued that during this period obstetric knowledge and techniques had not yet advanced to a stage where maternal deaths could be reduced. Not so. There were individual practitioners, general practitioners as well as obstetricians, who achieved excellent results by practising careful and conscientious midwifery. And there were institutions which showed that it was possible to achieve remarkably low levels of maternal mortality and a very high standard of maternal care judged not by the standards of today but by the standards of the time. Examples which come to mind are the nurse-midwives of the Queen's Victoria Jubilee Institute for Nursing the Poor in their Own Homes (usually referred to as the 'Queen's Nurses'), the Kentucky Frontier Nursing Service, the Chicago Maternity Center Outdoor Service in the USA, and the general standard of maternal care in the Netherlands and Denmark. But there were, between 1900 and 1940, large patches of very poor maternal care leading to thousands of unnecessary maternal deaths, which were potentially preventable.

In the UK there was a tendency for desultory antiseptic procedures to be combined with unnecessary interference in normal labours. An Edinburgh obstetrician, Milne Murray, complained of 'the ridiculous parody which, in many practitioners' hands, stands for the use of antiseptics—especially when we hear of forceps cases representing 30 to 70 per cent of the midwifery practice of some practitioners'. The same was true in the 1930s. Many reasons were given, some of which sound bizarre today. For example, civilization itself was blamed. It was widely believed that 'primitive' women from 'savage' tribes ('the Esquimaux and the Hottentot') always had quick painless labours and few deaths, but civilized women (which meant middle- and upper-class women) were incapable of delivering themselves without medical aid such as injections of morphine or heroin in the first stage of labour followed by chloroform anaesthesia and forceps delivery in the second. General practitioners who applied forceps under general anaesthesia in 50 per cent or more of their normal midwifery cases argued that it saved time, justified their fee, and that it was what civilized patients expected.

Apart from the conduct of birth attendants, the provision of maternal care by local authorities in England and Wales was characterized by indifference, inertia, and parsimony. The distribution of maternity beds and specialist obstetricians was extraordinarily patchy. In the 1930s a few English counties were well provided with clinics, specialists, and maternity beds, but some, such as Gloucestershire, had not a single obstetrician and so few maternity beds that general practitioners who encountered hair-raising obstetric complications had to deal with them as best they could in the patients' homes.

While the evolution of maternal care in the USA was strikingly different, there were many of the same faults. The standard of obstetric education was notoriously low. Home deliveries were condemned. Numerous US obstetricians indulged in what a British obstetrican called 'an orgy of interference'. Midwives were described with breathtaking hostility as 'filthy, ignorant, not far removed from the jungles of Africa, typically old, gin-fingering and guzzling, pestiferous and vicious'. In spite of copious evidence to the contrary from Europe, J. B. DeLee of Chicago said in 1916 that midwives were 'relics of barbarism . . . in civilised countries the midwife is wrong and has always been wrong'.

During the 1920s about 25,000 women in the UK and a quarter of a million women in the USA died in childbirth. By the end of the decade this scandalous state of affairs led to a series of investigations into standards of maternal care on both sides of the Atlantic. In retrospect one can see that before the Second World War wherever there was a country or a region in which there was a high proportion of home deliveries by trained midwives and a low amount of interference by doctors in normal labours, there was a high standard of maternal care characterized by a low rate of maternal mortality. That generalization was borne out by numerous national and regional studies.

Maternal Care and Maternal Mortality since 1940

If we now have some ideas on why there was such a poor standard of maternal care between 1900 and 1940—and at the risk of repetition I would stress that the single most important factor was poor obstetric education—we must turn to the reasons for the steep and continuous decline in maternal mortality from 1940 to the present. In part it was a result of the investigations of maternity in the inter-war period that led to a series of scathing reports, and thus to a sea-change in standards of maternal care between 1935 and 1950. In the UK, the Royal College of Obstetricians and Gynaecologists (founded in 1929) began to produce a corpus of trained specialist obstetricians and raised the standard of obstetric care in general practice. At the same time, a series of Midwives' Acts produced an army of well-trained midwives. But the single most important factor in the reduction of maternal mortality was the introduction of the sulphonamides in 1936–7, which were extremely effective in the treatment of puerperal fever. Between 1937 and 1945, about 70 per cent of the steep decline was due to this factor alone. Other factors were the introduction of ergometrine (a drug which, by causing tight contraction of the uterus, prevents bleeding after childbirth) and widely available blood transfusion (largely as a result of the war). During the Second World War the Emergency Maternity Service in the UK did more in a few months to improve the availability of high-standard maternal care to the whole population than local and national government had achieved in the previous twenty years, and the percentage of hospital deliveries increased from 24.0 in 1932 to 53.8 in 1946.

Post-war factors which contributed to the decline in maternal mortality included the availability (from about 1945) of penicillin, an integrated service of midwives, general practitioners, and obstetricians as a result of the National Health Service (NHS), and greatly improved obstetric education. Obstetrics changed from a speciality tinged with pessimism to a rapidly expanding discipline of central importance in medical education and medical care. This was broadly true in all Western countries, and may explain something which no one could have forecast in the 1930s: maternal mortality rates in the USA, England and Wales, and the Netherlands, which had been so far apart in the inter-war period, had, by the 1960s, converged to almost exactly the same level. Since the 1960s, improvements in maternal care, accompanied by continuing declines in maternal and perinatal mortality, have come about partly by the acquisition of new knowledge, but mostly by better training and application of obstetric care.

Maternal mortality is perhaps the most dreadful of all mortalities, for it comes 'out of the blue' in what should be a natural physiological process and a joyous occasion, and it robs the newborn baby of its mother and the husband of his wife. There were, and still are, differences in maternal mortality between Western countries, but the differences are minuscule compared with periods before the Second World War. Memories are short, and almost no one— including doctors and midwives—realizes that the conquest of maternal mortality since the mid-1930s is one of the most remarkable achievements of modern medicine.

Conclusion

Broadly speaking, the eighteenth century was a time of great activity in which the nature of normal and abnormal labours was established. In contrast, the nineteenth century was a period of relative stagnation and missed opportunities as far as obstetrics was concerned, apart from the introduction of anaesthesia in 1847 and of Listerian antisepsis in the 1880s. The first forty years of the twentieth century were marred by low standards of obstetric care. The dramatic and, above all, sustained fall in maternal mortality since the late 1930s has led to an ever-increasing public expectation that every delivery will result in a healthy and happy mother and baby. Childbirth, however, can still be a hazardous event. Expectations are not always fulfilled, and maternity departments are often criticized for too much technology and impersonal care. Ironically, the steep decline in maternal and perinatal mortality has been accompanied by an equally steep rise in malpractice actions against obstetricians to such an extent that the speciality feels deeply threatened and the practice of 'defensive obstetrics' is increasing. Although this is seen as a major problem in Western medicine, there is one disturbing fact which makes the dissatisfactions of the West seem trivial.

At least half a million women still die every year of pregnancy-related causes, but 99 per cent of these deaths occur in developing countries where rates and causes of maternal mortality are closely similar to those which afflicted Western countries in the early nineteenth century. There is no other health statistic in which the disparity between developed and developing countries is so wide. The provision of effective maternal care in developing countries must surely be one of the highest priorities in maternal care in the immediate future.

14 | Children in Hospital

J. A. WALKER-SMITH

BRITAIN lagged behind the rest of Europe in the provision of hospital care for children. When the Hospital for Sick Children in Great Ormond Street was opened in 1852, Dr Charles West, the inspiration behind its establishment, stated that neither in London nor throughout the whole of the British Empire was there a single hospital exclusively devoted to the reception of children, nor, with occasional exceptions, were children admitted to the numerous large (voluntary) general hospitals. This was because from the time they had first been established in the eighteenth century, the voluntary hospitals had devised rules on what kinds of patients should be excluded from in-patient care. Thus the voluntary hospitals refused admission to 'women big with child', cases of 'the itch', 'the pox', consumption, fevers, and incurable cases, and also children unless they required a surgical operation or had suffered an accidental injury. Although some of these rules were relaxed in the first half of the nineteenth century, the rules which excluded children were still applied. Sick children with medical complaints were not admitted.

On the continent of Europe it was quite different. The first children's hospital in Europe, the Hôpital des Enfants Malades, was founded in Paris in 1802. This was followed by the establishment of children's hospitals in Vienna (1837), in Hamburg (1840), in Moscow, Frankfurt, Prague, and Stuttgart in 1842, and in several other European cities in the 1840s. Britain and its Empire were late starters.

London, however, saw the development (admittedly on a small scale) of a quite different type of institution—dispensaries for sick children where parents could bring their children for what we would now call 'outpatient' advice and treatment. The first of these, the 'Dispensary for the Infant Poor', was established by Dr George Armstrong in 1769. It was a 'one-man' institution which faded away when Armstrong died in 1789. The second was the Universal Dispensary for Children, opened in 1816 by John Bunnell Davis at St Andrew's Hill. This was a much larger establishment than George Armstrong's. It grew rapidly. And, as the annual number of children seen at the dispensary increased, this institution changed its name a bewildering number of times, moved across the Waterloo Bridge to the south side of the Thames, and ultimately became known as the Royal Hospital for Children and Women. It finally became a children's hospital in 1856, when it admitted a few children as in-patients.

These dispensaries were of key importance in the development of medical institutions devoted to sick children, although Armstrong himself was against the idea of hospitals for children because he believed 'if you separate an infant from its mother or nurse . . . you will break its heart immediately'. John Bunnell Davis, however, was always in favour of converting his dispensary into a children's hospital but was prevented from doing so in his own lifetime by the intransigence of the governing body. But the underlying concept that sick children needed institutional care quite separately from adults was gaining ground in the first half of the nineteenth century. The children's dispensaries paved the way for the foundation of children's hospitals in England and underlined the need for specific requirements for children in hospital.

The Great Ormond Street Hospital, founded as we have seen in 1852 and still one of the most famous of its kind in the world, was followed by the establishment of at least six more children's hospitals in London by 1870 and another six in the provinces. By 1888 there were thirty-eight children's hospitals in the British Empire. The first in the British Empire was in Melbourne, and children's hospitals were established in Brisbane, Adelaide, and Sydney by 1880. Canada's first children's hospital was established in 1875 at Toronto. We now take up the story of the development of children's hospitals and the way children were cared for in hospitals from 1850 to 1990.

The Development of In-Patient Hospital Facilities for Children

Before (approximately) the mid-eighteenth century, the few hospitals which existed were primarily 'hospices', or refuges for the old, the poor, and those unable to look after themselves, whether through sickness, age, or poverty, or a combination of such circumstances. Thereafter, hospitals became institutions where adult patients were admitted specifically for medical or surgical care (or childbirth in the lying-in hospitals) and where—if they survived—they were discharged home as soon as they had been restored to health, 'improved' if not 'cured', these being the two terms one finds in the hospital registers alongside the names of the patients who were discharged.

A similar transition as far as children were concerned took place about a century later. Thus, before the nineteenth century children who were admitted to institutions were for the most part the abandoned or orphaned rather than the sick. Children's hospitals in the modern sense of 'hospital' were for the most part mid- to late-nineteenth-century institutions. They were founded for the same philanthropic reasons as the general hospitals—to provide medical care and cure for children, in the same way as the general hospitals catered for sick adults, in institutions such as the Great Ormond Street Hospital for children.

At the same time, however, some of the old-established general hospitals such as St Bartholomew's Hospital in London began to admit sick children to their wards, but not to departments with special facilities for children. Children were admitted to adult wards, where they were cared for in a disciplined environment with adults and children side by side. Both boys and girls were nursed in women's wards, but very young boys were sometimes nursed in

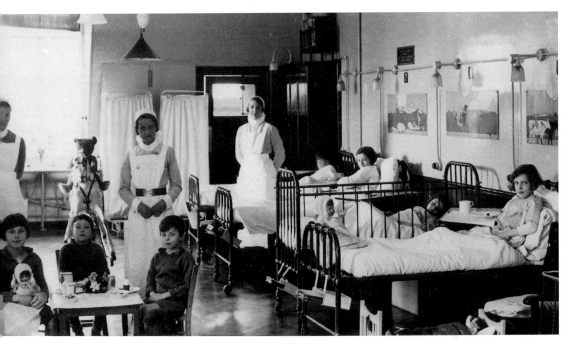

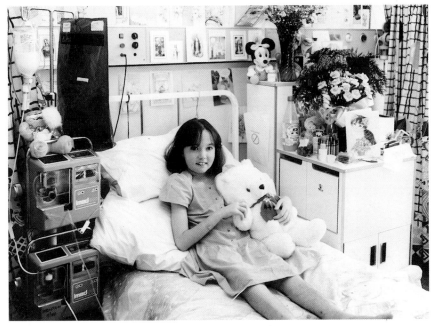

Children's ward at St Bartholomew's Hospital, 1930. There is still formality here.

Girl on bed with teddy bear in a modern children's ward (1980s). The relaxed informal atmosphere with many toys shows changing attitudes.

men's wards. This mixing of adults and children often led to the physical and emotional isolation of the child.

Astonishingly, this mixing of adults and children persisted at St Bartholomew's Hospital until 1930, when, for the very first time, wards specifically for children were opened. This delay occurred in spite of the fact that as early as 1877 the paediatrician Karl Rauchfuss, director of the children's hospital in St Petersburg, Russia, had shown that not only should children be admitted to children's hospitals but, most importantly, that these

223

should be constructed especially for the needs of children. He, like Charles West, was a great supporter of the need for independent children's hospitals. Apart from the question as to whether sick children should be admitted to hospital at all, however, there was from the mid-nineteenth century onwards a continuing debate concerning the question as to whether it was better for children to be cared for in children's hospitals, or in general hospitals.

Seidel asserts that the development of the children's hospital vacillated between the self-interest of the medical profession and the proper needs of children. The debate on the question of whether children were best cared for in children's hospitals or in general hospitals—like so many questions in nineteenth-century hospitals—hinged on the preconceptions, prejudices, and sometimes the self-interest of individual doctors and others involved in the care of children. For instance, on the grounds that children were unable to speak up for themselves, Florence Nightingale believed that they should be nursed alongside adults, preferably in women's wards. In fact, the main problem for the nineteenth-century child in hospital was the risk of cross-infection from other children suffering from infectious diseases, so that one of the arguments against children's hospitals was the high rate of cross-infection. The charitable institutions that preceded children's hospitals were all too aware of this problem, for, of course, hospital infection was the bane of all hospitals, but it was especially prominent in children's hospitals. A vivid example is provided by the medical report of the Benevolent Asylum in Pitt Street, Sydney, Australia for the year ending 30 June 1867.

The medical history during the year just terminated is peculiarly melancholy, as in other institutions devoted to the care of children, and as in the city and suburbs generally, a high rate of mortality has occurred amongst the infants and children in the Asylum from the prevalence of a very severe variety of epidemic measles . . . The houses at the time of the outbreak were overcrowded in all the children's departments. . . . In its progress the disease attacked every unprotected inmate, without distinction of age or other circumstance; women recently accouched and their infants, pregnant women, and children, all came under its influence and every variety of the

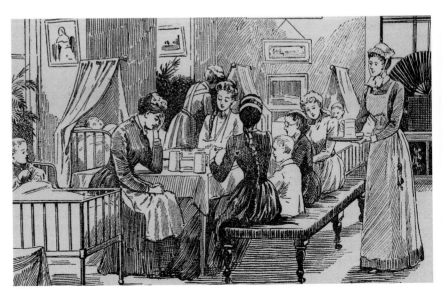

Tea time in Stanley Ward, St Bartholomew's Hospital, London, 1880, with children and women patients together. The ordered formality of the scene is clear. This is a disciplined environment.

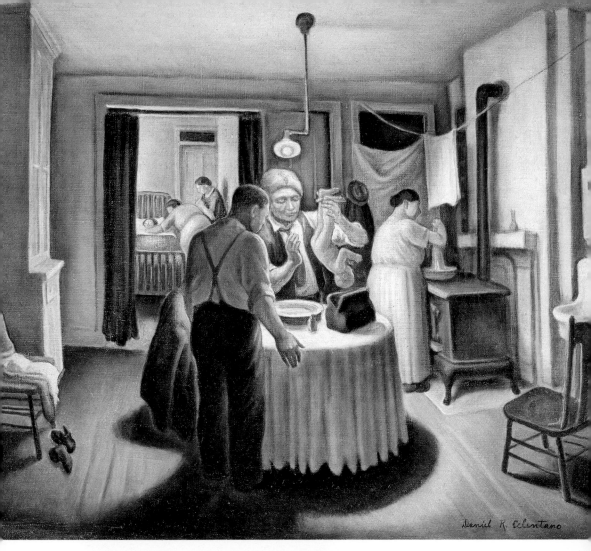

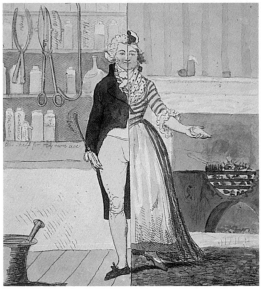

Daniel Celentano, *Just Born*. On the one hand this shows the 'hominess' and informality of a home delivery. But the date is 1939 and the danger of puerperal fever and the need for antisepsis and asepsis were well known. Yet, as happened nearly always in home deliveries, the doctor who acted as the birth-attendant did so in his shirt sleeves without wearing a mask, a gown, or sterilized rubber gloves, although these had become routine in most maternity hospitals.

This satirical etching of the early obstetricians, and the fact they were known as men-midwives, indicates some of the opposition to medical men meddling in midwifery, and also that the practice of midwifery by men was a relatively new phenomenon. Obstetricians thus preferred to refer to themselves by the French term 'accoucheur'.

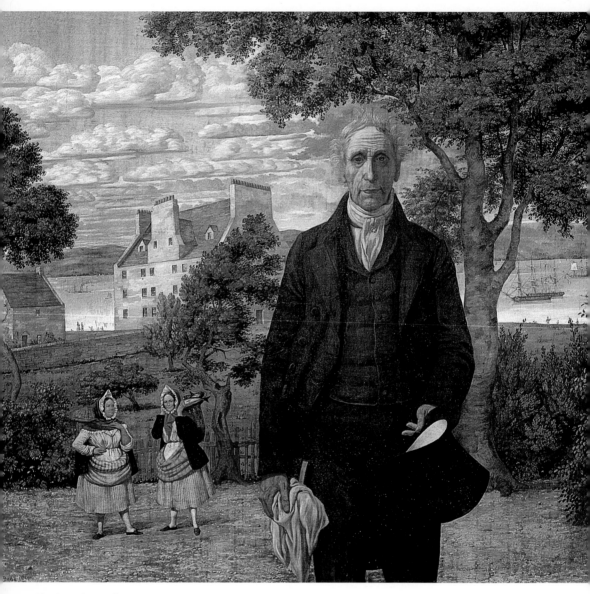

Sir Alexander Morison as portrayed by Richard
Dadd in 1852. Dadd had murdered his father but
was deemed criminally insane and placed in
Bethlem and then Broadmoor. Morison was
visiting physician to Bethlem and a collector of
Dadd's work. He appears here as a tired figure
in a strange landscape.

disease and its sequelae appeared. At the end of the month of April 250 patients were under treatment in bed. The foundling children who had been reared with much care and difficulty for the past two or three years and the children tainted with constitutional disease of scrofulous or syphilitic type suffered severely. In point of fact it may be stated that [out of] nearly all the deaths, at least three-quarters occurred among this class of inmate. . . . The disease swept away the majority of this class of children in the institution.

Thus the advocates of children's hospitals emphasized the need of isolation units for infectious diseases within a children's hospital. Karl Rauchfuss was amongst those who contributed to the development of measures for the control of infectious diseases of children within the hospital, and in this respect paediatrics was an example for adult medicine. But those who believed that children should be admitted to adult wards in general hospitals still argued that there would be less risk of exposure to infected children because the number of children crowded together would be diluted, and children were much less likely to acquire infection from adult patients.

However, there were other concerns related to children's hospitals. One of the disadvantages of independent children's hospitals was the academic and clinical isolation of their medical staff. Indeed, because of this isolation, a German paediatrician, Arthur Schlossman, advocated in the late nineteenth century the complete replacement of independent children's hospitals by large paediatric departments within general hospitals. In this way, he argued, the best care for children could be obtained by collaboration with other specialists. He did, however, recommend that all children under 14 years of age should be under the care of a paediatrician.

An alternative solution was for general physicians to care for child patients, whether they were admitted to general hospitals or to specialized children's hospitals. And this is what occurred in London. Several distinguished nineteenth-century English physicians such as Dr Samuel Jones Gee, who looked after children and adults, denied the need for paediatricians. There were, said Gee, two words he abhorred—'specialist' and 'consultant'. This sounds odd until one realizes that in the first two-thirds of the nineteenth century many of the élite physicians and surgeons who held appointments at teaching hospitals despised specialization. They accepted that hospital doctors should be divided into physicians (in the British sense), surgeons, and obstetricians. But that was as far as specialization should go. Those who advertised themselves as specialists in eye diseases, skin diseases, diseases of the ear, nose, or throat, and so on, were treated with scorn. The élite regarded them as so many upstarts who, having failed to achieve an appointment at a prestigious hospital, set out to attract the gullible public and make a name (and a large income) for themselves by outrageous claims of special knowledge and skill in one small branch of medicine. Men such as Gee would have been utterly horrified at the state of hospital medicine today, for he firmly believed that physicians should care for all medical complaints in patients of all ages. He set an example by caring for adults and children at St Bartholomew's Hospital and children only at the Great Ormond Street Hospital.

It was the views of men such as Gee that dominated the teaching hospitals of London, and the truth is that children's hospitals such as the Hospital for Sick

Children in Great Ormond Street and the North-Eastern Hospital for Children (later Queen Elizabeth Hospital for Children) flourished while they were staffed by these selfsame physicians. At the Great Ormond Street Hospital, Samuel Gee, W. H. Dickinson, and W. B. Cheadle served as honorary general physicians who were interested in the diseases peculiar to children. But the trend towards specialization was inevitable. This generation of physicians and indeed surgeons (such as Sir William Arbuthnot Lane) who were concerned with children only part-time was followed by the appearance of fully committed paediatricians and also eventually by paediatric surgeons.

In the first decade of the twentieth century Sir George Frederick Still, who was the first paediatrician in the UK to devote himself entirely to the care of children, became the Professor of Children's Diseases at King's College Hospital, London. Sir James Spence, a paediatrician who placed great emphasis on the welfare of children in hospital, later established an academic department of child health in Newcastle. Thus in the twentieth century the scene had changed so much that the medical care of children moved into the hands of practitioners who had devoted their professional lives to the needs of children. This transition was largely complete by the 1930s.

The Development of Specialization in Paediatrics

Dr Charles West believed that there were 'no surgical problems in childhood which demanded special skill or study'. However, by the early years of the twentieth century it was clear that surgical problems in children required very special skills, and the speciality of paediatric surgery arose. This recognition of the need for paediatric surgery was accompanied by the development of other specializations in paediatrics. The special emotional needs of children led to the development of child psychiatry, and after the First World War there was a progressive appreciation of the need for specialization throughout the whole field of paediatrics. Following the Second World War this trend accelerated. It became obvious that children required all the specialist care which was available to adults, but tailored to the specific needs of children. Furthermore, the specific and unique requirements of the newborn became understood, and so the special branch of paediatrics known as neonatal medicine arose.

All of this is an indication of the revolution that has taken place in the care of children in hospital since the mid-nineteenth century. In the 1850s sick children were often not admitted to hospital at all, or, if admitted, were cared for in an environment which was often unsuitable for children and almost totally lacking in the means of providing curative medicine. All that could be done therapeutically was to provide loving nursing care and the good nutrition that was so often lacking in the home. In contrast, children in the 1990s are admitted to wards or departments specifically devised for the needs of children as well as being able to benefit from modern medical technology.

Illustrations of children in hospital during the nineteenth century and early twentieth century reveal quiet and disciplined children, often on their own, sometimes with nursing or medical staff, but rarely accompanied by their mother or father. The placement of children in adult wards may have reduced the chance of cross-infection from the infectious diseases of childhood, but the

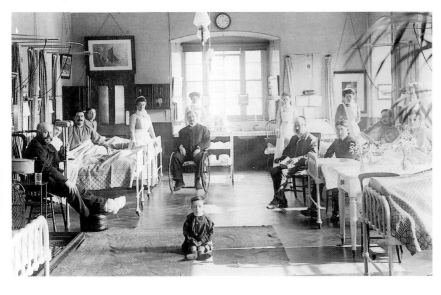

Lone child in adult ward,
1904. The isolation of the
disciplined child in this
adult environment is
obvious.

absence of other children led to social isolation in hospital. An example is a child patient at the North-Eastern Hospital for children in 1869. A little girl had been admitted to hospital with a brain tumour which was causing severe headache and convulsions. The only comfort that she was able to get was from holding tightly on to the nurse's hand. However, with other children to care for, the nurse could not remain all the time at the child's cot. The child's mother came in every day after work to watch over her dying daughter. The mother is reported to have said, 'While I work I pray the Lord to relieve my darling.' The child died a few days after admission. The high mortality of such seriously ill children when admitted to hospital led to an air of solemnity and a strong religious influence within the hospital community, as this example illustrates.

At the same hospital, which had been founded by the Quaker sisters Ellen and Mary Phillips in 1867, this religious aspect was reflected even in the Annual Hospital Report of 1874. It stated: 'Nor should we forget the medical staff, the Secretary, the Matron, the Dispensers and Nurses, and all those who are carrying on the work of the Hospital watched over by our Heavenly Father. It is on their care and solicitude that the pains and sickness of the suffering children depend for recovery, and the result of the past year calls for our sincere gratitude.' Benefactors were often influenced by such considerations. Some gave a benefaction in memory of a relative who had died in the hospital, marked by a sombre plaque over a hospital cot or bed.

The appalling mortality of children during epidemics of infectious disease in the nineteenth century was a major motivation for individuals such as the Phillips sisters to found hospitals for children. Ellen Phillips in particular had nursed children with cholera in the reeking cholera wards of the London Hospital during the severe epidemic of 1866 that had swept through east London. The wards had been heavy with the fumes of carbolic-soaked sawdust scattered over the floor and in sacks beneath each bed as a crude but essential measure of hygiene. The bed straw and the sack of sawdust under the bed had been burnt in an open space at the back of the hospital when a bed was emptied by death or discharge. A bonfire had blazed there each night throughout the epidemic. To those who had watched the leaping flames this was a never-to-be-forgotten sight. It symbolized the hell and suffering endured by patients in the wards where 'on every hand one or other would be dying'. This memory and all the terrible events of the summer of 1866 were seared into Ellen Phillips's mind and served to motivate her, and her sister, to found a hospital specifically for children. Inspiration to found another children's hospital following the cholera outbreak of 1866, but this time in Wapping, came also to a young doctor, Dr Nathaniel Heckford. He and his wife established a tiny children's hospital in a derelict warehouse in Shadwell in 1868, the year after the Phillips sisters had founded their hospital. The four beds rapidly expanded to forty, but the hospital, despite the obvious need for it, was in danger of extinction until visited by Charles Dickens. In his most emotional style he described the hospital as a 'Star in the East'. He wrote as follows:

A gentleman and lady, a young husband and wife, have bought and fitted up this building for its present noble use, and have quietly settled themselves in it as its medical officers and directors. Both have had considerable practical experience in medicine and surgery; he, as house surgeon of a great London Hospital; she, as a very earnest student, tested by severe examination, and also as a nurse of the sick poor, during the prevalence of cholera. With every qualification to lure them away, with youth and accomplishments and tastes and habits that can have no response in any breast near them, close begirt by every repulsive circumstance inseparable from such a neighbourhood, there they dwell.

Dickens's support was quite invaluable and the appeal was successful. Shadwell was to become one of the most successful children's hospitals in London, and the forty beds increased to 135.

However, despite the excellent standards in the hospital, social conditions in the slums around the hospital were very poor. The contrast between the social circumstances in which the children lived and the hospital environment could pose problems for the individual child. Children were sometimes reluctant to return to the misery and squalor of their homes after the comfort and care they had received in hospital. It is recorded at Great Ormond Street Hospital that occasionally children who were abandoned by their parents were sent to the Greenwich Workhouse or to an orphanage. Dr West in fact saw the hospital as motivating social change by drawing attention to the relationship between social deprivation and the need for hospitalization. But, when social conditions did eventually improve, it was sometimes found that children's hospitals were situated in areas from which the population had moved away.

Since the Second World War, the number of children's hospitals has steadily fallen. By the 1990s it had become the orthodox belief of the National Health Service (NHS) that children are best cared for in paediatric units in general hospitals. The Great Ormond Street Hospital has survived intact by adopting the role of a national referral centre. At the Shadwell hospital it became clear that an isolated small children's hospital could not survive, and the hospital, by then known as the Princess Elizabeth of York Hospital for Children, was merged in 1942 with the Queen's Hospital in Hackney Road, and renamed as the Queen Elizabeth Hospital for Children. This hospital itself came under threat in 1994, and it is planned by the end of the century to relocate most of its patients at Whitechapel as part of a general hospital.

Hospital Festivities

At the end of the nineteenth century, hospital authorities made a particular effort to lighten the lives of children in hospital with various annual activities. At the North-Eastern Children's Hospital the hospital authorities celebrated particular occasions such as New Year's Day, when children were given presents. Wealthy benefactors came to the hospital bearing gifts; indeed members of the Royal Family were frequent visitors to children in hospital.

By far the most vivid memories of my stay in hospital were: first, seeing the Queen's father [King George] drive past, the balconies were hung with flags and all of us out there at the time cheered like mad; above all, in spite of being in some pain, I still consider the best day of my stay was the Queen's [Princess Elizabeth] wedding-day, every little girl was given a small doll dressed as a bride—to me it was a really magic day. After all, in those days Christmas was really the only day we got presents.

At St Bartholomew's Hospital there has been a long-standing tradition that medical staff with their family, including their own children, would visit the children who were in hospital on Christmas Day. Nursing staff would ensure that all children received a present, and one of the medical staff would dress up as Father Christmas and distribute presents. By 1990, however, the scene had changed, with as few as possible children actually being kept in hospital for Christmas Day. This usually meant that only the more seriously ill children remained. So the possibilities for festive celebration were less than in earlier years, when the wards had often been just as crowded during the festive season

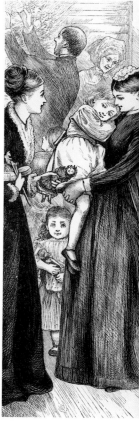

New Year's Day at North-Eastern Hospital for Children, 1873. Wealthy benefactors are shown visiting poor children of the East End of London.

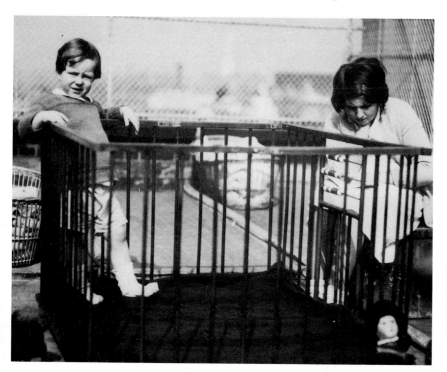

Children out of doors on the roof of St Bartholomew's Hospital in the 1930s. Outside the formality of the ward, the children relax.

229

as at any other time. Also by 1990 commercial organizations had begun to deluge the wards with toys. This was a great contrast to even a decade earlier at the Queen Elizabeth Hospital for Children, when second-hand toys were often received as gifts for the poor children in hospital. Indeed by the 1980s children in hospital were often surrounded by gifts as well as all the paraphernalia of modern hospital care. Through better education such modern children were much less fearful of the hospital environment than their predecessors had been. Of course all children, even with explanation and understanding, may still be somewhat fearful coming into hospital, but in the 1920s, for example, it could be a particularly worrying experience in a world of alien technology.

Children, Parents, and Hospital Visiting

The importance of the psychological support of a child's mother during investigative and also therapeutic procedures slowly came to be accepted. Photographs from the 1920s sometimes show that the child was accompanied by its mother during medical technical procedures. However, as late as the 1940s, family visiting of children was often banned, as the following memoir shows:

It was very upsetting for a small girl (as I was at the time) to find out that no visitors were allowed for the first two weeks. Coming from a large family, and being the youngest, I missed them a great deal. It was better when I was put out on the balcony. Mum used to stand on the pavement below and call and wave to me. However, when visitors were allowed, I remember the lovely new-laid eggs that Mum used to bring in from our own chickens in the back yard. Food was still rationed in 1947, as it was to be for some years to come.

Child in X-ray department, 1920s. The child's somewhat apprehensive encounter with alien technology is shown.

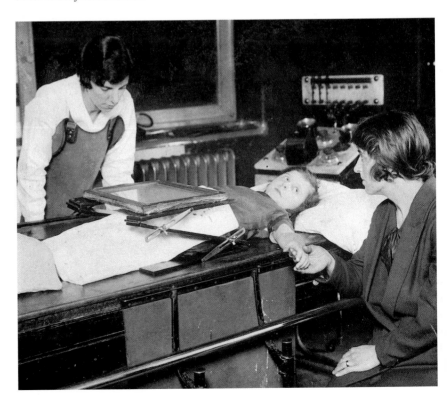

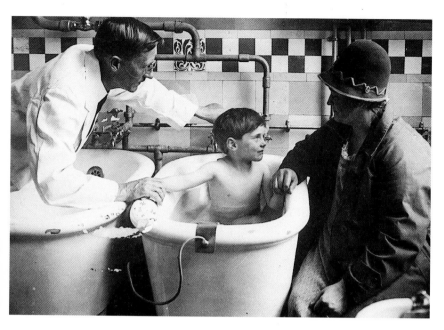

Although some of the nursing staff did what they could to cope with the emotional needs of children, the restrictions placed on visiting (which were especially awkard for working mothers) resulted in children suffering the misery of believing they had been deserted by their parents. Rules on visiting varied. In some children's hospitals there was a 'liberal' policy on visiting children in hospital. In others there was a rigid policy against visiting, often backed by senior nursing staff who opposed visiting on the grounds that 'It only upsets them and makes them cry', and also the belief that visiting could increase the risk of infection. To the disciplinarian element in the medical and nursing staff, the ideal children's ward was a tidy, regulated place full of quiet children whose parents were seen on admission but not again until the child died or was discharged.

In the 1950s and 1960s there was a concerted and successful attempt by some enlightened paediatricians, such as Dr Dermod MacCarthy at Aylesbury, who were in the vanguard of those responsible for the abandonment of the old strict, regimented approach to patients in hospital. Aided by the lay pressure group NAWCH (the National Association for the Welfare of Children in Hospital), they broke down the old and cruel traditions against visiting. Open visiting, and in some hospitals the provision of rooms for mothers who could stay and be near their children when they were seriously ill, led to an end of the awful sense of isolation to which children had been subjected in the past. By 1990 the child in hospital was a child who could have its parents with it virtually whenever it wanted, as accommodation for parents in hospital became generally available. The development of a more relaxed and sympathetic approach to in-patients and visiting—and this applies to adults as well as children—has been a feature of the post-war period. Paediatrics was at the forefront of this development.

15 | Medicine and the Mind

MICHAEL NEVE

FACED with such an enormous subject as the history of medical writings and practice on the mind, the student may be tempted, almost for convenience, to turn that history into a history of psychiatry. This temptation will be all the more attractive since this is what many psychiatrists, acting as historians, have done when turning their attention to the subject. As a result, this part of the history of Western medicine can end up as a form of endless retrospective diagnosis, with the proper contextualization of events and interpretations being sacrificed to the psychiatric categories employed by contemporary medical practitioners. The vital historical point about psychiatry is that it is a recent medical specialism (though many would dispute even that description) with a remarkable lack of consensus as to what clinical models actually explain the behaviours and beliefs under examination. The best psychiatries and the best histories of psychiatry share a common sense that this is only one among many approaches to the mysteries of medicine and the mind, and that the historical record clearly shows this.

As in many other aspects of Western medicine, the pursuit of a medical model of illness has led to the belief that certain behaviours and mental states are the result of diseases located in the brain. The history of medicine has shown the inadequacies of this, the medical model, as the basis for understanding the links between medicine and the mind. The pursuit of biological and materialist explanations has always been accompanied by the intrusion of other voices—voices that speak of the realities of the soul, or religious ecstasy, or visions of the Virgin Mary, voices (some of them modern) that whisper that the idea of mental illness is a myth, that the 'mind' cannot be diseased and that medicine cannot play a healing part in a benign way. Medicine and the brain— that is one thing. Medicine and the mind is more elusive.

The Missing Foundation Stone

The foundation of much of Western medicine is invariably located in the world of the ancient Greeks, with Hippocrates (c.450–370 BC) as a mythical founding father. Hippocratic writings and their doctrine of the humours and the healing power of nature have been hugely influential, not least because they provide a model of diseases as natural occurrences to be explained by material causes and cured by a visiting doctor. The simplicity and utility of humoral medicine survived the establishment of Christianity, but with certain modifications: the Christian physician was not permitted to regard the soul as a function of the brain. He was also not the final saviour of the sick. But the rise of Christianity did not diminish the stature of Hippocratic science. This is important with regard to the story of medicine and the mind, because Greek medical writing on mania or melancholia did not place these outside the humoral framework: there was no 'psychiatric' language for them and it would be a historical error to imagine otherwise. The equally influential writings of Galen (*c*.129–*c*.216) on spirits, or *pneuma*, associated with certain bodily organs maintained the Greek connection, which was that equilibrium could be reached by the medical use of opposites. Thus mania was a hot disease while melancholia was ultimately derived from the humour that was black bile. At the origins of the Western medical tradition, therefore, we have an integrated system of medicine and the mind where independent psychiatric categories are absent. This is one important example of the lessons to be learnt from avoiding a history of medicine and the mind based on a mistaken hunt for psychiatry's origins. Not least, the ancients in their drama and in their philosophy saw madness as something forced upon blind men by vengeful or laughing gods, a fate whose origins and outcome were apparently unconnected to medical views of mental illness. In the period up to Shakespeare at the very least, madness, however tragic, retained its connection to knowledge, a connection that would be jeopardized by subsequent medical and philosophical emphases on the place of Reason in a properly constituted human consciousness. An enduring legacy from the ancients was the naturalistic power ascribed to the passions and to styles of life: sedentary scholars were prone to melancholy; first love was often close to madness.

Christian doctrine on sin and salvation accompanied this materialist framework and never replaced it. Indeed, some Christian writings endorsed a surprising and historically very specific claim that some madness (being thought mad by non-believers, for example) was a good in itself, a proof of true Christianity. This historical theme of the virtue in a life that others thought mad, because of its disdain for the world and its deceptive glories, is an aspect of the history of madness that is often overlooked.

Madness and Civilization

Difficult to locate in the classical world, the foundation stone for a systematic understanding of diseases of the mind can be found within the later period of the European Enlightenment of the eighteenth century. This was the intellectual fruition of a great number of ideas too complex to summarize easily. The essential parts were the views among the educated European élites that extreme forms of religious belief and (often accompanying) beliefs in magic and witchcraft were rendered primitive and mistaken by the rise of science and philosophies that paid tribute to Reason and not the occult. Indeed, the priority given by the educated to doing away with ideas of demonic possession and the entire structure of accounts of disturbing behaviour based on

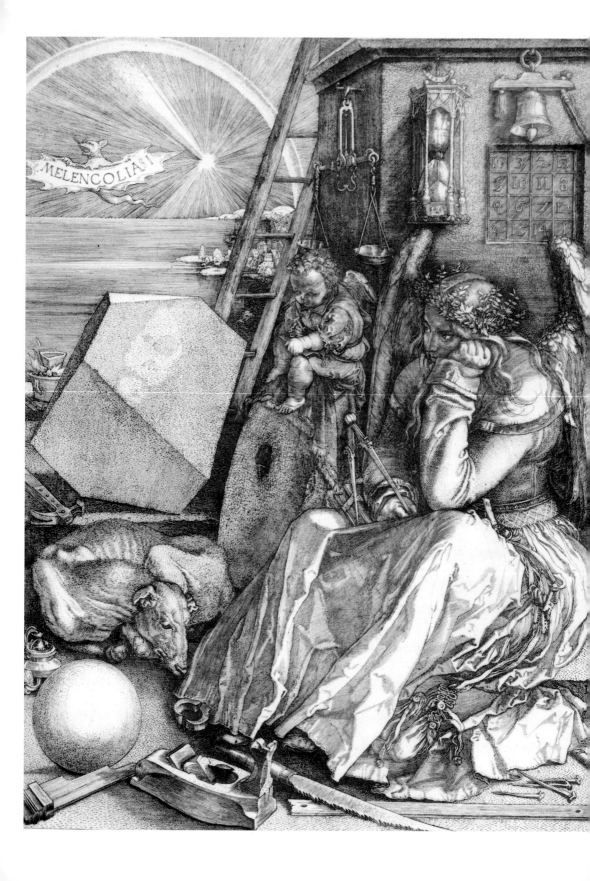

demonology was a fundamental basis for the generation of rational and even scientific accounts of medicine and the mind.

The most famous claims for a new separation of body and mind were those of René Descartes (1596–1650). Descartes equated mind with the soul, and claimed that the mind endowed human beings with rationality, morality, and immortality. The influence of his philosophy within medicine was complex, since one side of his equation could be seen as endorsing outright materialism—everything but the mind/soul was a machine and could be treated as such. But his dualism and those like it marked a real break with humoralism and integrated accounts of medicine and the mind.

This famous engraving of *Melencolia* by Dürer (1514) is a vivid illustration of what would now be called depression.

Writers such as Thomas Willis (1621–75) worked within the Cartesian tradition and shifted attention to medical and neuroscientific studies of the brain. He proposed that animal spirits made many neurological activities possible and that they existed between bodies and minds, being influenced by both. By the late eighteenth century, the previously missing foundation stone for a secular psychiatry can be detected. For example, mania and melancholia prior to then had been seen not as diseases of the mind but (on ancient principles) as diseases of the body. The soul of a madman (echoes here of Shakespeare's Hamlet) was immortal and incorruptible, even in the most furious bouts of manic lunacy. It was when doctors began to argue that this *soul* should really be seen as the *mind* and that this mind could be deranged that we are at the beginnings of a world where psychiatry as an independent discipline would be possible. An object of medical research—the mind—was made or discovered in the eighteenth century, and minds and not just bodies could now go mad, or be judged irrational and found wanting.

Although not universally accepted, the influential writings of John Locke (1632–1704) on the environmental explanations for mental capacities and insanities provided a further rationale for new psychiatric therapies: the disturbed could be reformed and re-educated and shown new mental pathways, pathways unknown to the conventional religious writer or the constrained and often illiberal views of moral philosophy. The final theoretical addition to this new programme was that of the Edinburgh physician William Cullen (1710–90), who defined insanity as a form of dynamic nervous disorder, originating in the brain and the nervous system and presenting as deluded imagination. The crucial point for Cullen was that mental disorder was grounded within neurophysiology, but not all specific cerebral traces could be physically detected. There was room, therefore, for both corporeal and moral factors in the causes of mental illness, and the new kid on the block—the mad-doctor or alienist or doctor of psychological medicine—was entitled to pay attention to both. The Enlightenment in medicine created not souls, not bodies experiencing humoral imbalance with specific behavioural signs, not individuals in the grip of authentic visions, but minds that could be diseased. It also created places where men and women with these minds could be studied and detained.

The Asylum

The Enlightenment medical model endorsed by Cullen and other authors had important implications. Patients could be seen as suffering from any number

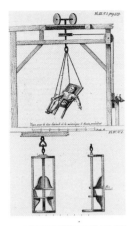

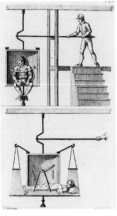

A variety of restraints and treatments (1818–26). The growth of both real and imagined shock therapies from the early nineteenth century was meant to accompany the kinder and more humane procedures of moral management. The full history of the response of patients to compulsory shock treatments, up to the twentieth century and its innovations, has never been fully told.

of medical conditions, with the trained doctor as the proper authority as to how to classify and treat those 'diseases of the mind'. But even more important, the doctor could employ new kinds of encounter with patients which were designed to reach the patient's mind and thereby impose discipline and sanity. The patient could be managed by moral means, by the careful but imaginative use of non-physical, managerial methods. Methods such as a theatrics of fear, or staring, or a dynamics of promises, rewards, and some mild punishments were all deemed by the psychiatrist as a major advance on previous methods of allegedly brutal physical treatment of the insane. It would be no exaggeration to say that the mad-doctor was himself the essential agent of cure in the battle of wits, needing in the words of one historian of psychiatry 'the acting skills of Garrick and the virtuosity of Machiavelli's prince'. The meeting of medicine and the mind was quite literally person to person, with the doctor as the forgiving if frightening father and the patient as the unhappy child whose insanity was medically understood and who could play a part in the drama whose plot was his or her own recovery.

The single most influential author on these themes was the Frenchman Philippe Pinel (1745–1826), who used his experience in Parisian custodial institutions to supplement his other work on clinical medicine in a famous *Treatise on Insanity, in which are Contained the Principles of a New and More Practical Nosology of Maniacal Disorders*, translated into English in 1806. Pinel summoned the ghosts of the Hippocratic past in laying out his theme: that the patient should be morally managed, the physician paying detailed attention to each case history and in particular to the disturbances in the passions. Post-mortems on the brains of lunatics did not reveal detectable abnormalities (exactly as Cullen had said), and this required the Enlightenment doctor to concentrate on moral management and to summon the other great classical power, the healing power of nature. This could be properly done only in the asylum. The asylum had to be designed, administered, policed, and inhabited to allow the staff to dramatize and also to provide a narrative for each individual patient. Pinel even retained the simpler classical divisions of melancholia, mania, idiocy, and dementia to provide a final link between the new Enlightenment understanding of diseased minds with the ancient understanding of how these might best be classified. The simplicity that had been one of the hallmarks of the Hippocratic system was here put to novel and distinct use in the asylum, where new kinds of patients met, feared, and were supposedly to be cured by new kinds of doctor.

Not that this new kind of doctor was to have an easy passage. In England, in the city of York in the last years of the eighteenth century, the Northern Quakers mobilized opposition to the ill-treatment and subsequent death of one of their number in the local York Asylum. The Asylum was presided over by a physician and was exposed in various disturbing ways, leading the Quakers to finance their own asylum, the York Retreat. The main founder of the Retreat, William Tuke (1732–1822), was a merchant with a well-formed distrust of the medical profession of his day, and his involvement was maintained by his grandson Samuel, who published a *Description of the Retreat* in 1813. The Retreat came to embody a critique of the secretive and brutal ways in which the insane could be treated. This also raised the deeper question whether doctors—as against caring laymen—were the right people to look after the insane at all, given the York Asylum example. Was moral management actually safe in the hands of the medical profession, for all the theoretical rationales that the profession could muster? At an important moment in the formative years of the organized psychiatric profession, the medical claim to appropriate moral management was doubted, however briefly. But the real possibility had arisen that the combination of medicine and the mind was not a relationship that needed the mediation of doctors; that the Enlightenment model was one that both legally and practically could be best employed by humane entrepreneurs financing staff brought together by a common religious purpose and without full medical education. Even at the Retreat, when proper accord was given to the physician, the importance of his role was to do with common qualities of good sense and kindness as much as medical expertise.

A major part of the story of psychiatry in both the UK and the USA in the nineteenth century was the incorporation of management into the medical domain, but there are echoes of the York initiative and the claims for lay expertise right up to the present. The part to be played by the family in dealing with alleged lunacy is the consistent theme: whether to admit to a problem, or allege a lunacy, in order to put away a difficult relative, or to seek medical help and yet remain involved in the custodial and the healing process—these elements make up much of the social history of madness, and much of it remains out of historical sight.

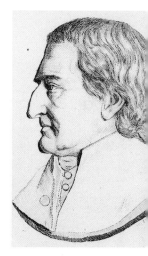

William Tuke with other members of his family is famous for the introduction of the humane treatment of the insane, at the Retreat in York.

The part played by relatives in the hospitalization of difficult family members is seen by some historians as a fundamental issue. For some historians, the use of secular medical descriptions of behaviour (as against religious or existential) allowed families, especially of the European nobility, to control troublesome individuals by means other than resorting to the criminal law. From this perspective, the mixture of custodial and healing aims at the heart of psychiatry is reinterpreted as pure coercion, a new way of using the relationship of medicine and the mind to promote ways of securing economic interests by applying fake disease models and avoiding the religious and legal difficulties that would otherwise pertain. This coercive ambition (especially important in the writings of Michel Foucault and Thomas Szasz) then extends into policies taken up by the State. Both in the period of the absolutist monarchies and then, less overtly, in constitutional regimes, and finally and most horrifically under modern totalitarian systems, the psychiatric system is seen as collaborating with the political to incarcerate the opposition.

The claims and counter-claims around false incarceration are as long as the history of psychiatry itself, and have particularly come to light as the stories and experiences of alleged lunatics themselves have been historically examined. Other accounts stress a less conspiratorial reading of the evidence: that many families found the admission of family madness very difficult, especially among the respectable classes, and the existence of discreet mad-doctors a source of relief. The essential dispute here rests on the reality or otherwise of the disease model of the mind that reached its maturity in the medicine of the Enlightenment and its social uses: few historians disagree that the visibility of lunacy and its place in medical classification and disease categorization were always strongest and most easily achieved among the pauper lunatics in large public institutions rather than the wealthy in more agreeable and less accessible private houses.

Museums of Madness

The history of the modern asylum displays shared characteristics in both Europe and the USA. By the middle of the nineteenth century, the asylum was the province of a now professionally organized medical corps, but one that had uneasy relations with more established parts of the medical profession. Psychiatrists worked in both the public and the private sectors—that is to say, in institutions for pauper lunatics as well as in more select houses for the affluent. Drawing on a variety of sources, the theoretical aim was to establish somaticist or biological/materialist explanations for mental disease, focusing on the brain but always retaining a place for the additional causal effects of personal unhappiness, business misfortune, loss of children through early death, and so on. The work, for example, of the German academic psychiatrist Wilhelm Griesinger (1817–68) was famous for the rallying cry 'Psychological diseases are diseases of the brain' and its firm hostility to earlier idealist or Romantic German psychiatric writing. But Griesinger was equally interested in the unconscious and in dream analysis. University psychiatry was developed outside the asylum and thus outside the harsh world of boredom and violence that asylum staff often inhabited, but the key task, to develop an organic psychiatry that allowed for behavioural and secondary mental characteristics, was all the more pronounced. As we shall see, this materialist mission was eventually to lead to proposals, many of them turned down, of a wedding between psychiatry and neurology. But even this wedding had its earlier versions, most notably the interest taken among psychiatrists in the phrenological teachings of Franz Joseph Gall (1758–1828) and J. C. Spurzheim (1776–1832).

In a bold attempt to detach the understanding of mental functions from philosophy and to root it in anatomy, Gall proposed that the brain was the organ of the mind; that the brain was composed of several parts, each of them constituting a distinct mental faculty, the size of the individual part directly indicating the power or lack of it for the faculty in question. Even when found wanting by medical men, which was the case by the 1850s, phrenology had a great impact in the general plan to locate medicine and the mind on that altar of orthodoxy—the brain. *Brain* was the name given to a British psychiatric and neurological journal from 1878, and it is worth noting that one of its founders, James Crichton-Browne (1840–1938), was deeply influenced by the educational and social aims of phrenology. Mainstream medicine and the mind continually sought the extension of organic explanations for mental illness while holding to non-restraint and moral management as the proper form of government in the asylum itself.

Before looking at the actual experience of the asylum for those on the receiving end of the theories of an emergent psychiatry, it is worth examining some of the ways in which the theories sketched here were extended, with real implications for ideas on mental life in general. Was unusual human creativity, for example, in fact linked to certain kinds of madness? Was it possible to

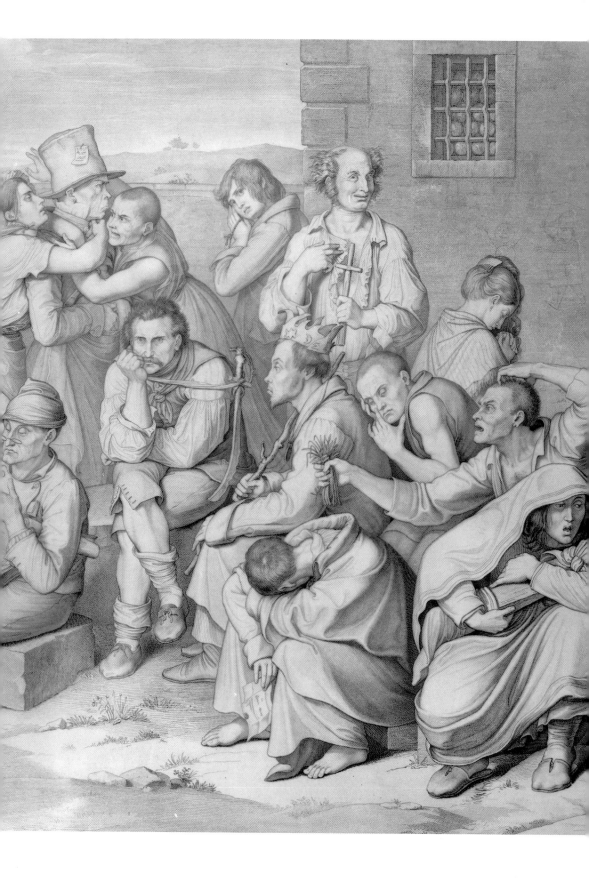

be only partially insane, to be wholly recognizable as sane except with regard
to one particular area, an area that could nevertheless lead to the overthrow of
the healthy mind and culminate in acts of violence? And what about the possibility that people could be morally insane—that is to say, have nothing broken or diseased within their capacity to reason, in the sense of 'knowing what
they were doing', and yet be insane because their moral faculty was lost and
broken? They pick up a gun in the full knowledge it is a gun, with bullets, but
the moral restraint to desist from using it has gone, making them mad. Did the
asylums see such new objects of psychiatry's attention amongst its troubled
multitude?

One clear way of investigating this story of the growth of psychiatric explanations for medicine's understanding of the mind is to examine the first early
appearances of the notion of criminal insanity. Deployed by a number of
skilled US and European doctors and lawyers from the late eighteenth century,
the case for deeming certain persons brought to trial as criminally insane and
thus needing treatment not imprisonment or execution was a major topic in
both legal and psychiatric circles by mid-century. In Britain in 1843 the argument was brought to a head in the trial of Daniel McNaghten, a Glasgow wood-
turner who had tried, and tried unsuccessfully, to murder the Prime Minister
Sir Robert Peel. Instead, McNaghten had shot and killed the Prime Minister's
private secretary. At the trial a strong case was made that the accused was in
the grip of a partial insanity that might lead to a 'partial or total aberration of
the moral senses and affections, which may render the wretched patient incapable of resisting the delusion, and lead him to commit crimes for which
morally he cannot be held responsible . . .'. Finally the jury brought in a verdict
that found the defendant insane at the time of the act, and McNaghten was
sent to Bethlem and eventually to a new kind of hospital, Broadmoor, for the
criminally insane. In ways that are not hard to recapture in current debates on
capital punishment, this verdict caused a great deal of public shock. Was it
really true that McNaghten had not known that what he was doing was wrong,
was against the law of the land? Even if he was convinced that the Tory Party
and its minions, the metropolitan police force, even at one time the Church of
Rome were all out to get him, why should he be excused an act of murder and
escape execution? The House of Lords was asked to bring some clarification, to
sort out what one historian has called two incommensurable discourses: the
legal (wherein human agency is voluntary and responsible) and the new med-
ical/psychiatric (wherein human agency is often governed by forces outside its
control and is in the proper sense irresponsible).

The attempt at clarification by the Law Lords was known as the McNaghten
rules, and the confusing nature of the rules tells a great deal about the relationship between medicine, psychiatry, and the law in the middle of the nineteenth century. If he is to be defended on the grounds of insanity the accused
must have been 'labouring under such a defect of reason, from disease of the
mind as not to know the nature and quality of the act he was doing; or, if he did
know it, that he did not know he was doing what was wrong'. To put it more
simply, the rules fell between two stools, neither ruling out the possibility of
the effects of mental disease nor letting go of the need for defendants to be
judged as to whether they could tell the difference between right and wrong at

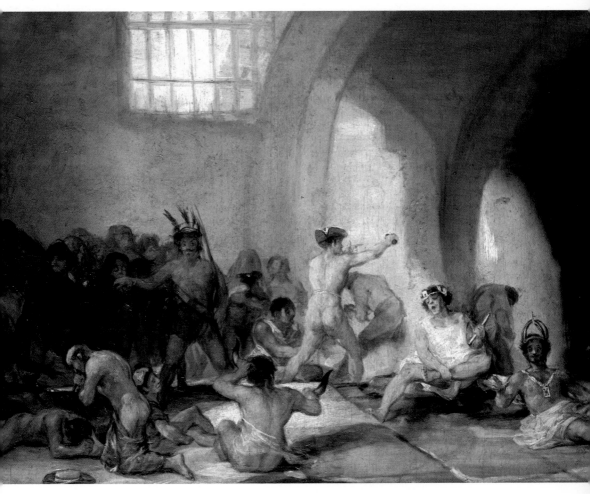

The Madhouse, by Goya. A powerful portrait of both personal and social hell, Goya is both bringing a hidden work into sight and giving a warning about the destiny of the isolated Romantic imagination.

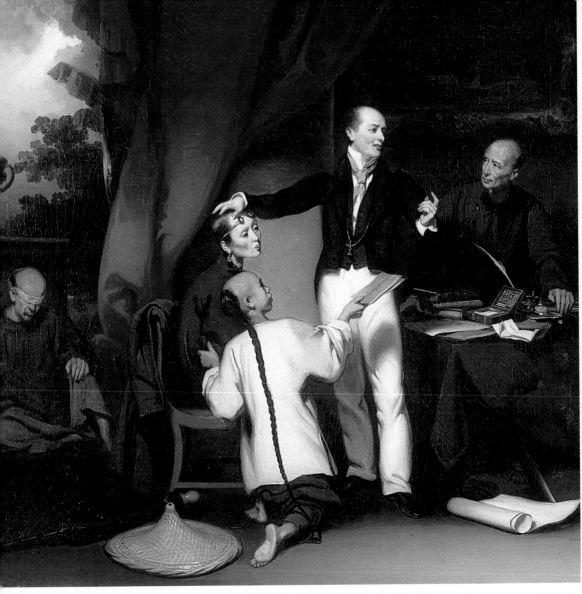

Thomas Colledge treating a Chinese patient at the opthalmic hospital he founded in 1828 in Macao, China. Colledge was an East India Company doctor who began treating Chinese patients and went on to found a hospital and dispensary. In the 1830s he worked with the American medical missionary Peter Parker and was a founder of the Medical Missionary Society in 1838.

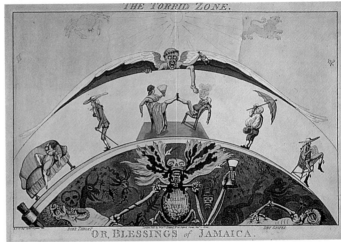

THE TORRID ZONE.

OR, BLESSINGS of JAMAICA.

The Torrid Zone. *Jamaica: Languorous noons in the hells of yellow fever.* European colonialists had an ambivalent view of the tropics: it was a region that might produce great wealth and pleasure; yet its environment was also threatening and dangerous, not least because of diseases like yellow fever which were new to western medicine.

the time of the act. The full case for psychiatric illness was not accepted, because the moral element was retained: the legal lay down with the medical, causing confusion for many decades. The full nature of this confusion can be easily summarized. Daniel McNaghten was convinced that there was an organized conspiracy, led by the government, to persecute him. At the time he attempted to kill the Prime Minister, he knew that the act was wrong but this was as nothing compared to his delusional conviction. He was found not guilty by virtue of insanity, but the catch is this (one of the first paradoxes in the nineteenth-century dispute between law, medicine, and the mind and their various claims to authority): under the rules to which he gave his name, Daniel McNaghten would have been hanged.

The general world of the asylum did not, therefore, see criminal lunatics, at least from the mid-1860s, because they were granted their own hospital, Broadmoor. But a general accumulation of a variety of unfortunates, many of them poor, did have one striking historical effect: a silting-up of the institutions themselves and a very early death for the optimism and ambition behind the theories of moral management and the hope that the asylum as a second home, a place for the 'domestication of madness', would bring reasonable rates of cure and discharge. This dream faded, even in the lifetime of the most famous of the English moral managers, John Conolly (1794–1866). Conolly's name both in Europe and the USA was synonymous with non-restraint as a system and with the promise that architecture, discipline, and courtesy might combine to bring reasonable rates of cure. Especially in the USA, the sheer difficulty of keeping this ideal alive in actual asylum practice was swiftly realized, and a mournful, but all too real, possibility loomed into view. The asylum was in fact much like the poorhouse. The asylum was in real terms a place where the theories of medicine and the mind meant very little, where restraint, ill-feeling, and subdued violence were the order of the day. It was, for all that, a place that was difficult to leave, because the outside world was now unmanageable and hostile. A museum, a place where new and startling behaviours might be sighted and written about by doctors (females masturbating in shared quarters, females uttering endless obscenities, males convinced they were Napoleon, males soliciting attendants) but where the first promise of environmentalist reform and re-education was failing. Museums of madness, full of refugees from agricultural depression, or ex-slaves in the USA, or those who could not succeed in the arbitrary and heartless political economy of the UK, the first industrial nation. If all the work to promote a scientific and usually secular psychiatry had resulted only in a population that might as well be in the workhouse, was there another explanation, another foundation for medicine and ideas of the mind, more scientific and also more realistic because more pessimistic? If so, how might psychiatry reflect this sombre mood in its contribution to medical philosophy?

The Tyranny of Organization

In ways that might be thought to have echoes of classical ideas of cruel fate, the nineteenth-century life sciences generated powerful theories of biological evolution that proposed a natural explanation for human nature and how that

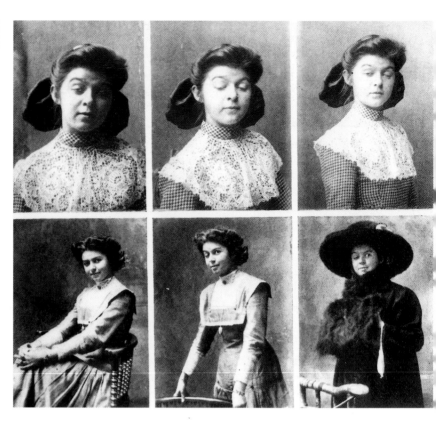

The ocular manifestations
of hysteria in a
photograph from 1912.
The growth in the imagery
of the hysteric,
photographic or
otherwise, was a
representation of the
patient which at the same
time displayed the expert
understanding of the
observing physician. Here,
the eyes have to be read
and interpreted as part of
the wider representation
of the signs of hysteria.

nature was shaped by heredity. Individuals were not merely related to animal ancestors, they were constituted out of familial pasts that made heredity the determining factor in the character, the skills, and the disposition to illness in the present generation. Ghosts were seen as the authors of the script being acted out to descendants whose strength or weakness was determined to a large extent by forces beyond individual control. In the words of the pessimistic British psychiatrist Henry Maudsley (1835–1918), 'We may rest assured of this, that infirmities of mind are transmitted from parent to child by a law as sure and constant as is any physical infirmity.' Maudsley was unusually pessimistic and came to doubt the efficacy of much asylum practice. But the central theme in the life sciences and in medicine both before and after Darwin was that no one could escape the tyranny of their organization, their unasked-for hereditarian legacy.

There were, of course, varying degrees as to how far a pessimistic hereditarianism was fully accepted within differing national psychiatries and indeed within different parts of the medical profession. In general, those involved in public-health initiatives and then in the various movements under the banner of mental hygiene stressed the environmental causes of apparent pathologies and their dependence on bad diet, bad housing, and bad planning: these could be altered if the political will existed. On the other side of the nature/nurture divide, the appeal to social and thereby changeable causes for illness or maladaption was refuted. Especially in Darwinism, the frail, the chronically mentally ill, the tuberculous—all these were the objects of natural selection and a minimum of interference was required in order that the forces of selection might do their work, leaving a stronger general population.

But, whatever the disagreements, these arguments took place under the shadow of an old but now biologically approved 'scientific' idea: degeneration. Some individuals, some families, maybe some types of human being were forms of arrested development, caught in the grip of hereditary taint. The case for degeneration could be made within a French psychiatry influenced by Catholicism or it could come out of Darwinism—the crucial point for the asylum doctor was that the optimistic aspects of moral management had to be exchanged for a bleaker prospect for psychiatric therapies which none the less demanded the presence and the skill of the trained medical psychiatrist. The asylum might become custodial and (generally) non-curative, but its continuing contribution to social health was in some respects all the more important. The sad procession of familial degeneration, accumulating across the generations, had to be mapped and then supervised by the same figure who had previously placed his hopes in moral management. Henry Maudsley the pessimist was the son-in-law of John Conolly the optimist, and their proximity was also the proximity of one dream of the asylum turning very quickly to something else.

This shift in the social role of the asylum coincided with an even more extended application of psychiatric analyses to human character and behaviour. The differences between male and female natures were now placed within an evolutionary framework which stressed antipodean difference and new hierarchies. Female life was defined by cycles of reproduction and its attendant dangers, while female sexual practices not aimed at reproduction were deemed abnormal and morally perverse. The natural female life was therefore domesticated and vulnerable: it was fecund and yet passive, emotionally sensitive and yet confined to the home, not the market place or the political arena. Above all, and especially for Darwinians, it was not a life where sexual selection was an active female possibility. Human evolution depended on males competing among themselves and to the victor the female spoils: women waited to be asked. In French biomedicine and psychiatry, a particular emphasis was made on the difference between male and female brains and their capacities, an approach stimulated by the work of Paul Broca (1824–80) on cerebral localization and on anthropology. The left hemisphere was less developed in the female, containing as it did the site for the more advanced capacities.

In Britain the model was more evolutionary, especially in the influential work of John Hughlings Jackson (1835–1911). Jackson used the language of evolution and its opposites and was most well known for his discussion of one disease widely observed in the asylum world, epilepsy. But, as with degeneration debates in general, whatever the differences of explanation involved, all sides had their agreements. One was that deviations from the naturalistic account of the normal life—domestic and reproductive for women, political and external and aggressive for men—could lead to madness. Men without will, full of introspective gloom and physically feeble, might become sexual inverts and melancholics. Women without homes, seeking the solace of alcohol or sex without responsibility, might become manic, obscene, and violent. These are almost the clichés of nineteenth-century ideas of deviance. Less noticed until recently was one great implication of this gendered view of medicine and the mind: that, because the female brain was less developed or evolved, women by definition could not practise the very activities—the very sciences—that constructed these accounts of their biological difference. They were to be objects and not subjects, studied by the male practitioners of medicine and the sciences until such time as these bastions of educational privilege were entered. But, of course, for many psychiatrists, the desire to enter these bastions was itself a form of mental disturbance. Being female was itself close to being a malady, in the very tight definitions of biomedical normality that a great deal of the psychiatry of the nineteenth century endorsed. An account of medicine and the mind written by women, and a psychiatry that took its cue from that, was a long way off.

Finding the Patient

There is a multitude of psychiatric diagnoses that come into fashion and are then gone, and the only reason for noting this is to remind ourselves about the fashionability of diagnostic criteria, a feature of medicine that the history of medicine and the mind displays very clearly. Does masturbation lead to insanity? Hardly a nineteenth-century doctor thought that it did not. Was the constant attempt to escape from slave plantations a sign of mental disturbance? Was it a reason to ask medicine to cast its eye on the mind if a wealthy landowner decided to pay his agricultural workers more than the amount that seemed rational to political economists? Was it a sign of mental illness to have constant cravings for sexual relations with members of one's own sex? Of all the many examples that might be explored, one stands out in indicating the ambitions of psychiatry in the period from the 1840s to the present.

Hardly an American or British psychiatrist or psychoanalyst has not written on the case in question, the customary attempt being to solve a mystery that has eluded previous authors. This is the case of Hamlet and his various relationships but especially that with Ophelia. The use of Ophelia as a type of unfortunate young woman, driven mad by a love that is cruelly abused, was sufficiently widespread for versions of Ophelia to be posed in asylum photographs. As for Hamlet himself, the key point that psychiatric medicine wished to make was that his famously adopted mad style, his 'antic disposition', was not the theatrical riddle that previous critics and previous audiences had seen. The adoption of madness was actual madness; the character became trapped in the part and could not escape. He suffered from insane hallucinations, he was abusive to his seniors and to his girlfriend, who then committed suicide. His own suicidal longings were pathological. His melancholy did not display the sad wisdom of a prince who knew the corruption of the state, as the Jacobean audience might have thought and as admirers of the prince in the period of European Romanticism had also thought. No: he was exactly the morally destructive, abusive kind of young man, full of fantasies and a pathological lack of will, who played at being mad because he did not know that he was mad. Hamlet belonged in the asylum. Other accounts—that he longed for his mother, but did not realize it, is the most famous—are not nearly as widespread in the psychiatric literature as the writings that 'solve' Hamlet's madness. And medicine and the mind could, at a very tricky moment in the history of the psychiatric profession, come up with a new founding father, to be placed alongside Pinel and Conolly: William Shakespeare, the first psychiatrist. The history of retrospective diagnoses of Shakespearian characters is a potted history of the profession's ideas of itself.

Heroic Remedies, Desperate Cures, and Fringe Counter-Attacks

It would be fair to say that the organicist drive within mainstream psychiatry became even stronger in the period from 1880 onwards than it had been previously. The work of Karl Wernicke (1848–1905) on aphasia and on cerebral localization and concepts of cerebral dominance was the most famous European example, and the utility of this approach was borne out when, for example, the psychiatric signs of secondary and then tertiary syphilis became understood. Asylum populations had large numbers of alcoholics and syphilitics among them: it was perfectly proper to be dubious about their chances of avoiding their fate (until at least the arrival of Salvarsan in the late 1910s and then penicillin in the 1940s) while explaining that fate in strong materialist medical terms, whether exposing the diseased philosophy of the syphilitic Friedrich Nietzsche (1844–1900) or simply tracking the decline of an unknown pauper.

Dr Egas Moniz was the first medical practitioner to carry out a pre-frontal leucotomy, in 1935. In 1949 he was awarded the Nobel Prize for his discovery of the therapeutic value of leucotomy in certain psychoses.

There did, however, arise certain problems within asylum practice at the century's end. Medical science had undergone a bacteriological revolution in those years, with new laboratory-based identifications of the typhoid bacillus, the tubercle bacillus, the cholera vibrio, and the diphtheria bacillus among others. From the 1880s there had also been a growth in the use of what one historian has called 'fantasy surgery'—surgical operations on patients who presented with certain signs but for whom the actual physical site for the cause of distress was invisible. None the less it was thought they would improve if certain body parts (ovaries, colons, appendices) were shortened or removed. Psychiatry had not kept up with this and had also not kept up with the clinical sophistication of neurology. Neurology had joined with psychiatry in places— Wernicke's work was an example—but too often the academic had become divorced from the practical and the harsh realities of the asylum seemed distant from the advances in clinical medicine.

The new century saw some startling attempts to rectify this awkward situation, culminating in the treatments of the 1930s—insulin shock, metrazole shock, electric shock, and then finally psychosurgery. The inventor of the pre-frontal leucotomy, Egas Moniz (1874–1955), was awarded the Nobel Prize for Medicine, and, along with that of other doctors, his reputation testifies to the rapidity of these new interventions entering the mainstream. It is clear that by the time electroconvulsive therapy (ECT) was first employed in 1938, the relationship between medicine and the mind had reached a new dividing-point and a historically significant crossroads. What was to be the status accorded those therapies that stressed the functional nature of mental disorder as against the biological or organicist, whose methods now included direct action on the brain itself? How would psychology fit with psychiatry and how

245

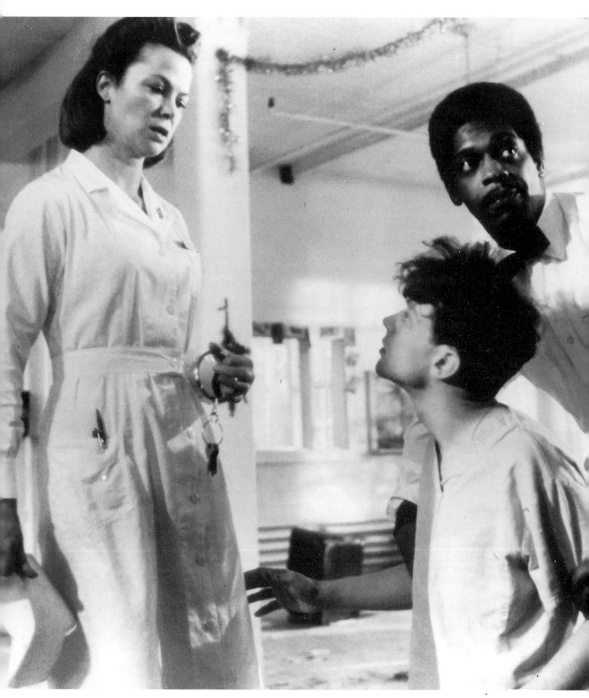

Scene from the satirical film *One Flew Over the Cuckoo's Nest*, which attacked some of the most brutal aspects of the treatment of the insane.

would psychiatry fit with neurology? And where would spiritualism fit in, or strange esoteric *fin-de-siècle* religious cults? And what, finally, of the asylum itself, that huge building on the edge of town, behind the bushes and out of most citizens' ken or even their interest?

The possible misuse of psychosurgical and electroconvulsive procedures is still debated, and the careers of those who favoured them (as against psychotherapeutic or other techniques) are seen as either realist and heroic or

246

cruel and destructive. For historical purposes, no career shows up the contra-
diction better than that of Sigmund Freud (1856–1939).

It is often forgotten that Freud started his career as a neurologist and a very anti-idealist one at that. He was a product of Viennese hard-line organic neuroscience who broke away entirely into the alternative world–the world where talking in the fullest sense, the most open and unsecretive sense, can alter the state of the patient's body. Psychoanalysis is based on an absolute neurophysiological materialism that also holds that the way into that world is through the verbal news that the patient brings, unknowingly, from his or her unconscious. In that sense Freud completed a defection from the hunt for the physical basis of mental illness in the brain that had started in the late Enlightenment with F. A. Mesmer (1734–1815) and been extended by the French neurologist J. M. Charcot (1825–93). The history of ideas of animal magnetism and then the use of hypnosis by Charcot in examining hysteria culminated in Freud's sexual theory of the origin of neurosis, to be understood by talking to an invisible listener in a darkened room. The theme of classical connections to the ancients was not missing even here: many male talkers were to discover that they were experiencing the very things experienced by Oedipus–a longing to kill the father and marry the mother.

It need hardly be added that in psychiatric cultures where the hopes of moral management were not entirely dead, such as the UK, this journey into the basement of the individual life was seen as a fraudulent misapplication of true principles. The slow accumulation of evidence that Freud and his followers were quite as capable as other doctors of damaging patients' lives, often women patients, reinforced this hostility. Hope, according to these practitioners, could return only by diversion, by physical exercise, and by drug therapy. This last point was reinforced with the arrival of new tranquillizers in the mid-1950s, such as chlorpromazine, this being followed by other psychoactive drugs, including anti-depressants and then lithium for the treatment of manic depression. This important series of developments gave impetus to the neurophysiological research project in Western medicine and in turn spurred on the research project for a genetics-based understanding of mental disorders, usually running in families. The distance between these approaches and the psychoanalytic is great, and current psychiatric orthodoxy can rightly point to its ability to combine the functional and the biological without losing sight of the main goal–the organic understanding of mental disease. In that sense the academic aims of much nineteenth-century psychiatry have been realized, thanks to the advances in psychopharmacology.

Care in the Elusive Community

The history of medicine and the mind displays a wealth of conditions and diagnoses that are jettisoned almost as quickly as they are invented. And the task of proving the etiology for mental disorders is not easy–the status of disease is not granted to ailments that have an unproven etiology, and in *Diagnostic and Statistical Manual 3*, for example, they are named as syndromes or disorders. In the same edition of this influential manual, produced in 1980, homosexuality was removed as a mental disorder. This is but one example of the history of

changes in classification, but the historian might be allowed to wonder what Plato or the ancient philosophers would have thought of its being there at all! It is not impossible that schizophrenia, itself coined in the early twentieth century to clarify confusions relating to the category dementia praecox, may one day have served its turn and be replaced by a newly coined and preferably classical-sounding name.

And beneath all these alterations of language, suffering continues and needs assistance, exactly as the Quakers knew in York in the 1790s and the families of the distressed have known through historical time. The admission of strange and difficult behaviours to outsiders is as much part of the story as the cynical use of psychiatric interventions to see off annoying members of families. Current policy in both Europe and the USA is to cut down on the numbers inside the large asylums and deliver them into the 'community'—quite often back to the family, if there be one. The difficulties and dangers of this policy have brought yet another change in the history of mental-health policy and attitudes: that the asylum, so long the dreaded Victorian dustbin full of the unwanted and the dangerous, and so often the target of the anti-psychiatry writings of the present century, should not be closed, should not be traded for care in the community which does not exist.

According to this view, the asylum may have to be revived, but revived in the light of the understanding and the knowledge that looking at the history of medicine and the mind can bring. In particular it must be recognized that mental disorder is real, even if concise watertight definitions of mental disorders, along the lines of definitions of organic disease, are virtually impossible. The study of medicine and the mind combines a fascinating variety of claims to understanding but also historically based responsibilities for care and support. It may well be that the best conjunction between theory and practice is one that asks for the shredding of the claims to expertise, many of which have produced cruelty, false diagnosis, involuntary incarceration, and, when put to political use, outright terror to promote social conformity. The historical lesson may be that the less that is claimed for certainties of medical knowledge in this shifting landscape, the less esoteric the diagnostic terms, the more the lay community will be able to understand, tolerate, and cope with mental disorder. The history of medicine and the mind teaches us about the varieties of religious experience, the varieties of psychiatric attempts at the solution of mental disorders, and the varieties of failure. The historical understanding for these very failures should be seen as enlightening and instructive elements in the continuing attempts to understand and care for those suffering from mental disorders.

16 | The Spread of Western Medicine

MICHAEL WORBOYS

A WORLD survey of medical ideas and practices in AD 1000 would have found three 'great systems'—the Chinese, Indian, and Western, though the latter would have been more appropriately termed 'Mediterranean', as it was based largely on Greek, Roman, and Islamic ideas. Alongside these systems was a myriad of 'little systems' and folk beliefs, specific to local communities or regions. The 'great systems' all worked with similar humoral models of bodily function and were broadly equivalent in their therapeutic aims and efficacy. There had been contact between them, but each remained quite distinct, embedded in the religion, culture, and politics of its society. A similar survey undertaken today, as the next millennium closes, would find a single predominant medical system—Western medicine. While having roots that are traceable to its forebear, modern Western medicine shows little or no resemblance to its earlier form. What is historically distinctive about the Western medical tradition has been the revolutionary changes that have taken place in its ideas and practices, especially since the eighteenth century. This is not to say that Chinese, Indian, and other systems have remained static, but that they evolved more slowly and have probably changed most in the last 100 years in response to the claims of modern Western medicine to be the world orthodoxy. These other systems persist today and some thrive, though now as 'traditional' and 'alternative' systems, or as lay beliefs.

From the Renaissance, Western medicine began to diverge from other systems in its beliefs and organization. However, it was not until the end of the eighteenth century that humoral ideas were abandoned and replaced by a view of the body as made up of parts—organs, tissues, and cells—where disease is due to structural abnormalities or physiological malfunctions. Defined in this way, the body became subject to ever more invasive and interventionist procedures, seeking to repair, correct, or remove the sources of disease. The training of modern Western medical practitioners has become more science-based, with professional standing dependent on knowledge rather than status. Indeed, the defining characteristic of modern Western medicine, especially to its critics, has been its reductionism and materialist approach, treating the disease rather than healing the whole sick person.

Since the organized medical profession in almost every country in the world now not only practises but itself develops modern Western medicine, it has been argued that *cosmopolitan* or simply *modern* medicine are more appropriate terms. However, the term Western medicine remains valuable historically as it was in Europe, and latterly North America, that this now dominant medical enterprise developed, and from these regions that it was spread to the rest of the world. That said, Western medicine was not and is not a single entity and it has to be remembered that it has changed over time, and that in any period ideas and practices varied between different national and professional groups.

The spread of Western medicine across the world over several centuries is a huge topic; hence this chapter makes no attempt to be comprehensive. The approach taken is to concentrate on the contexts in which the Western medical tradition spread, on the main agencies involved, and on the ways in which it was received in non-Western societies or those in the process of Westernization. We can identify three major ways of looking at changes that have occurred across the world and the centuries. First, there was the change from the position before 1800, when there was an exchange of ideas between the largely non-Western systems of medicine, to the modern situation, when Western medicine has become the dominant, monopolistic form of medical theory and practice. Secondly, there was the change from the passive, or even accidental, introduction of Western medicine as an adjunct to European exploration, settlement, or colonial rule, to deliberate and active attempts to impose Western medical traditions either as part of imperialism, or later as part of the modernization of independent states. Thirdly, there are the changes which were initiated by non-Western societies themselves when they appropriated Western medicine and adapted it to their own environment and purposes.

This chapter is divided into three broadly chronological sections which define the main context of change: settlement, imperialism, and modernization.

Settlement

European explorers usually took a surgeon or physician along with them to look after their health. Medical services were much in demand, as these ventures typically saw high rates of sickness and death from injuries, malnutrition, and fevers. Whilst early explorers, soldiers, settlers, missionaries, and traders took it for granted that their medicine, like the rest of their culture, was superior to that which they found in other societies, they were willing to swap ideas and remedies with local healers. Working in remote situations, with few resources and often confronted with unfamiliar diseases, Western practitioners had little to lose and a lot to gain from such exchanges. As noted already, Western and other traditions shared similar humoral models, and it was sometimes suggested that indigenous therapies might be better suited to local diseases. Therapies, which could be assessed empirically and given new rationales, were exchanged more easily than ideas, which in all systems were closely linked to religious and other beliefs.

Healers and lay people in other continents also sought to learn from and use European practitioners and were particularly impressed by the technical skills of Western surgeons. However, the openness of other cultures to Western medicine varied greatly in space and time. Until this century, the developed medical traditions in Asia provided a formidable barrier to Western medicine, and in China and Japan this was linked to a powerful political resistance to Western influence more generally. This meant that the activities of those very few Western medical practitioners who became resident in missions and trading stations in East Asia were controlled and that they contributed little to the diffusion of Western medicine locally.

Western medicine was carried to the Americas, Australasia, and southern Africa as an integral part of European settlement of these lands. Settlers also carried with them European diseases, such as smallpox and measles, against which the indigenous peoples had no immunity. This led, especially in the Americas, to the decimation of the indigenous population and contributed massively to the destruction of their societies. The sense that the New World was a hostile place was reinforced by the high death rates amongst settlers, though this was due more to insanitary conditions than exposure to new diseases; the exception was yellow fever, which seems to have spread to the Americas from Africa with the growth of Atlantic trade. Following humoral ideas, it was argued that European bodies were ill-adapted to the new environments in which they found themselves and that their balance and operation were upset by it. Medical practitioners felt powerless in the face of such forces and largely offered the standard regimes and treatments of the Western canon, or variations on this. However, experience taught that in a generation or so Europeans became 'seasoned' or acclimatized, and, more surprisingly, that the general health of settlers became better than that enjoyed back in Europe. The change was such that the New World was soon experienced as a healthier and more productive environment, where Europeans might flourish free of the corrupting influences, physical and moral, of the Old World. The relatively low numbers of qualified practitioners amongst migrants, together with the scattered pattern of settlement, meant that organized medicine was even less accessible than it had been in Europe. This reinforced the already strong tradition of self-help medical care and led to a greater tolerance of lay and other non-orthodox healers in these new societies.

In North America, Australasia, and elsewhere where new European-style societies were re-created, the full range of Western medical institutions was eventually established. Practitioners in these new countries modelled their hospitals and training programmes on those in Europe, yet they continued to regard their practice as derivative, and Europe remained the main source of knowledge and professional legitimacy. In some cases, as in Australia and New Zealand, medical dependency followed political ties, but elsewhere, most notably in Canada and Latin American countries, the geographical position and growing cultural power of the USA created linkages that broke with historical and political ties. As new countries, such as the USA, moved towards political independence, there were parallel moves to throw off the yoke of direct European medical control; the establishment of local medical organizations was often an integral part of wider nationalist activities. None the less,

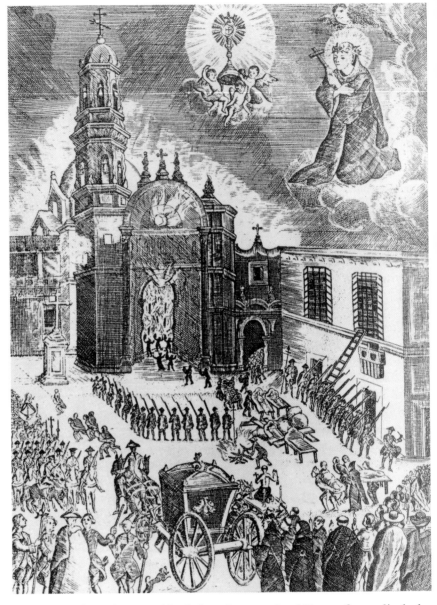

**Hospital de San Juan de
Dios**, Mexico, 1766. In the
New World, hospitals were
established on the pattern
of European institutions,
being primarily places of
Christian charity. They
were refuges for the poor,
orphans, the aged, and
travellers as well as the
sick. This engraving of the
hospital burning down
offers a rare glimpse of
the sick inmates, all of
whom appear bed-bound
or disabled. The social
and political importance
of the hospital in the town
is shown by the presence
of the army and the local
nobility.

Europe, and from the 1880s North America, remained Meccas for medical education, postgraduate experience, and research, and to this day they continue to draw practitioners and scientists from across the world.

Imperialism

In areas of European settlement, broadly similar mechanisms of transferring Western medicine operated, with broadly similar results. However, in countries that resisted settlement, or were deemed unsuitable, Western medicine spread in a number of quite different ways. While there was still some passive carriage by the medical personnel who supported military, administrative, and trading ventures, the new departure was the deliberate transfer of Western medicine as part of wider political, economic, or social policies. European imperial powers transferred medicine to colonial territories as a 'tool of empire', to protect and consolidate their control. The rulers of independent countries who wished to modernize their culture and economy often chose to adopt Western medicine as part of programmes of changing beliefs, remodelling institutions, and seeking economic transformation. Non-governmental agencies were also involved with the active dissemination of Western medicine; individual practitioners, missionary medical organizations, philanthropic foundations, and international medical organizations all played a role.

Formal and informal European imperialism in Africa, Asia, and South America was concentrated in tropical regions where disease played a major part in deterring attempts at European settlement. Until the end of the nineteenth century most medical work in these areas concentrated upon protecting and maintaining the health of Europeans. With practice confined to enclaves and with so few practitioners, Western medicine did not reach the indigenous peoples to any great extent. This was evident in perhaps the most lucrative of all imperial ventures—taking African slaves to the Americas. This trade initiated yet another global exchange of pathogens, further massive losses of life, and new disease ecologies on both sides of the Atlantic. Despite this, for many decades the health problems created by the slave trade were ignored; shortfalls in number due to deaths and disabilities were compensated for by taking yet more Africans from ever deeper into the continent. Only during the second half of the eighteenth century, and then for reasons of economy as much as humanitarian concern, were efforts made to maintain the health of slaves. These included the establishment of hospitals and, most importantly for the number of lives saved, preventive inoculation against smallpox.

This procedure is often claimed to be one of the great triumphs of Western medicine, as it eventually helped to eliminate smallpox from the world. However, inoculation was practised in Asian and Islamic countries before being introduced into Europe from Turkey in 1717. What changed following its adoption in Western medicine was that it was more widely diffused through European networks of power, and then was refined and made safer, with cowpox lymph replacing the use of material from actual smallpox cases. Further innovations followed, notably using lymph from animals rather than taking it from person to person, which made the technique much easier to use, even in remote areas. This story shows both that Western medicine, especially before the nineteenth century, did learn from other systems, but also that exchanges facilitated the development and improvement of knowledge and technique.

The protection afforded by inoculation against smallpox was of minor value to Europeans in the tropics, as they continued to suffer mortality rates which were much higher than those by then current in Europe and in areas of European settlement in the New World. Deaths from disease hindered military campaigns, and, in several cases in the West Indies in the eighteenth century, over two-thirds of the men were lost to disease. There were variations between stations, and in one or two places, notably Tahiti, European health improved in tropical climes. The main source of European deaths and ill health were so-called 'tropical fevers', probably what we would now differentiate as yellow fever, malaria, typhoid, cholera, and amoebic dysentery. These fevers were seen to be due to either the direct weakening effects of heat and sunlight, or the indirect effects of climate on the production of disease poisons that spread through the air as miasmas. Western medical opinion was generally pessimistic about the possibilities of curing fevers—which were thought to have to run their course—and put more stress on prevention and avoidance. It was assumed, with little or no real evidence, that the indigenous peoples of the tropics did not suffer from such afflictions to the same degree, as they were acclimatized to the tropics and lived in harmony with the local environment. Medical beliefs were important in creating and sustaining ideas of race and racial difference, especially differential mortality and the accumulation of anatomical data. Later in the nineteenth century, when the idea of the healthy Noble Savage was abandoned, other medical ideas meshed with Social Darwinism to support ideas that coloured races were degenerate, licentious, indolent, polluted and polluting, and hence dangerous carriers of disease.

The first deliberate attempts to spread Western medicine to the indigenous population of colonial and other territories were made by medical missionaries. Jesuit orders had missions in China and America from the sixteenth century; however, the limited medical services that they had were there to look after the health of the brothers, not to serve local communities or to help spread Christian beliefs and ideals. Indeed, like other Europeans in strange lands, Jesuit brothers had been eager to learn from other medical systems and were responsible for many of the earliest translations of texts between traditions. Medical services became an integral part of the evangelical armoury only with the new wave of mainly Protestant missionaries in the nineteenth century. The first medical missionary in Africa was John Van der Kemp from Holland in 1799, while in China it was an American, Peter Parker, who arrived in 1834. The full integration of medical services into missionary activity took place after mid-century, with the exploits of Dr David Livingstone, who was not medically qualified, in Central Africa. His travels, or more exactly the popular reporting of his adventures, caught the imagination of the Anglo-American public, brought in money to support similar ventures, and inspired religious-minded medical practitioners to emulate his exploits. There were many motives behind this work, as the aims of the Medical Missionary Society in China, founded in 1838, testify. They were variously: to allow Christian philanthropy and service; to diffuse the benefits of Western science and technology; and, above all, 'To cultivate confidence and friendship, and introduce the Gospel of Christ in place of heathenism'. The wider missionary movement had mixed feelings about medical work and worried that saving of bodies would take precedence over saving of souls, so it was usually incumbent on the medical missionary to build a church before a hospital.

Although Christian missionaries were active across the world, it was their work in 'Darkest Africa' that attracted most attention. They generally claimed complete cultural superiority and demanded total conversion to their faith and its values. Undermining the influence of other faiths, particularly the power of superstition and the hated 'witch doctors', was where missionaries felt Western medicine would be valuable. Whatever happened with conversions of faith, in medicine it appears there was no simple nor total conversion

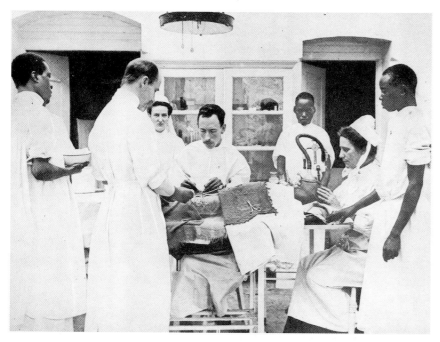

Albert Cook, a Christian Missionary Society doctor, operating at the Mengo Hospital, Uganda, *c*.1900. From the point of view of other cultures, major surgical operations, particularly the removal of tumours and cataracts, were the most impressive and distinctive features of modern Western medicine at the turn of this century.

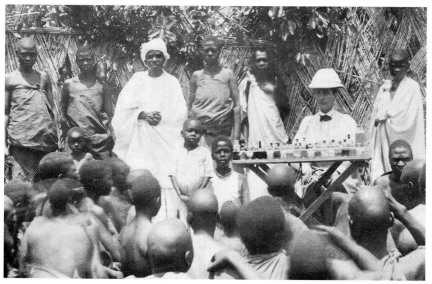

Mrs Cook dispensing medicines on safari, *c*.1900. Many missionary doctors were accompanied by their wives, who helped in both their clinical and spiritual work. Besides founding mission hospitals, doctors visited remote villages to dispense medicines and the scriptures. The Western pharmacopoeia, which still mainly consisted of plant- and mineral-based drugs was more readily transferred across cultures than other features of Western medicine.

to Western medicine amongst Africans. Rather, they operated what is now termed 'medical pluralism'; that is, they used different healers for different purposes and moved between healers, and hence systems, to obtain the best care and treatment. This was not, and is not, very different from the situation within Western societies, where patients have regularly sought second opinions and where alternative healers and remedies have always been available. In their selective use of Western missions, Africans were particularly impressed by the skills of Western surgeons, and operations to remove tumours and on the eyes—especially operations for cataracts which often allowed the blind to see again—were especially favoured. The dramatic quali-

255

ties of the latter, as well as the biblical resonances, were not lost on missionaries. It should be noted that medical missions spread Western medicine in the context of spiritual and moral values, a position quite different from that in Europe and North America, where its development was increasingly linked with materialism and secularization.

Until well into the twentieth century, the scale and orientation of medical missionary work in colonial Africa and Asia meant that it touched more people than the services provided by the colonial governments, although it is important to recognize that many places, especially in smaller settlements and in remote rural areas, were untouched by missionary or state provision. In countries like India and China, where the scope of evangelism was much more limited, medical missions still helped to shape Western medical institutions. The first Western medical school in China was set up in Tientsin by the missionary J. K. MacKenzie in 1881, with financial assistance from the local Viceroy Li Hung-chang, and the London Missionary Society aided the foundation of the Hong Kong Medical College in 1887. In India from the 1880s, women medical missionaries initiated a number of projects concerned with the health of Indian women and the training of women for medical work.

From the early nineteenth century colonial states also began to use Western medicine in their management of subject peoples in limited and often temporary ways. The initial motivation of such moves was to help control epidemics that threatened European health and trade. As such, vaccination for smallpox and sanitary measures to control cholera were often seen by the indigenous population not as health measures, but as another form of imperial domination, and they were often a site of conflict—as exemplified by resistance to attempts to control pilgrimages. Over the nineteenth century, Western medicine also seeped out of its colonial enclaves in a number of other ways. Western doctors established private practices and treated anyone who could afford their services. Those seeking such services were largely the local élites, for whom Western medicine was associated with political power and cultural improvement. A number of universities and colleges in India established medical schools to teach the small numbers of (wealthy) local students and any Europeans who were unwilling or unable to afford a European education. A small, yet increasing, number of students from Africa, Asia, and South America obtained medical qualifications in Europe and North America. Many returned home, not only to practise, but also as apostles of Western medicine, and many sought to build their own institutions along Western lines.

During the nineteenth century European medical practitioners increasingly dismissed other 'systems' as primitive and dangerous. This new attitude derived in part from new medical ideas and in part from wider political policies that demanded the imposition of Western language, culture, and technology on subject peoples. The result in medicine was that Western practitioners moved from a tacit acceptance of pluralism to a position where they sought a dominant, if not monopolistic, position wherever they practised. Western medicine increasingly based its claims to exclusivity on its preventive and therapeutic effectiveness, its power to describe and classify diseases, its grounding in testable scientific truths, and its overall progressiveness, especially its openness to critical evaluation, revision, and improvement.

Other systems, along with older Western beliefs, were dismissed as dogmatic, speculative, and ineffective. They were described by Westerners as offering mere metaphorical descriptions of disease, whereas the new Western medicine gave literal accounts, grounded in observation and investigation. In Arab-Islamic countries, the new Western medicine displaced medical systems that were based on texts rather than observation, though there were sufficient similarities in approach and institutions for there to be a relatively smooth accommodation with Western medicine.

For most of the eighteenth and nineteenth centuries, Western doctors who went to practise overseas went with increasing confidence in their powers, but with no special training or knowledge. However, the adaptation of Western knowledge to new conditions and new diseases was often very difficult, though practitioners were able to draw upon a growing literature on the diseases of particular regions and of the tropics more generally. Many diseases, such as smallpox, proved to be common across the world, but others, especially fevers, were very variable or highly specific, like Delhi boil and Pali plague. All fevers seemed to become more intense in tropical latitudes, a phenomenon that was attributed to greater heat and higher levels of putrescent matter in the air. On top of this, the insanitary lifestyle of the 'primitive races' threatened Europeans, who kept their distance in segregated settlements when and where they could.

Tropical pestilence began to be tamed from the mid-nineteenth century, seemingly when the dictates of European sanitary science and hygienic discipline were imposed on colonial troops and applied to European settlements.

Cholera vaccination of the Third Gurkhas in India at the time of the 1893 epidemic. Government inquiries into the health of the Indian Army in the 1860s precipitated both reforms in military hygiene and the expansion of a civilian public health service in India.

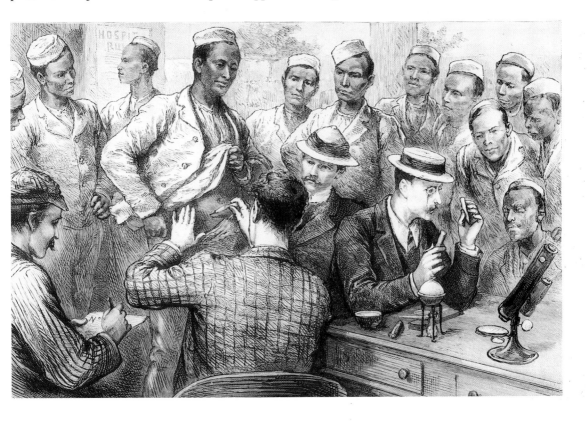

At the end of the century, in the context of the 'new imperialism' that had led to the scramble for Africa and calls for the greater exploitation of colonial resources and labour, the much improved position was still said to be inhibiting economic development, trade, and administration. In addition it was argued that the existing corpus of Western medical knowledge was deficient for Africa, India, South-East Asia, and Latin America. The answer to this was to establish a new and special branch of theory and practice, to be termed tropical medicine, to be taught to those working in colonial medicine. Imperial governments and other organizations accepted the idea and rapidly invested in the new specialism. Schools and laboratories were founded in Europe and in the colonies, to instruct and carry out research on vector-borne parasitic diseases, such as malaria, sleeping sickness, yellow fever, and schistosomiasis.

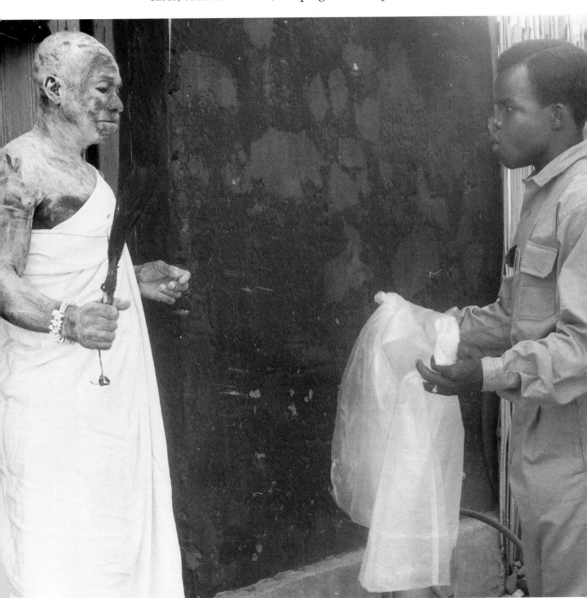

With hindsight, it is evident that few of these diseases were unique to the tropics: malaria was still prevalent in Europe and North America, and yellow fever was still an occasional visitor to the North. The common characteristics of these afflictions did not lie in their pathology or etiology; it was simply that they were the diseases causing most problems for imperial governments. They were all poorly covered in Western medical training and yet they offered exciting research opportunities to the new breed of medical research scientists. That those living in tropical countries, both colonized and colonizers, suffered from a wide range of diseases and that most of these were the same as those found in Europe was lost sight of in colonial medical policy.

The form in which tropical medicine was developed meant that, for much of the twentieth century, what we now term the Third World or developing countries received a skewed form of Western medicine. The medical policies and campaigns, first of colonial governments and then of agencies like the World Health Organization, directed their attention towards a relatively limited range of largely parasitic diseases. Furthermore, these agencies sought to control these diseases by what are now known as 'vertical' control methods—that is, programmes that dealt with a single disease at a time and relied on direct interventions against the parasite or its vectors, such as mosquitoes, tsetse flies, and snails. They were programmes devised and run by Western experts. Increasingly they used advanced medical and other technologies that were imported directly from Europe and North America, with no linkages into the local community, economy, or culture. The most ambitious of these schemes, the eradication of malaria, was proclaimed by the World Health Organization in 1957. The programme drew heavily on post-Second World War optimism about the power of science and technology, and its ability to accelerate the social development, if not the industrialization, of all poor countries, many of which seemed to be held back by low standards of living and poor health. Malaria was to be eradicated by the destruction of mosquitoes by DDT spraying, undertaken by teams that moved through towns and villages. Initially there were successes, as in Sri Lanka, where malaria seemed to have disappeared. In the longer term, the high economic and environmental costs of the programmes, the failure to provide the infrastructure to sustain the campaigns, and the absence of other preventive policies led to the resurgence of the disease and the abandonment of the policy goal by the World Health Organization in the 1970s. The flaws of such attempts to deploy advanced Western medical ideas and technologies in Third World countries are now seen, by both local health agencies and Western advisory bodies like the World Health Organization, to lie in their failure to involve and mobilize the local population, together with their reliance on outside expertise and resources. In the last quarter of the century, policy-makers have argued that Third World countries and their peoples would benefit more from so-called 'horizontal' health policies that aim to develop an infrastructure of institutions that can deliver sustainable health care and treat the full range of illnesses. In other words, Third World countries would perhaps gain most from creating institutions and practices very similar to those found in primary health care in modern Western societies, rather than from policies that assume they have quite different needs. Arab-Islamic countries had followed Western patterns from the late

Attempts at the global eradication of malaria were largely based on spraying with the insecticide DDT, an example of the transfer of technologies from industrialized countries to modernize third-world countries. The ideology of such programmes in the early 1960s is illustrated by the contemporary notes on this photograph: 'Centuries versus Progress—The strongest tool is understanding!! The young man explains how we will cover the fetish charms with the plastic sheet he's holding, so the insecticide will not touch the natives and reduce their potency. This is one problem among many that intercepts the work of United Nations Agencies . . . who are aiding in the struggle for progress in the interior of new African nations.'

nineteenth century, under either French or British influence. These did not change with political independence, nor with the economic independence that oil revenues brought many states, nor have they been much affected by the growth of Islamic fundamentalism because of the high priority that the faith gives to the preservation of life.

Modernization

In those countries that remained independent, notably Japan and China, Western medicine was seen as an integral part of Western power and its alien culture, not as politically neutral science or benign welfare. Yet, there was an ambivalence towards Western science and medicine, which was also seen more positively as an important factor in Western material supremacy, and something which any country seeking to resist direct Western control, or to modernize, would have to embrace. Similar assumptions were made after 1945 by ex-colonial states seeking economic and social development and true independence. In both cases the decisions to adopt Western medicine were taken by the rulers or élite groups, often as a means to consolidate their own position as much as to improve the health of the population as a whole.

Until 1867 Japan had proved particularly infertile ground for Western medicine. It had been practised only in isolated missions and Western trading ports such as Nagasaki, and in the face of such an overtly anti-Western regime there had been very little local impact. Yet, following the fall of the Tokugawa Shogunate in 1867, the restored Meiji government decided to adopt Western medicine as part of their broader programme of modernization, which was also aimed at resisting foreign control. In the struggles leading up to the Restoration, the medical adviser to the Meiji forces was the British surgeon William Willis. His assistance on surgery, wound management, and military sanitation was seen to have played an important role in the success of the campaign, and Willis played a role in the formal decision, in March 1868, to foster Western medical training and practice. An early and successful test came with a major smallpox epidemic in 1871, against which vaccination appeared to be successful. After this time, Kanpo, the Japanese variant of traditional Chinese medicine, while not banned, no longer enjoyed State support, and, as its legitimacy waned, it subsided into folk practice.

Adopting Western medicine was no easy matter. The whole infrastructure of institutions had to be built from scratch, and it was accepted that the training and deployment of personnel would probably take at least a generation. Also, there was not just one version of Western medicine to emulate. From the viewpoint of the Japanese rulers, two main versions were on offer: first, British hospital-based, clinically oriented medicine that had a partial foothold in the country because of the position of Willis and Britain's strategic position in the region, and, secondly, the German university-based system that gave greater prominence to scientific training and laboratory work and which at that time was assuming the position of world leadership. The latter was chosen, and in 1877 the first German School of Medicine was opened in Tokyo. When asked to provide candidates for key posts, German authorities offered military doctors, who they assumed would fit more easily into Japanese culture and whose military rank would give them greater authority than their medical expertise.

The rate of expansion of places in Western medical schools was slow and for a long time the quality of the training was relatively poor. It was not until the 1920s that the number of medical schools reached double figures, by which time student enrolments each year had just reached 1,000. Paradoxically, it was from this time that Kanpo began to attract new practitioners and followers, often amongst those who had studied Western medicine and found it . deficient because of its focus on disease rather than the whole sick person. This revival of traditional Japanese medicine continued after 1945, though by the late twentieth century it is surely a quite new form of practice, as it has been separated from the older religious and other meanings and is often offered as an adjunct to Western medicine.

The spread of Western medicine in China followed a similar pattern to that in Japan, with initial contacts through individuals, missionaries, and traders. However, China saw greater missionary activity and this had a longer-term impact, especially on medical education. The decision to adopt and develop Western medical training and institutions was again political. It followed various crises and wars in the 1900s, the plague epidemic in 1911, and the establishment of the National Government in the same year. In 1915 the role of the Christian Medical Missionary Association as the leading professional agency promoting the adoption and spread of Western medicine was taken over by the newly formed National Medical Association of China. The greater openness of the new regime allowed the building of close links with the USA: for example, Harvard University joined a cooperative venture in medical education in Beijing in 1912 and the Rockefeller Foundation played a leading role in the development of the Union Medical College from 1914. In subsequent years medical colleges opened in cities across China, though Western medicine remained a largely urban phenomenon and its impact elsewhere was limited, even though the Nationalist Government invested in the development of rural health services in the 1920s and 1930s. This policy was aimed to improve the health of the population, to make medicine and hygiene a force of modernization, and, perhaps, to impress the Rockefeller Foundation, which was looking to invest in public-health measures in China.

The Rockefeller Foundation, founded on the strength of John D. Rockefeller's personal fortune to promote human welfare and economic modernization through scientific and medical research, came to play a leading role in the development of medical education and rural health services in China and in many other countries. From supporting the reform of medical education and hookworm eradication schemes in the USA, the Foundation's work gradually extended through Latin America to South America, Asia, Africa, and Europe itself. Its health programmes were again disease-centred, with yellow fever and malaria receiving a lot of investment and being linked to attempts to establish model rural health schemes that it was hoped local governments would take over and extend. The Foundation's work in medical education aimed to raise standards generally, to promote research, and to advance the subject of hygiene. In South America, Rockefeller officials arranged and paid for US professors to work in medical schools and championed the estab-

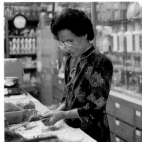

Traditional Chinese medicine is essentially a creation of the twentieth century, having been remade in reaction to Western medicine, yet paradoxically in many ways modelled on its professional organization and practice. This two-way flow of influence and interaction was evident in the refinement of acupuncture in the light of Western anatomy and the attempts to find the active agent in many traditional drugs. In contemporary China the two systems coexist and patients often receive combined therapies.

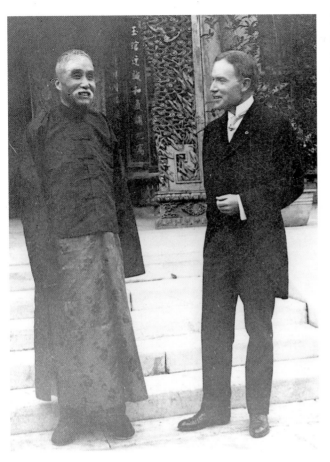

lishment of full-time posts in medical schools so that laboratory-based, research-oriented medical scientists could take over medical training from part-time clinicians. Rockefeller Foundation policy was to create institutions from which élite, research-minded practitioners would emerge who would spread Western medicine both in their work and by trying to emulate the best practice they had experienced in their training. This 'top-down' approach to the spread of Western medicine paid little attention to the appropriateness of science-oriented approaches to non-Western societies, nor to the infrastructure necessary to maintain Western medical practice. Thus, with yellow fever in South America and Africa, Rockefeller grants bought technical successes in understanding the complex etiology of the disease and in developing a vaccine, but there were major problems in translating these achievements into saving lives. This policy—and later the post-colonial medical and research training programmes—underestimated the pull of Western institutions and lifestyles to

John D. Rockefeller II and Hsu Shih-chang, at the Winter Palace, Beijing, in September 1921. The Rockefeller Foundation's work was directed by its permanent staff and expert committees, but both John D. Rockefeller I and his son played an active role as statesmen, especially for major initiatives such as the medical education programme in China.

those whose training made them professionally mobile. The result was that, rather than aiding its spread across social and geographical boundaries, these programmes often helped to lock Western medicine into élite, urban institutions that were oriented more towards the international medical research community than to the health of local peoples.

There have been many attempts to counter such tendencies and to diffuse Western medicine to all social levels and all parts of countries. The most well-known was in Communist China, where 'bare-foot doctors' were trained and used to take medicine to the rural masses. From 1949 the Communist government had an ambivalent attitude towards Western medicine. On the one hand, it was seen as essential to modernization, whilst, on the other, it was clearly a product and bearer of capitalist culture. Various ways of meeting this contradiction have been tried, but the most significant was to seek a synthesis of Chinese medicine, stripped of its feudal associations and mysticism, and Western medicine, without its bourgeois ideology. Thus, practitioners in both traditions were required to have ancillary training in the other. In the short term this policy tied up students and doctors in additional training and led to a shortage of practitioners across the country. Part of the problem was that the government had ambitious plans to bring basic health care to every citizen. The answer to both problems was the creation of the cadre of 'barefoot doctors'—that is, medical personnel trained with basic skills and knowledge who could cope with minor illnesses and recognize the more serious complaints that needed the attention of fully qualified doctors. The innovative feature of this scheme, which was run down at the end of the Cultural Revolution, was its attempt to avoid the creation and diffusion of a carbon copy of hospital-oriented modern medicine.

Conclusion

In probably every country in the world, modern Western medicine is the legally and culturally dominant form of medicine at the end of the twentieth century. Its knowledge and social relations, especially professional self-regulation of qualifications, practice, and ethics, backed by State licensing and international corporations, now seem the inevitable way in which medicine has to operate. The seemingly inexorable spread of modern Western medicine has had as much to do with Western global economic and political power as with specifically medical influences. However, it would be wrong to conclude that modern Western medicine has swept all before it. The US anthropologist Charles Leslie made the perceptive observation in 1976 that, 'The health concepts and practices of most peoples in the world today continue traditions that evolved during antiquity.' Thus, there are many parts of the world, especially amongst the rural poor in Third World countries, which modern medicine has still not reached. Even in Western countries, lay beliefs about the body, disease, and its treatment, particularly minor illnesses that constitute so much of our experience of disease and do not involve organized medicine, continue humoral ideas as we 'catch colds', 'starve fevers', and link illness to personal misfortune. In addition, certain of the most advanced and technically sophisticated forms of modern medical practice are under attack for being dehumanizing and ethically suspect, while alternative systems and therapies, such as homoeopathy, naturopathy, osteopathy, and faith healing, seem to attract increasing numbers of devotees. There is even some evidence—notably the incorporation of methods like acupuncture and chiropractic into orthodox practice—that, at the end of the second millennium, Western medicine may itself be moving to a new form of medical pluralism.

17 | Unofficial and Unorthodox Medicine

MARGARET PELLING

THE scene is late seventeenth-century London, near Tower Bridge. John Wilmot, second Earl of Rochester, satirist, poet, and libertine, having disgraced himself at court by over-indulgence in horseplay with his friends, has disguised himself as 'the noble Dr Alexander Bendo', Italian mountebank, apparently with entire success. Dressed in an old overgrown green gown

lyned through with exotick furrs of diverse colours, an antique Cap, a great Reverend Beard, and a Magnificent false Medal sett round with glittering Pearl, rubies, and Diamonds of the same Cognation, hung about his Neck in a Massy Gold like Chaine of Princes mettle, which the King of Cyprus (you must know) had given him for doing a signal Cure upon his darling Daughter the Princess Aloephangina, who was painted in a Banner . . .

Bendo presided over a laboratory of henchmen 'dress't like the old Witches in Mackbeth', producing medicines for a gullible public. Although they had between them Latin, French, and Italian, they spoke gibberish, 'since our Mystery (as all Trades else) flourished but under the deep recesses of Concealment and Secrecy'. It was therefore not appropriate to do anything in English, except laugh. His enemies, Rochester gloated, thought he had been exiled to France, and all the time he was selling to them, their wives and children

Washes, Paint, Powders, Oyntments, Plaister's Balsomes Anodynes, Philters, Salves, Troches, Antidotes, Amuletts, Electuaries, Charms, Apocems, Elixirs, Causticks, Oyls Spirits, Sulphurs, Vitriols, Pills, Potions, Essences, Salts Volatile, & fixt, Magisterialls, Pastills, Lozinges, Opiates, Sudoroficks, diureticks, Tinctures, Chimicall Preparations of all Sorts, with Specificks and Nostrums innumerable.

The services Bendo advertised also included 'Predictions, casting Nativities, Interpretations of Dreams, solving of Omens, Responses to horary Questions, illustrations of Signs and Tokens, Judgements upon Moles, Wenns, Warts and natural Marks, according to their severall Kinds...in various parts of the naked Body'—and the resolving by astrology of anxious questions to do with valuables mislaid, whether a wife or a husband would survive the longer, the sex of an unborn child, what kind of spouse a person would marry, and whether ships had been lost at sea. Rochester claimed that Bendo's bills—that is, advertisements—used only 'clean words', avoiding the 'bawdy' of many physicians' bills. To modest women Bendo offered the assistance of Mrs Bendo, who would visit them at home, where they could show her their bodies in privacy. Mrs Bendo was, of course, also Rochester in disguise. The satiric earl, royalist on his father's side and highly religious if not puritan on his mother's, did not omit also to make a virtue of his deception. The charade was aimed not at illiterates but at 'persons without virtue or sense, in all stations'; the moral was that 'the Politician is, and must be a Mountebank in State Affairs, and the Mountebank no doubt, (if he thrives) is an errant Pollitician in Physick'. Only trial—that is, experiment—could reveal the difference between the valiant and the coward, the wealthy merchant and the bankrupt, the politician and the fool, since virtue in this world could be so exactly counterfeited. The only exceptions were the select few who were already in the know.

Mountebanks, Charlatans, and Quacks

Rochester's Bendo epitomizes the stock figure of the mountebank, who was a literary and dramatic creation as well as a lived reality for Western Europe. Rochester was well-read, with a wide experience of the world, including a visit to Venice, which was famous for its mountebank practitioners. The word 'charlatan', which originally emphasized loud public boasting as much as deceit, entered the Italian vernacular in the early sixteenth century, possibly as a borrowing from the Middle East. The definitive literary representation in English was Ben Jonson's comedy *Volpone* (performed 1605–6), although Jonson's style was classicist and highly sophisticated rather than popular. 'Mountebank'— *monta in banco*, according to an Italian–English dictionary of 1598, referring to the use of raised platforms or temporary stages—is also of Italian derivation, and of similar date. 'Quack', an abbreviation of quacksalver, is more obscure, but probably derives from sixteenth-century Dutch, and also refers to the practitioner's powers of speech. Medical buffoons were an integral part of *commedia dell'arte*, the itinerant Italian popular comedy which flourished from the sixteenth to the eighteenth centuries, in which stock characters were represented by actors wearing masks and fantastic clothing. With its long traditional history, and possible roots in classical sources, the *commedia* shows (like Rochester) the hazards involved in dividing popular and élite culture, and the difficulties of distinguishing between the street in the theatre, and the theatre in the street. Although the mountebank performing on a stage in the open, accompanied by musical instruments (especially drums), intriguing animals such as monkeys, parrots, or snakes, and the clown or zany who often acted as his foil, might appear to be the regular practitioner's polar opposite, the *commedia* emphasized that the main difference in human life was not between the good and the bad, but between the ideal and the reality. As Abraham Cowley put it in 1663: 'a cowardly ranting Soldier, an ignorant charlatanical Doctor, a foolish Cheating Lawyer . . . have always been, and still are the Principal Subjects of all Comedies.' Often, as Rochester maintained, one could tell the difference only by results.

Rochester's Bendo belongs to a favourite theme in Western Christianity, the moral implications of human gullibility. Faith was essential for salvation, but

gullibility was dangerous, because it supported the wrong sources of authority. The quack could serve as simply one more example of human folly, but
medicine itself did not escape suspicion, because it appeared to give priority to
the body, rather than to the soul. Hence the Physician of Chaucer's *Canterbury
Tales* was proud of his classical learning, and did not read much in his Bible;
Chaucer, a man of cosmopolitan background, did not see it as appropriate to
contrast this apparently respectable figure with an obvious quack. Instead, he
combines physical with spiritual quackery in the figure of the Pardoner, an
appendage of the pre-Reformation church. Following the Reformation, the
quack is more obviously a lay figure, but often appears as a foreigner, signify-
ing religious and political unreliability. He—such figures of false authority are
very rarely female—is often depicted as raised above his audience, in profile
like a bird of prey, looking Jewish, 'Egyptian' (gypsy), Eastern, satanic, or otherwise alien. In addition, the foreign quack often apes (and thereby carica-
tures) the dress, manners, language, and superiority of the social élite, in an
attempt to pervert the natural allegiances of the people. Figures of this type—
or literary and pictorial representations of them, usually by artists of a bourgeois level of society, producing primarily for an audience of the middle and
upper classes—have a very long history in Western society, surviving into the
present day. After the peasants' revolts of the Reformation, when the new religion and its anti-authoritarian message seemed to subvert the social order by
appealing primarily to the peasantry and the artisan class, gullibility is often
depicted as something natural to the lower orders. An example particularly

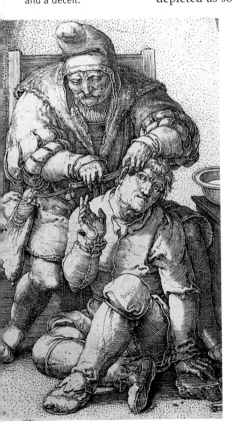

common in northern European art is the motif of the peasant
having a head operation to remove stupidity. (It is worth noting,
however, that 'head operators', pretending to remove stones or
other foreign bodies, were allegedly also active as a recognized
variety of quack in the medieval Middle East.) The cunning oper-
ator can sometimes simply look like an artisan, rather than an
outsider, and the foolishness of the victims is usually underlined by some visual reference to their being robbed of their
money. However, the itinerant practitioner also became suspect in pre-industrial Europe, along with other itinerants, as a
result of crises of poverty, war, and social dislocation.

In later centuries, the fact that the mountebank performed or
sold his goods in public could be enough in itself to suggest that
such figures survived because of popular support, or popular
ignorance. This is particularly true in societies where privacy
became a value for the rising urban middle class, such as England and Holland. The College of Physicians of London, founded
in 1518, had appropriated by the early seventeenth century a set
of attitudes by which its members contrasted their own rich but
sober dress and demeanour with the colourful public displays
of those whom it regarded as empirics. Although hostile to
secrecy among illicit practitioners, the College adopted a model
of practice which, if it did not encourage contact between practitioner and patient, certainly disparaged medicine as it was
practised in the street and the market place. It should be noted,

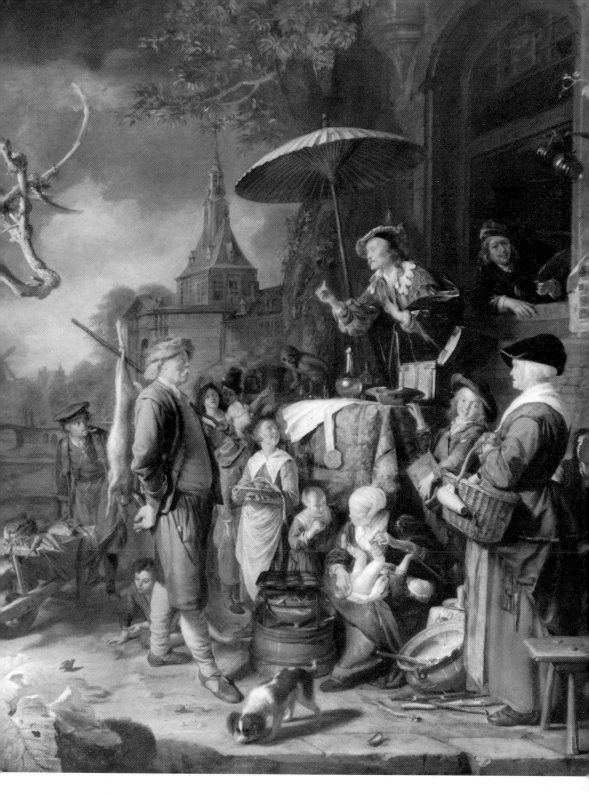

A favourite subject of seventeenth- and eighteenth-century painters, especially in northern Europe. The quack, a dramatic but precarious figure, in almost gothic surroundings, seeks to impress a village audience, who are partly aware and partly taken in. The portrait of village life given by such artists was more likely to be satirical than literal or sympathetic.

267

however, that the College was frequently aiming not at the mountebank but at the barber-surgeon and the apothecary. In the pre-industrial period both of these crafts were carried on in a semi-public manner, in shops open to the street. Apothecaries placed their drugs and spices on display, and their shops were located in busy places, such as shopping streets or near public water sources. Barber-surgeons' shops were marked by signs, poles, and (when not prevented by city authorities) basins of blood; they attracted and distracted their customers with music, food, drink, and news. Patients in danger of death were subject to semi-public discussion and inspection by the elders of the barber-surgeons' guild.

Medical treatment was not therefore a private matter—unless sufferers had particular reasons for not wanting their condition to be known, in which case they were the more likely to be beguiled by a quack. The practices of apothecaries and barber-surgeons were merely typical of what was still expected of artisans in general—that they should work openly (while protecting the skills of the craft), and be recognizable in public by the clothing and accoutrements suitable to their trade. The morality plays sponsored and performed in the streets by the craft guilds faded with the Reformation, but the companies of early modern Europe continued to dress up for ceremonies in public. In general, physicians sought to distance themselves from craft organizations, although in the city states of continental Europe the physicians were far more integrated into civic life than they were in London. In repudiating the quack, the London College was also seeking to repudiate the artisan. Rochester's Bendo lodged with a goldsmith, and left puzzled carpenters and apothecaries behind him when he vanished. Rochester was typical of his time and social class in equating the 'mystery' of a trade with the disingenuous secrecy of the quack. The craft guilds collapsed under capitalism earlier in England than in (for example) Germany, and something of this is reflected in changing attitudes to people who bought and sold in the streets. Marcellus Laroon's 'London Cries' were a late seventeenth-century version of a traditional European genre of 'characters', often satirical but also socially comprehensive, including a wide range of status and occupation. Increasingly such character portraits concentrated on the lower levels of society, depicting the street seller as poverty-stricken, disreputable, or picturesque. Among these was usually included the mountebank.

It would be wrong, however, to suggest that increased social stratification necessarily broke the link between the irregular practitioner and the social élite. The monarch's public body might demand a highly regulated approach to medicine; his private body was often tended by an extraordinary range of practitioners, female as well as male. When it came to illness, fertility, or childbirth, the élites of European countries reserved the right to employ whom they pleased. This might suggest that quacks belonged to traditional, pre-industrial societies, and that they would consequently fall

The mountebank's pose, his clothes, and his animals are all designed to attract attention as he sells phials of medicine. Laroon (originally Lauron) was born in The Hague, the son of a French face painter and landscapist who moved to London after the Restoration.

victim to 'modernization'. The Enlightenment, which stressed the perfectibility of man and the interrelationship of physical and spiritual life, brought with it attempts to regulate medicine in the public interest and to suppress popular healers. The travelling mountebank began to be seen as parasitic upon a primitive state of society and as an object of interest which by the nineteenth century had become antiquarian, reformist, or anthropological. Any attempt to assess the actual effects of these developments depends on arguments about the timing and depth of the division between popular and élite culture, and the relationship between religion, magic, and science. Some would argue that the mountebank left the streets only to reappear in 'the media'—that the decline of both magic and religion is more apparent than real, even in the most industrialized of Western societies, and that 'magic' merely updates itself to accommodate science. Others suggest that the quack takes on a new lease of life whenever a *laissez-faire* approach to economic affairs is instituted. Examples are eighteenth-century England, and late nineteenth-century Germany—and, possibly, 'post-modern' Western society generally. This argument assumes a level of prosperity among the middle and upper classes, with medicine becoming not only an aspect of consumption, but also a kind of leisure activity. The emphasis is not on need, but on consumer demand and consumer choice.

Eighteenth-century England, the 'first industrialized nation', was notorious for its quacks partly because of the outburst of forms of communication—newspapers, advertisements, improved transport, outlets such as booksellers—which helped to create 'quackery' as a form of social commentary. This can be seen as another variation on the theme of the relationship between London and the provinces, in which England provides a strong contrast with the city states of many countries of continental Europe. The comparatively low social status of even physicians in Britain also gave scope to the view of the wits that all medicine was more or less quackery. The famous eighteenth-century quacks were not 'low life', but they were often foreign, or assumed foreign airs and mysteriousness. The type tended to shift from Italian to German, possibly in compliment to the Hanoverian monarchy. Such quacks did not sell in the streets, but continued to advertise themselves by visible eccentricity or public display, combined with nascent advertising techniques. Some quacks had a more shadowy existence as the names behind proprietary medicines, although lending one's name to a patent medicine was not yet definitive of irregular practice. Many of these names had a traditional appeal, rather than reflecting a desire for the novelties of commercial production. This suggests a rather less optimistic view of medicine as a source of security in the face of change. The eighteenth-century quack is known mainly by his advertisements and by records of the impact of his personality; much less has been discovered about his business or about his customers.

How Typical was the Mountebank?

The mountebank, although medical, was one in a range of characters in a long-running morality play, both symbolic and real, which touched on fundamental religious and political issues. Attitudes to the mountebank could be

Mountebanks, Charlatans, and Quacks

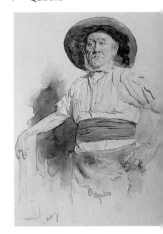

A positive image of a French blacksmith healer, stressing natural authority as well as the dignity of labour. The late nineteenth century was a pioneering period for folklorists as well as a period of anxiety about national strength and national identity. Of those dealing with animals, blacksmiths were perhaps the most widely credited with healing powers.

serious, or frivolous. But to what extent was this colourful figure representative of 'unofficial' or unorthodox medicine?

That the mountebank existed, and was more or less ubiquitous in Western
Europe, seems certain, although not yet fully investigated historically. It
seems equally obvious that there were well-known forms of fraud practised in
the East as well as the West, their standard character determined by common
needs and fears—the disabling (and impoverishing) effect of blindness being
perhaps the best example. However, it cannot be assumed that even all mountebanks were frauds. Setting aside the placebo effect, which might ensure a
positive outcome even though the intent was to deceive, there are major historical problems in sorting out the practitioners of previous periods according
to sincerity or effectiveness. Assured efficacy in medicine was extremely limited until very recently, and the current trend towards 'evidence-based' medicine is one reminder of how much medical treatment has still to be given
without a clear understanding of how—and even whether—it works. Historians
agree that medicine gained in status in most Western countries before, not
after, it acquired an effective knowledge base, and it can be argued that the
major improvements in life expectancy in the so-called developed countries
over the twentieth century are not primarily due to medicine at all, whatever
medicine's role in maintaining such improvements.

From the historian's point of view, the historical record—especially with
respect to literary sources—is largely the creation of interested parties, and has
to be balanced accordingly. Many of the features which seem to define modern
Western medicine—full-time practice with a vocational image, an assumption
of almost universal respect among the public based on a unique ethical commitment, domination of purpose-built institutions such as hospitals, dissocia-
tion from commercial values, registration of qualifications, a confidential
relationship between patient and practitioner—are themselves historical
developments belonging to particular places and times, and cannot be applied
retrospectively to distinguish good practitioners from bad.

The role of itinerants is a useful case in point. As already suggested, itinerancy in the modern world lacks respectability; specialization in medicine, on
the other hand, is a feature which has become more than respectable at the
end of a long history of ill repute. 'Specificks' were inevitably among the litany
of Bendo's commodities. Official medicine embraced a 'universal' ideal. As late
as the nineteenth century, élite physicians and surgeons in teaching hospitals,
even if they themselves were known for particular abilities, disparaged specialization as a form of quackery. Specialists can be seen as 'failed consultants'
even in the twentieth century. However, the available evidence suggests that
in the pre-industrial period, and even later, itinerant and other specialists performed a valuable role in making available unusual and urgently needed
skills, in particular couching for cataract, cutting for stone in the bladder (an
agonizing condition much more common in the past than it is today), palliat-
ing deformities such as hare lip and conditions such as fistula and rupture,
inoculation for smallpox, tooth-pulling, and bone-setting. The need for these
services ultimately prompted some of the earliest specialist hospitals. Such
skills were often passed on in families or by informal apprenticeship; in this
respect, some unofficial medicine was in reality more dynastic than regular

medicine. However, there were also itinerant practitioners who were formally qualified according to the standards of the time.

In addition to specialists, medicine was practised by a great many other 'wanderers', because it was an art that was both portable and in universal demand. Pre-industrial society was far more mobile than conventionally assumed, although permission was often required for travelling; medicine could justify, excuse, and finance a journey. It was an obvious resort for those exiled for religious or political reasons, who could be highly learned; it was also a plausible cover for diplomacy and spying. For ethnic and religious minorities, such as Jews or Quakers, medicine was an acceptable means of livelihood as well as a pursuit compatible with ethical philosophies. Thus, although medical corporations (like other craft organizations) attempted to restrict the entry of 'strangers', itinerancy does not of itself define the unacceptable practitioner, even in more urbanized societies.

None the less, the real issue in defining unofficial or unorthodox medicine is not the grave physician on the one hand or the visible itinerant on the other, but the huge area of practice in between. Both physicians and mountebanks were tiny minorities, satisfying a minute proportion of the demand for medical care. Historians have made much progress in recent years by a rejection of two assumptions: first, that a high level of mortality or morbidity induced an indifference to minor ailments and even to the survival of infants, family, and friends; and, secondly, that the bulk of populations before the present day had no access to medical services worthy of the name. If medical polemic is put to one side, and more respect paid both to community sanctions and to actual practice, then pre-industrial Western societies are revealed as using the services of an extremely wide range of practitioners, most of whom would, according to other medical groups or to modern criteria of professionalization, be seen as 'unofficial'. Official medicine is defined, even in the present, by ignoring the question of whether or not it meets the extent of need. One example of this is that official medicine has always preferred to avoid 'less-developed' rural areas, so that rural practitioners tended to be unofficial almost by definition. The most striking example, however, relates to the role of women.

Women and Health Care

The level of illness in society is still often measured in terms of the uptake of medical services. However, it is generally realized that this is a very inadequate measure of either the state of health of a population, or of its consumption of medical care. One historical constant, at least for Western societies, appears to be that the family was, and is, the first port of call for advice about illness. A second is that most such advice, and the bulk of primary care, was, and is, provided by women. Moreover, any investigation of human relationships tends to confirm that it is women who more frequently monitor and take responsibility for health. The historical record produces much evidence in letters and diaries that men were also concerned with health questions, and it is important to notice this; but the evidence is skewed, because of higher literacy and record survival among men than among women. Health care, like child care, seems perennially to have been a female responsibility, even when due

A Netherlandish triumph
of avarice, with hay the
symbol of worldly gain.
The haywain is drawn
onward to damnation by
devils and demons,
complacently followed by
the great and the good.
Others are led into
violence and other sins.
Among those who have
managed to stuff hay into
their pouches is a quack
(centre foreground).

allowance is made for such exceptions as the few truly all-male institutions (monasteries, some ships) and the major phenomenon (until the twentieth century) of male servants. This broad base of the health-care pyramid, where it is recognized, is inevitably classified as unofficial rather than official medicine.

Women have also played a role outside the family. Historians are increasingly having to modify the idea that there was a 'golden age' of women's work, when women shared more equally with men in forms of production organized within the household, and were given some standing in public life as a result of their occupational status. Instead, it appears that women's work has always been lower paid, and of lower status than that of men, and that women's access to the world of work outside the household has been primarily a function of adverse economic conditions. In medicine, as in other occupations, isolated examples can be found of women who gained some form of official recognition from a ruler, a guild, or a university; but historians are having to conclude, even for the medieval period, that these are the exceptions that prove the rule.

Unofficially, however, women's role in medicine outside the household was considerable, although often very difficult to document historically. The most detectable examples are the noblewomen and gentlewomen who treated their dependants and advised their friends. Contemporaries justified this as an aspect of either religious duty (particularly proper to women) or *noblesse oblige*. Sometimes, but not often, a noblewoman's interest in medical matters was seen as an indication of intellectual attainment, especially in the classical languages. Some educated women, like many educated men, became learned in medicine as a result of searching for a cure for their own illnesses. (Rochester, who, according to Samuel Johnson, 'blazed out his youth and health in lavish voluptuousness', became terminally ill in his early thirties, and may have been another example of this.) This was undoubtedly something which happened at all levels of society, as it still does today, especially in the context of psychology or alternative medicine. Lower down the social scale, the wives of ministers or clergymen could provide medical advice, particularly in rural areas, their practice justified in part by the absence of regular practitioners. Among artisans, the widows of barber-surgeons and apothecaries had some rights to practise, and other women defended their knowledge of physic or surgery by citing a father, brother, or even uncle. Occasionally women worked in some kind of partnership with male practitioners, as did 'Mrs Bendo', attracting female patients with the promise of female modesty and female expertise. Others developed a speciality (for example, 'purging ale') out of the very great overlap between medicine and the production of food and drink. As long as the management of purging, vomiting, and sweating was seen as a fundamental aspect of the medical task, women had a kind of entrée which was only superseded by the mass production of proprietary medicines. Faith in laxatives, or in the effects attributed to laxatives, continues in the present day. 'Cunning women', who were found in towns as well as in the countryside, were seen as having a peculiar understanding both of human behaviour, and of natural powers, including those that were invisible or 'occult'. (There were, of course, also 'cunning men'.) These practitioners were asked to use 'white magic' or 'natural

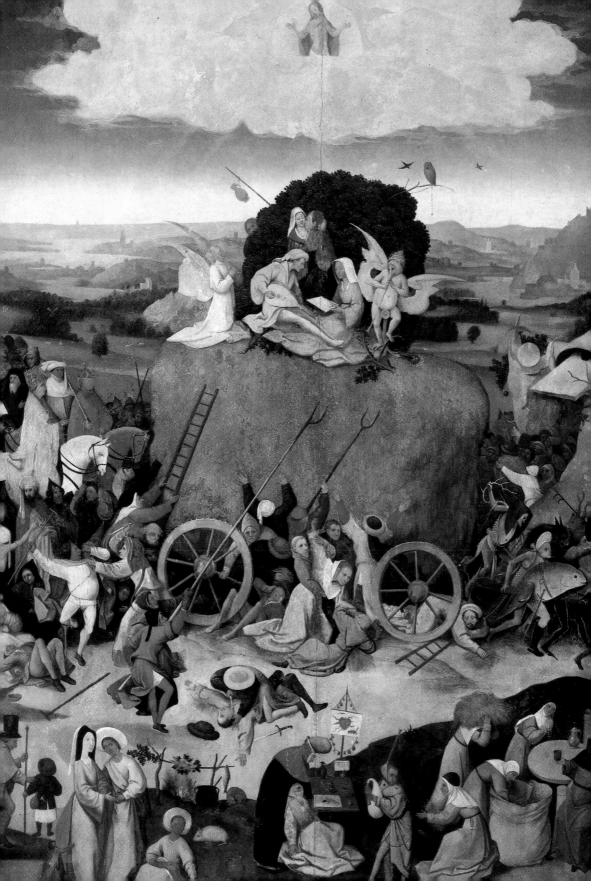

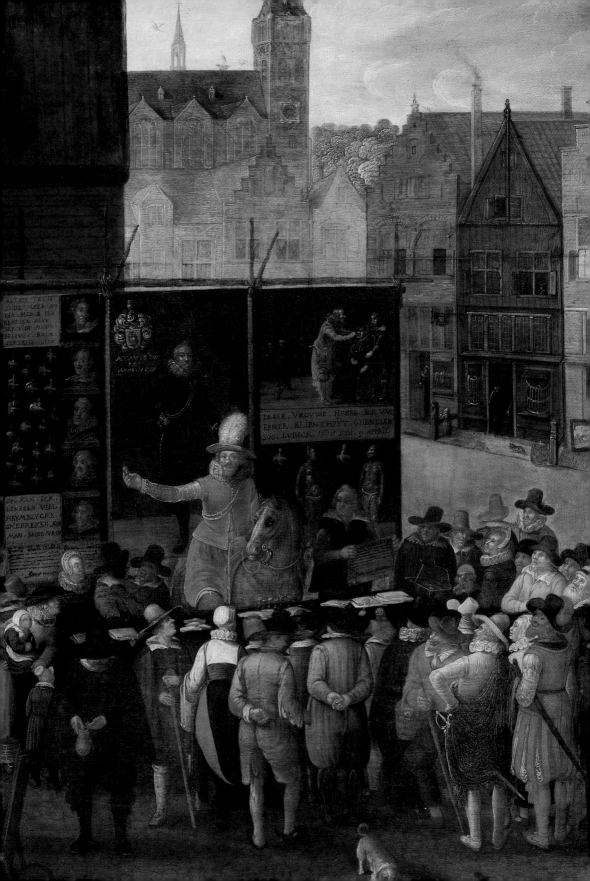

astrology' as a means of finding answers to the kind of questions invited by Rochester's Bendo. They could be described, retrospectively, as experts in the management of uncertainty. The same could be said of one of the most highly prized attributes of the physician: his skill in prognosis.

Because medicine, more especially physic, involved skills, behaviour, and substances which were closely associated with the world of women, unofficial medicine inevitably reflected the complications of gender relationships as expressed at a given time or place. Women practised medicine, and were a source of influence, experience, and expertise. Occasionally a male practitioner or natural philosopher placed it on record that his source of information was a woman, and some writers praised the prudence and judgement of mature women or midwives, while many male practitioners were prepared to tolerate (especially if they could guide) the activities of medically inclined gentlewomen, who normally practised without charging fees. Generally speaking, however, official medicine is notable for the vehemence of its rejection of female practice (reserving particular distaste for 'old women'), up to and including the admission of women to medical schools in the late nineteenth century. Official polemic often suggested resemblances between female and popular or folkloric practitioners—they were particularly active in rural areas, they were often paid in kind or not at all, they pandered to popular

Trappings of nobility (*facing*): the central detail, shown here, is an itinerant surgeon, well dressed and mounted, who draws a good crowd in the street. At left, a man sharpens tools and instruments. The surgeon is backed by a vast painted display of his credentials, while his man holds up one of his written and sealed testimonials. The whole picture includes (pointedly) a painter's shop, a school, various low-life street-sellers, and a disabled beggar.

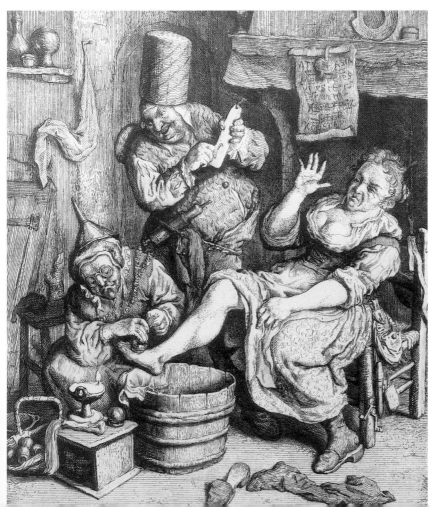

An old woman bleeds a younger by cupping; on the chimneypiece is a barber's basin. 'Fat Piet' sharpens the lancet in readiness and makes lewd remarks about 'clystering' the patient when she faints. The image echoes many others where an older female attendant is an accomplice in sexual activity, but also underlines, at the plebeian level, the perceived connections between medicine and sex.

superstition, they were illiterate and ignorant, and they encouraged the worst tendencies of the poor. This hostility is sometimes difficult to understand, given the automatic and almost total exclusion of women from qualifying institutions such as universities and guilds. It can be attributed in part to the knowledge that lay people, even educated lay people, took little notice of formal qualifications, but partly also to the need for male practitioners to distance themselves from the low-status connotations of the world of women and of women's work. Critics frequently implied that women were particularly prone to flock to irregular practitioners, which can be seen as an oblique reflection of the greater role of women in organizing, assessing, and consuming medical care. Although in periods before the present century sufferers frequently consulted practitioners through relatives or friends, rather than going themselves, it seems also to be true then as now that women were more likely than men to consult practitioners on behalf of other people, whether asked to do so or not.

Midwives provide an excellent illustration of the complexities of the division between official and unofficial medicine. Midwives were probably the most ubiquitous, as well as the least visible, of practitioners; they were often the first branch of medicine to attract supervision (initially by lay or ecclesiastical, rather than medical authorities), but were among the last to be professionalized in the modern sense. Because of their vital role in the welfare of new souls, in human continuity and self-perpetuation, and the legitimate descent of power and property, 'official' midwives—those designated by a ruler, or a ruling élite—appear from a very early date. Midwives employed by the town or the parish, especially on behalf of the poor, were common throughout Western Europe. None the less, midwives largely remained outside institutions, they were judged as much on character as on skills and formal education, and they continued to learn by an informal mode of apprenticeship in which men played little or no part. Midwives were also subject to sporadic campaigns of vilification, of which the most widespread example in Europe was the notion of the 'midwife-witch'. Recent research has shown that those prosecuted as witches were very seldom midwives, and that a more likely target for persecution was the monthly nurse, who spent more time than the midwife in the household with the newborn child. However, the myth was generally believed, probably because of the importance of the midwife's functions and her ambiguous role in the community as both a repository of important secrets and a public functionary obliged to provide evidence on a range of moral and legal questions including virginity, impotence, and the paternity of illegitimate children.

Worlds of Difference

'Official' midwives, it seems, do not look very much like what is usually understood as 'official' medicine; and nearly all female practitioners had no official status at all. Official medicine also excluded most of those, men as well as women, who practised in rural areas or treated the poor. However, until the advent of nationwide health systems, official medicine was more exclusive even than this. As other contributions to this volume will show in greater detail, the bulk of regulation of medicine in Western Europe has been the responsibility of craft organizations. In this context medicine has had no ethical pretensions which have not been shared by other occupations. Although the guilds were concerned both to supervise training and to maintain the standard of practice, they had the related function of regulating the entry of 'strangers' to the craft. Official medicine in one town or region was consequently unofficial medicine in another, regardless of the level of expertise, and the criteria for acceptance could include family connections, religious affiliation, or legitimate birth. Such regulation was strong or weak according to broader social and economic factors, and local barriers were often easily penetrated. In any case, the need for most to work as they travelled, and the tradition of journeymen travelling to gain experience, led to a widespread custom whereby any 'stranger' could practise unmolested in a town for a specified initial period (often one month). Many young surgeons travelled widely as a result of either choosing, or being obliged, to gain experience on board a ship. Generally, there were as many forms of official sanction as there were sources of authority, and these were often played off one against another. A medical practitioner might plead the support of the crown, a local noble, the Pope, a bishop, a university, a town council, a guild, a medical corporation, or two or more of these. Attestation often took the form of patronage, being given on the basis of character, or successful cures. Local discretion combined with remote authority made it possible for mountebanks to deceive some by displaying a welter of parchments hung with seals; at the same time, distinguishing true claims from false was far from easy, even for those able to interrogate in Latin, the lingua franca of scholarship. One qualified person does not infallibly recognize another, even in the twentieth century.

Not surprisingly, the exclusiveness of official medicine also extended to intellectual matters. Two institutions which pressed hard for intellectual conformity were the London College of Physicians and the Medical Faculty of the University of Paris. Each regarded the Galenic corpus of texts as canonical. On this basis, the London College claimed, in the early seventeenth century, the right of (at most) forty practitioners to monopolize the practice of physic in a city of 200,000 people, and attempted to enforce its claims through fines and imprisonment. However, although the medical corporations managed to establish an ideal of uniformity in medical philosophy, this remained an ideal, rather than a reality. One reason for this was that medicine continued to be seen as an aspect of man's relationship to both God and the natural universe. Rival cosmologies could have very practical implications. Rochester's Bendo, for example, offered chemical remedies which echoed the conflict between the classicist followers of Galen and the experimental followers of Paracelsus, who was a religious as well as medical reformer of European importance, adopted as patron by a wide variety of political groupings into the twentieth century. Many Paracelsians were at least as well educated as members of the London College or the Faculty of Paris, and in general it cannot be assumed that orthodox can be separated from unorthodox medicine on the basis of the social or intellectual standing of the different adherents. However, much unorthodox medicine had a religious, philosophical, or political dimension which implied a challenge to the status quo, at least until some kind of accom-

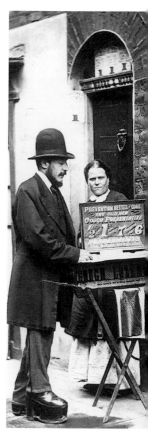

Respiratory conditions, including 'consumption', continued to be a major problem in industrial towns. Although posed, this photograph provides a vivid image of the 'respectable poor' of later nineteenth-century London. The salesman, himself disabled, may have been Jewish.

275

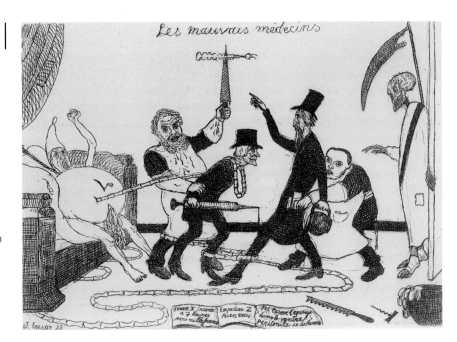

Les mauvais médecins

Ensor drew on older satirical traditions, but also shows concerns typical of nineteenth-century public health reformers. The 'bad doctors' are tied up in a tapeworm, of which they have triumphantly extracted the head. Death has to remind them that in so doing they have killed the patient. Like their accomplices (surgeons? butchers?), they are interested only in their fees.

modation was reached. By the nineteenth century, Western medicine was sufficiently institutionalized, in universities and hospitals, for rival medical philosophies to appear as 'alternatives'. The best-known examples are homoeopathy, mesmerism, hydropathy, and medical botany. Some of these systems took a holistic or vitalist approach to mental and physical well-being, and can look like a nostalgic, 'back-to-nature' response to industrialization. Their apparent point of origin was often the European countryside, or rural America. As against this, it needs to be recognized, first, that rural areas were often also neglected areas; secondly, that these alternatives drew strength from the unresolved religious and political conflicts of previous periods; and, thirdly, that the scientific world-view was itself a fruitful source for many forms of unorthodox medicine.

In most Western countries, convincing definitions of official medicine, and thereby of unofficial medicine, were ultimately produced not by medical corporations but by the State. 'Official medicine' emerges particularly clearly whenever a growing and healthy population is seen to be a national asset. This view could be strongly held by both absolutist and revolutionary regimes, and might involve either the creation of medical corporations, or their abolition. Similarly, popular healers could be enlisted in the State's service, or suppressed. Those sympathetic to reform could be highly critical of the individualistic, profit-making basis of orthodox medicine, which is often seen as indifferent to public-health issues. Before the twentieth century, the most thorough attempts to ensure the extension of medical services to entire populations were made under the absolute monarchies of Prussia and of post-revolutionary France. By the end of the nineteenth century, many European countries had embarked on systems of national insurance which first defined the national version of official medicine, and then ensured its survival by securing an income to its practitioners.

18 | Medicine, Politics, and the State

JANE LEWIS

DURING the twentieth century, the domestic issues that we might loosely categorize as 'welfare' issues—matters concerning employment and unemployment, health, housing, and education—have become the stuff of 'high politics'. This has happened gradually. In the UK, the government spent more time discussing the problems of ruling India in the 1930s than it did mass unemployment. But post-war elections have been won and lost on social policies. Health care has become both big business and a major political issue. The National Health Service (NHS), set up in the UK in 1948, is one of Europe's largest employers, and while it was no secret that, while Prime Minister during the 1980s, Margaret Thatcher wished radically to change its form, the political threat any such action would have posed to the Conservative Party allowed the NHS to survive as a universal, tax-based service, free to all at the point of delivery. In the USA of the 1990s, it was widely accepted that health-care reform could make or break the Democratic Presidency. The spectacular growth in size and complexity of Western health-care systems has been underpinned by the fundamental assumption that personal health care delivered by a doctor to a patient, especially in the hospital, is a worthy endeavour that should be widely available. In Europe, one of the hallmarks of the post-war welfare regimes was the way in which the relationship between economic growth and social provision was seen as positive. Early growth theorists stressed that the accumulation of physical capital was basic to growth, and human capital theorists extended discussion to individual human capital. The period of the 'classic welfare state' (from 1945 to 1976) was characterized by a commitment to full employment, social security that redistributes (although the extent to which this actually happened is debatable) and enhances social consumption, and social services (education, health, housing) that may be regarded as social investments. These kinds of beliefs ensured an overwhelmingly large role for the State in the provision of health care in all European countries. In many, the State had in any case been an active provider of health care throughout the early part of the century via health insurance schemes and Poor Law systems. Even where the State did not become a significant actor early on, as in the USA,

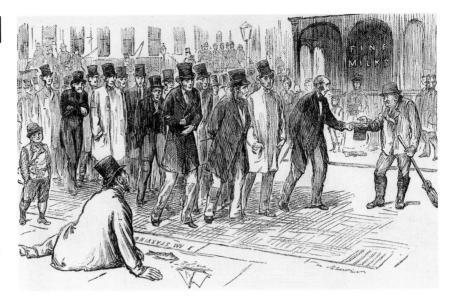

A *Punch* cartoon of 1875 with the caption: 'Out of work and starving physicians'. *Punch* mocks the way that the medical profession is always complaining that there are too many doctors, and that they are underpaid, and beset by 'bad debts'.

the belief in the progressive power of scientific medicine to cure was shared by policy-makers and consumers, as well as by the medical profession itself, and, when the gaps in the private insurance market became too large in the 1960s, the State stepped in to fill them.

The Cost of Western Medicine

It has been the strength of the consensus regarding the value of Western scientific medicine that has made it such a difficult political issue. Western medicine has become increasingly expensive, and the main debate in the twentieth century has been about how much of it can be afforded. In the case of the USA, alarm bells started to ring when nearly 10 per cent of gross domestic product was being spent on health care in the late 1970s, even though less than half of that was public money. European health-care systems, especially in the UK, have absorbed a far lower percentage of gross domestic product, but the concern about costs has also been great; indeed, in the case of the NHS, it has been present from the beginning. At some point, it is feared, spending on health care must become detrimental to growth, rather than assisting it. Raising the question of how much a country can afford to devote to health-care spending leads to a fundamental conflict between doctors, who are imbued with an absolutist ethic of treatment, and the utilitarian concerns of policymakers, who must consider not just the welfare of individuals but the collectivity, and who must juggle priorities. The views of the recipients of health care are much harder to distinguish. But there is evidence to suggest that a majority want the kind of care that they are told, by the medical profession, is best, even though as individuals they may remain sceptical or even fatalistic about the treatment they receive. However, on the whole, populations will rally to the defence of a local hospital that faces closure, and politicians have found it very difficult to find acceptable ways of limiting spiralling costs. It is the search for these that has dominated the story of late twentieth-century health-care systems. This chapter begins the story in the early twentieth century by examining the growing emphasis within medicine on the importance of personal health care and, in the case of Europe, the growing role of the State in providing such services before the First World War.

By the end of the nineteenth century, Britain had an extensive Poor Law medical service which provided both domiciliary medical relief and hospital beds. However, from a political point of view, the decision to expand the role of the State in 1911 by introducing a National Health Insurance scheme was to prove crucial because of the way in which it shaped the pattern of relationships within the health-care system. The UK followed Germany in adopting the insurance model, but the USA did not follow this path, despite the fact that the Progressives' rhetoric regarding the relationship between health and national efficiency or vitality was remarkably similar to the dominant strain in the British debate.

As health-care systems matured, so the battle for control between providers and financers also became fiercer. Until recently the medical profession has succeeded in wielding most power, and its success has been intimately related to the privacy of the patient–doctor relationship and the control over resources that it gives to the doctor, as well as to our faith in the profession and our belief that we should obey doctors' prescriptions for fear of what will happen if we do not. The question of the precise relationship between the health status of a population and the amount spent on medical care (as opposed to housing or the relief of poverty) was raised in the UK during the 1930s and

Several illustrations in this chapter show various aspects of poverty and the obvious ill-effect on the health of the nation. This one, entitled 'Evicted: Living in London, *c.*1901', shows the dire poverty and despair of the poor turned out of house and home with all their furniture.

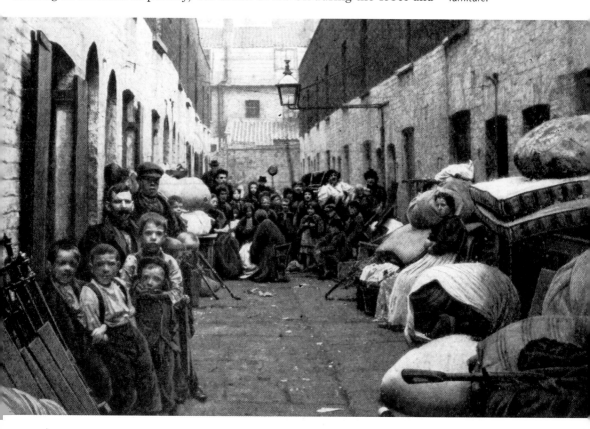

1940s by those outside the medical profession and again, much more force-fully, in the 1970s, when it helped to tip the balance of power away from the medical profession for the first time in the history of modern health-care systems.

During the 1970s it was frequently observed that, while the percentage of gross domestic product absorbed by health care was twice as high in the USA as in the UK, this was not reflected in superior outcomes (measured by mortality rates). Indeed, the UK, with by far the lowest health-care costs, managed to achieve mortality rates that were no higher than average. The doubts raised about the efficacy of high-tech modern medicine were new and, together with concern about its cost, have fuelled radical reforms to health-care systems that have increased the power of managers over doctors and have sought to shift money from the acute, hospital sector to community care.

The Move towards Health Insurance in the Early Twentieth Century

By the early twentieth century much more regard was being attached to the medical profession and to personal medical care. The reasons for this are com-plicated. Traditionally it has been thought that the rise in the status and power of the medical profession was intrinsically related to its increased ability to cure the patient, with the dissemination of the germ theory playing a particu-larly important part. However, M. Jeanne Peterson has argued that Victorians did not judge occupational status by efficiency, and that increasing secular-ization and more concern about physical health, human life, and productivity provided a social environment in which knowledge of the human body, even in the absence of effective treatment, began to be significant. Such an envi-ronment permitted the independent authority of the physician to grow. Paul Starr has identified a complicated conjuncture for the USA, including the growth of the market for medical care as incomes rose; the standardization

National Health Insurance
was introduced in 1911,
providing free medical
care for workers with an
annual income below a
certain level. It was
introduced by Lloyd
George of the Liberal
Party which advertised the
benefits of the new form
of health insurance.

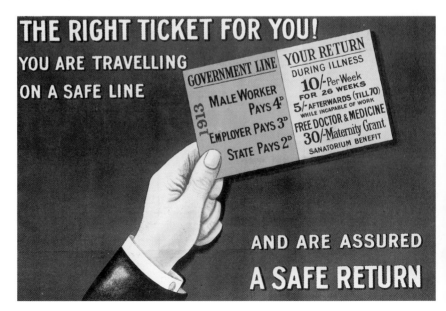

and expansion of medical education providing additional legitimacy for the profession; and the rise of new structures of dependency, such as insurance, replacing the doctor's reliance on lay patronage and thereby tipping the balance of power and authority in favour of the profession rather than the lay person. Undoubtedly the increased interest in medical care was a product of much more than suppliers creating their own demand or professionalization internal to the profession. Changing attitudes to health and disease, the high premium attached to health, and changing market conditions, as well as changes in the training and organization of the medical profession (legitimated by scientific advances) all played a part.

Nineteenth-century health policy had focused primarily on questions of 'public health', and the standard accounts have concentrated on the heroic battles for sewerage and clean water, and against infectious disease. 'Slum' and 'fever den' were terms used interchangeably in the urbanized UK of the late nineteenth century. Both they and their inhabitants were feared as agents of infection before it was understood precisely how this occurred, and State intervention went furthest in matters of public-health policy, largely because of the threat diseases such as cholera and smallpox posed to the whole community. Vaccination against smallpox was the only measure that central government made the obligatory responsibility of local authorities. The focus of nineteenth-century health policy was pre-eminently environmental. All dirt was considered dangerous and public-health Acts were often a filter for broader social reform, especially in respect of housing standards. All sorts of social questions concerning poverty were packed into the fear of urban degeneration and physical deterioration.

But from the beginning of the twentieth century more emphasis was placed on what the individual should do to ensure personal hygiene. The campaign to reduce infant mortality in the UK provides a good example of this. In the late 1900s epidemiological studies of the problem conducted by medical officers of health employed by local authority public-health departments revealed the death rate to be highest in inner city slums and to be closely correlated with poverty and poor sanitation. Yet government officials and public-health doctors tended to view maternal and child welfare in terms of a series of discrete personal health problems, to be solved by the provision of health visitors, infant welfare centres, and better maternity services. Before the First World War, the bulk of their attention was focused on health education, encouraging mothers to breastfeed and to strive for higher standards of domestic hygiene. Clinic work was seen as a new kind of personal preventive clinical medicine. Thus, once it was realized that dirt *per se* did not cause infectious disease, the broad mandate of public health to deal with all aspects of environmental sanitation and housing as the means of promoting cleanliness disappeared. Germ theory made it possible to concentrate attention on the individual and made a direct appeal from mortality figures to social reform more difficult.

The shift to personal health-care services must also be related to the movement for national efficiency and the debate about the relationship between poverty and sickness. Ill health was viewed primarily as a barrier to national efficiency, both industrial and military. Nineteenth-century proponents of public-health reform had stressed the idea that sickness causes poverty (result-

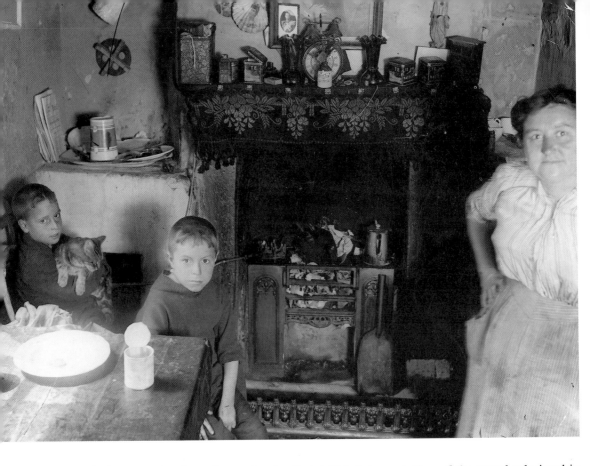

The photographer's caption for this vivid illustration of domestic poverty was 'Distressing scenes in the East End. All the food in the house—a little butter, sugar and a nearly empty tin of milk. July 25, 1912'.

ing in a charge for the State). This interpretation of the vexed relationship between poverty and ill health was also dominant in the early twentieth century, but the solutions offered were rather different. The Fabian socialist strand of opinion in the UK favoured building upon the 'personal preventive' services of the local public-health departments to promote hygienic habits among the poor. In this view, a choice had to be made between two existing forms of State provision—the Poor Law medical service and the public health service—if more people were to be brought into the ambit of personal medical services and the health and welfare of 'the race' thereby improved. Opinion generally could see little mileage in expanding the Poor Law medical service. The Poor Law was, by definition, a deterrent system. It tested an applicant's destitution before providing relief, whether in the form of medical services or of money. Any increase in efficiency or humanity would merely tempt more people to pauperize themselves in order to obtain medical relief. Hence the search in Britain for new ways to extend the coverage of personal health-care services.

The National Health Insurance Act of 1911

Starting from a similar concern with national efficiency, the Liberal Government of the period 1906–14 enacted a rather different model of health reform based on State insurance. The National Health Insurance Act of 1911 was financed by contributions from employers, employees, and the State, and provided sickness benefits and limited access to medical care in the form of a 'panel' doctor (general practitioner). Lloyd George, who was primarily responsible for the Act, was clearly worried about the level of physical fitness, remarking that a C3 population would not do for an A1 empire. But the main aim of the legislation, in common with most early national insurance schemes, was to prevent poverty due to sickness. The UK scheme, like most of its European counterparts, was first and foremost an income maintenance system. It offered cover mainly to the male workforce; only 10 per cent of married women were employed full-time in insurable occupations, and the scheme did not cover dependants, despite the strong anxiety about the health and welfare of infants. In the UK context, national insurance represented a way of taking a particular section of the population outside the Poor Law in the name of promoting national efficiency. The legislation nevertheless offered an entering wedge for the provision of health care by the State, and the question of who was to be covered for which medical services was hard fought by the medical profession. By offering a relatively high capitation fee to those prepared to participate in the panel-doctor scheme, Lloyd George was in the end able to detach the often rather hard-pressed general practitioners from their much better-off consultant colleagues and gained their consent to the reform. In addition, general practitioners found the idea of control by a national insurance scheme a somewhat lesser evil than control by mutual aid societies, such as friendly societies and trade unions, who had operated their own schemes prior to 1911 (often referred to as 'club practice') and who had exerted considerable control over the doctors they employed.

Lloyd George was much influenced by Germany, where the Sickness Insurance Law had been passed as early as 1883 by Bismarck and is still in the 1990s the basis of German health-care policy. The German scheme was financed by employers and employees alone and from the beginning offered more generous medical benefits, including hospital care. There was no active professional association of doctors when the law was passed, so Bismarck did not have to contend with the interest-group politics that beset Lloyd George almost thirty years later. In Denmark, the medical profession gave its active support to the medical insurance scheme established in 1892, seeing it as a way to more secure incomes and feeling less threatened by the fact that it was a voluntary scheme. It remained voluntary until the Second World War, but achieved greater coverage during the inter-war years than either the UK or German examples.

Thus, while insurance was the preferred model for extending health-care services in turn-of-the-century Europe, the schemes took significantly different forms. In all countries except the UK the coverage and scope of the schemes were gradually extended, and insurance has remained the basis of the vast majority of late twentieth-century continental European medical systems.

Remarkably little attention has been paid by historians to the attraction that insurance held

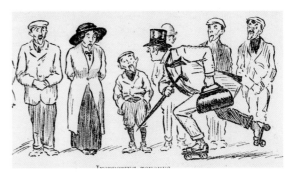

A doctor on roller skates inspects tongues in this 1912 cartoon. This was the year after the introduction of National Health Insurance, and suggests that those general practitioners who provided care for the scheme (the 'panel doctors') were so rushed that they were only able to spend a few seconds on each patient. Roller skates could speed them up!

for European governments. In the UK, the young Winston Churchill waxed eloquent about the 'magic of averages' whereby the lucky worker could count on
getting ninepence for fourpence (because of the contributions also made by
employers and the State). Certainly insurance offered a self-policing system of
welfare provision that proved popular with people and governors alike. Having paid in so much, the contributor had the right to draw out so much. Insurance avoided tests of means or, more unpleasantly still, destitution. But more
important was the opportunity insurance was perceived to offer in terms of
protecting or incorporating the private sector, and stimulating and rewarding
continuing voluntary effort. In Germany there were no fewer than 19,000 sickness funds comprising employers and employees in existence in 1885, and in
the UK, too, the administration of national health insurance was left to trade
unions, friendly societies, and commercial companies. In Denmark the State
eschewed compulsion altogether. With the advantage of hindsight, it seems
that the role of the State would inevitably prove decisive, but this was not necessarily how it appeared at the time.

The USA and the Second World War

That said, it has to be explained why the USA did not follow the European
example in respect of either health or unemployment insurance. This question has dominated accounts of the rise of modern welfare states, and an enormous range of answers has been offered. Among the most convincing in
respect of health insurance has been, first, the relative strength of the American Medical Association compared to its European counterparts, a factor that
continues to be relevant in the late twentieth century. US doctors succeeded in
controlling the non-statutory forms of insurance that developed in the USA in
the form of Blue Cross and Blue Shield as well as the commercial companies.
Whereas in the UK national insurance provision increased the power of doctors (as well as the influence of clinical medicine and the hospital) by securing
their incomes and liberating them from 'club practice', in the USA, the profession was already strong enough to resist State insurance.

A second factor is the nature of the US State and bureaucracy. In most European countries expert administrators established a monopoly of information
which they then used to further welfare expansion. Given this, the relative
lack of an established independent bureaucracy in the USA assumes considerable importance. It is also important to think about the larger framework
within which policy was being made. In the USA, the larger goals of the Progressives were to attack the monopoly and corruption associated with the
State. Suspicion of the State was widespread. Women's groups experienced
considerable success in lobbying for maternal and child welfare services,
which were also staffed by women, but the kind of State involvement
demanded by an elaborate national insurance scheme did not command
widespread support. Indeed, the USA showed a marked reluctance to engage in
social spending, although it nevertheless promoted the growth of the health
industry through indirect and direct subsidy to medical education, hospitals,
research, and, eventually in the 1960s, vulnerable groups in the population via
Medicare and Medicaid. Less convincing is the stress some analysts have tried

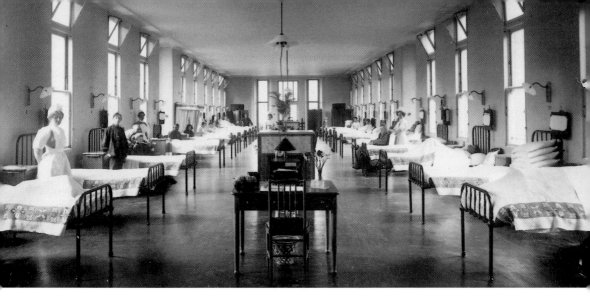

A ward in King's College Hospital in April 1914. The voluntary hospitals (so called because they depended on voluntary subscriptions from the public) were the pride of the UK, especially the large teaching hospitals. This picture illustrates the cleanliness, tidiness, and air of regimented efficiency of a well-run ward under the eagle eye of that powerful and authoritarian hospital figure, the ward sister.

to put on the demands of organized labour. The American Federation of Labor certainly opposed national insurance (chiefly because it did not guarantee universality and threatened to subordinate workers to a State they did not control—in other words, because it was an insufficiently radical measure). But British trade unions were not enamoured with the idea either. They offered sickness benefits of their own and feared that State interference in health provision would subvert their relationship with their members.

The UK national insurance system created a structure which ensured doctors a large measure of professional autonomy and control. The major concern of the majority was to ensure that any extension of State provision did not call this into question. In particular they looked with suspicion upon the salaried, public health department doctor, fearing that this might yet prove a model for future reform. The attitude of doctors, anxious to defend independent practice, together with the vested interests of those administering the scheme and the reluctance of the Treasury to increase public expenditure during the years of the Depression, meant that health insurance was not significantly extended in any respect during the inter-war years. Compared with many other European health insurance systems, that of the UK appeared limited. During the Depression, sickness benefits were cut. Furthermore, the prestigious, voluntary, non-profit hospitals, which included all the big teaching hospitals, were experiencing acute financial difficulties while determined to remain independent. Government firmly resisted calls from social investigators to examine the relationship between mortality, income, and levels of nutrition and the extent of morbidity, especially among women after childbirth, which it felt could only result in demands for more public expenditure on both benefits and medical treatment. By the beginning of the Second World War, access to health-care services was perceived as being profoundly unequal and inadequate, while administratively the system was characterized by muddle.

The effect of the war on social policy has been accorded great significance in the historiography of the British welfare state. Certainly war 'tests' medical services in particular, and as early as 1939 the Emergency Medical Service was introduced in order to coordinate hospital care. The impressionistic survey of attitudes towards welfare policies carried out by G. D. H. Cole in 1942 showed health care to be people's first priority and recorded strong negative feelings about the inadequacy of the panel-doctor system. In 1944 a Government White Paper proposed the setting-up of a National Health Service. The medical profession successfully fought against a salaried service for general practitioners and control by the local authorities, but in 1946, when the NHS Bill received the royal assent, a comprehensive, universal service was introduced (in 1948) in which hospitals came under the control of the State. The American Medical Association spent some $1.5 million campaigning against what it termed 'socialized medicine' in 1949, the first full year of the service's operation. Although substantial changes in health-care systems took place in many countries following the Second World War, the idea that there was a causal relationship between war and the development of social policy in the UK has been criticized; moreover, such a causal relationship cannot be established in other countries. Nevertheless substantial changes in health-care systems took place in most places following the war. The Swedish health insurance system, which was built around regionally elected agencies, mostly funded by local taxation, and which had developed relatively slowly, became compulsory in 1947 and rapidly expanded. The German system reverted to the pre-Nazi insurance scheme, which became virtually universal in coverage, albeit that status dif-

Sleeping inside a New York mission, under the notice on the wall 'How long since you wrote mother?', is another illustration showing homelessness and poverty, this time in the New World.

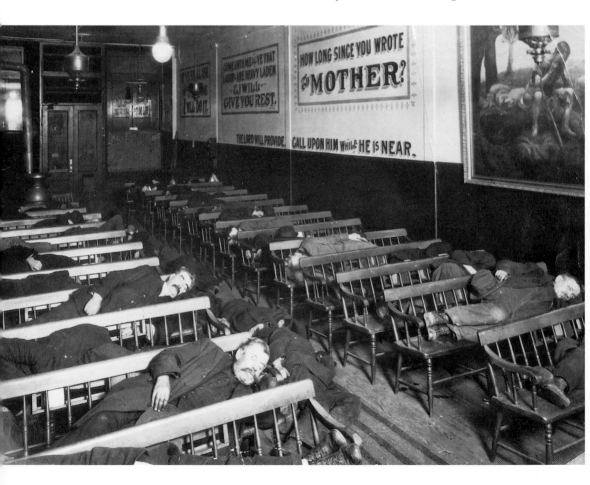

ferentials were preserved between the different sickness funds, with white-collar workers often being eligible for rather more and better treatments than blue-collar workers.

All the European schemes were as much attached to a model of health care that gave the dominant place to hospital medicine as was that in the USA. Nor was the consumer of medical care given any great voice in the new national systems. While the post-war European systems were very differently organized from the fragmented US provision, founded as they have been on an ethical imperative to achieve equity, all Western health-care systems have experienced an explosion in costs because of demographic changes and the rapidly increasing proportion of elderly people in the population, advances in medical technology, and rising labour costs. As a result, all have experienced major reform. It is also true that the US State has become more involved in health-care provision for pragmatic as much as ethical reasons. Thus in the late twentieth century there are some signs of convergence in Western health-care systems.

From Medical to Managerial Domination

Since the 1980s, the issue of spiralling costs and the question mark hanging over the relationship between the provision of medical services and health status has resulted in doubts about the efficacy of scientific medicine and about the role of the State in making it more widely available. In the 1980s and 1990s government has attacked the issue of spiralling costs by attempting to reduce the power of the medical profession. In the UK this contrasts with both 1911 and 1946, when the profession's autonomy was reinforced. Furthermore, this pattern is common both to northern Europe and to North America.

In fact, concern about costs marked the NHS from its inception. Charles Webster has estimated that public expenditure on health-care services amounted to 3 per cent of gross national product in 1939 and that the introduction of the NHS resulted in only a small rise to 3.5 per cent, readily explained by the backlog of demand for particular services such as dentures, the increase in nurses' pay, and inbuilt inefficiencies such as the overpayment of dentists. This is in line with the view of Richard Titmuss and Brian Abel-Smith, who reported in 1956 that, when the changing age structure of the population and inflation were controlled for, the net diversion of resources to the NHS had been relatively insignificant.

William Beveridge, whose 1942 Report provided a blueprint for post-war social-security reform, one of the underpinning assumptions for which was a national health service, assumed that by making access to all health services universal the NHS would raise health standards and thereby eventually reduce the demands on the service and hence costs. Unhappily this did not prove to be the case. By the mid-1970s, the service was absorbing 6 per cent of public expenditure and, more significantly in terms of the future, the hospital sector's share of total costs had risen from a half to two-thirds. This was still significantly lower than other systems: in Sweden 6 per cent of GDP was being absorbed by hospitals alone by the 1970s. The most effective early critics of the NHS stressed that the demand for health care was infinite, while pointing out that resources were finite. Many of these critics went on to argue, in a manner not dissimilar from right-wing critics during the 1980s, that the rational consumer would demand all he could while refusing to supply through higher taxes. It followed that the options for government were to ration demand strictly (allowing only so many days in hospital and so many visits to a GP), or to abandon State control of the health system in favour of the market. Given that rationing of this kind would be politically unacceptable, this amounted to a demand for a market system in health care, something that was refuted by Titmuss, who argued powerfully that health care was not a consumer good like shoes or refrigerators. The need for health care was uncertain and unpredictable and the consumer was usually ignorant of his or her needs, unable to estimate their cost, and unlikely to learn by experience.

During the 1960s and 1970s governments pursued first rational planning and then managerial reform in an effort to control costs. Only towards the end of the 1980s have both US and northern European governments converged upon the idea of 'managed competition' or 'quasi-markets' as a solution to the problems of health-care systems. The NHS put all hospital doctors on salary at the price of giving them freedom of action. During the 1960s there were attempts to involve doctors in management as a way of reconciling clinical autonomy with managerialist goals, but these were in the end unsuccessful. Similarly, grand attempts to achieve greater coordination between health and social services ended up as mere exhortation.

In 1974 the service was reorganized as a result largely of the Treasury's desire to gain more control over spending by the Department of Health and Social Security. It was widely believed that the planning efforts of the 1960s had been frustrated by the tripartite nature of the NHS, whereby general practitioner, hospital, and public-health (community) services were administered separately. The reorganization aimed to unify the service, increase central control, create a more effective consensus, interdisciplinary, management structure, and make possible a better planning system. When this failed to hold down costs in the hospital sector, two further reorganizations followed, in 1982 to simplify the bureaucracy by removing one tier in the administrative structure, and in 1984 to identify 'general managers' for each level of the service in the hope that they would be better placed to make firm management decisions than the consensus management teams created in 1974. Decisions would be taken, not by management teams composed of the different health disciplines, but by professional managers.

In the USA, in keeping with historical tradition, State intervention to contain costs took the form of increased regulation. In the early 1970s the Federal Government facilitated prepayment schemes in the form of 'health maintenance organizations', which united insurer and provider and hence ended the open-ended commitment of third-party payers. Pre-payment schemes of this kind were viewed as an alternative to both the fee-for-service medicine practised in the USA and further centrally financed medical care. States also began regulating hospital rates, particularly for Medicaid patients. During the 1980s government began to use 'diagnostic-related groups', whereby reimbursement rates were predetermined according to an average fee schedule. Insurers also insisted on strict resource management within clinical regimes, which, as one British commentator has put it, made the UK medical audit look like 'a teddy bears' picnic' by comparison. These initiatives, like their UK counterparts, were intended to promote the power of managers over that of the medical profession.

The effort to curb the autonomy of the medical profession has been strengthened by a series of studies suggesting that medical services have played very little part in raising the health status of populations. Ivan Illich went so far as to argue that modern scientific medicine has had positively iatrogenic consequences. Thomas McKeown's historical work on the decline of mortality in Britain showed that curative medicine came a poor third, after rising living standards and public health, in accounting for the decline in death rates. Western governments were able to take up this research in arguing for a shift in resources from the expensive acute sector to preventive medicine, community care, and the 'Cinderella' specialities such as geriatrics and psychiatry. In the USA this research also had the effect of invalidating arguments for improving access to medical services through a national insurance scheme.

Nevertheless, in the 1990s the Clinton Administration once more put forward a plan for universal health insurance. The ethical argument was not new, although it had strengthened in proportion to the increase in exclusion from provision. By the mid-1980s one-sixth of those under 65 years of age had no insurance cover and a quarter were either under-insured or not insured. The percentage of the poor receiving Medicaid remained constant during the 1980s, but the numbers of poor increased significantly. The arguments for national health insurance were also pragmatic. Since the early 1980s it has been argued that such a reform would yield savings by eliminating some medical services and holding down costs. In the USA it seems that there is a growing consensus that the limit to expenditure on medical care has been reached. In particular, health-insurance premiums have served to increase wage-bill costs. In view of the history of the USA's fragmented health-care provision, with the large role played by the private sector, it is not surprising that President Clinton began to talk about insurance in a framework of 'managed competition', a hybrid of free-market forces and regulation. It is considerably more puzzling to explain why northern European governments have also moved towards competition in their latest efforts to reform health-care delivery systems.

In the UK, broadly speaking, the NHS could be rated successful in terms of the outcomes it has achieved (albeit measured rather crudely by mortality rates) for very low cost. In large measure, the effort to inject market mechanisms into the NHS can be attributed to the ideology of successive Thatcher administrations. It is well known that, before her review of the service, Mrs Thatcher had studied the US system. In addition, it was the work of an American, Alain Enthoven, on the NHS that proved particularly influential in policy-making circles in the mid-1980s. Indeed, the vast majority of British policy initiatives during the 1980s were in some measure US imports. However, other northern European governments have also been moving in a similar direction, particularly the Netherlands and to some extent Sweden and Denmark. This means that we must look for deeper structural pressures for change in the form of rising consumer expectations, the need to maximize productivity in

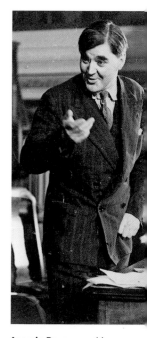

Aneurin Bevan speaking at a meeting of the National Council of Civil Liberties. The role of Bevan in the introduction of the National Health Service is well known. That Bevan succeeded in winning over most of the medical profession was in no small measure due to his vivacity and charm which are vividly shown in this picture.

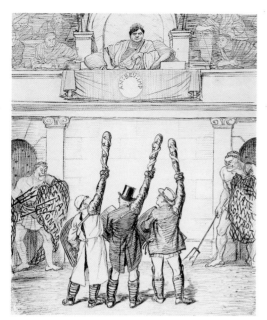

Members of the BMA dressed as gladiators, conceding the introduction of the National Health Service to Aneurin Bevan, dressed as Nero. This, perhaps, was the way that Bevan was seen by the members of the medical profession who opposed the introduction of the NHS in 1948.

what are predominantly service-based economies, and the collapse of working-class support for social democracy. The forms of market mechanisms that have been introduced differ considerably, although all share the characteristics of a 'quasi-market'. This differs from 'real' markets in that the supplier is not necessarily out to maximize profits, nor is it necessarily the consumer who exercises choice in purchasing. Consumer purchasing power is not expressed in cash either, because purchasing is still financed by taxation. In the Dutch reforms, more competition has been introduced between insurers and between hospital specialists and general practitioners, with money following the patient. In the UK reforms, competition has been introduced on the supply side. A purchaser/provider split has been created with two sets of purchasers, district general managers and general practitioner fundholders. Given the historical divide between general practitioners and consultants in British medicine, giving the former purchasing clout represents a real shift in power within the profession. Providers have become 'trusts' and compete for contracts. The changes in the UK have been part of a paradigmatic shift in welfare provision since 1988, which has sought to separate the finance and provision of all social services. It is not possible to see these changes primarily in terms of cost-cutting measures. The introduction of market mechanisms will certainly force up administrative costs. But they have succeeded in giving managers real power over the system at last in the hope that they will increase productivity and quality.

In many respects, the move towards markets is as much 'a jump in the dark' as was Bismarck's plunge into health insurance in the late nineteenth century. They have been justified in large measure by a rhetoric that emphasizes a better deal for the recipients of health care. However, while government by contract might improve the position of the patient as consumer, it does not serve to empower him or her as citizen. There is no sign of any significant increase in patient participation in health-care systems. Nor is it clear that the fundamental issue of how much modern health provision should be restricted or rationed—namely, the question of how much should be spent on whom, and for what medical purposes—will be easy to solve.

If there is a finite amount that states are prepared to spend on health care and if medical technology gets ever more sophisticated, how are choices to be made between 'new hips and new hearts'? There have been signs, particularly in the UK and the USA during the 1980s and 1990s, that government would like to do less. Even in the 1960s, the then British Cabinet Minister with responsibility for the NHS commented that it was inherently unsuitable for administration by a politician. However, the problems of access to, and the allocation of, health care are amongst the most central political issues of the late twentieth century and are likely to remain so.

19 | The Patient's View

ANNE DIGBY

TRADITIONALLY, the history of medicine neglected the past experience of patients and sufferers in favour of the history of institutional development, the control and conquest of diseases, and the achievements of medical practitioners. Since the 1970s the patient as a forgotten element in the history of Western medicine has been succeeded by the patient as an increasingly researched, but problematical, part of a more complex analysis. There is no overall shortage of material on past patients, since recorded lay perceptions and experiences of sickness are legion. But uneven coverage amongst different social groups has left the top and bottom of the social hierarchy much better served than those of the middling groups.

The affluent, literate, sufferer has left subjective accounts of ailments and treatments in letters, diaries, and autobiographies from which can be derived impressionistic anthologies. Some, like Sir Walter Scott, recorded their ailments reluctantly: 'My journal is getting a vile chirurgical [surgical] aspect. I shall tire of my journal if it is to contain nothing but bile, plasters and unguents.' Others noted every ache and pain, like the hypochondriacal John Wyndham, who gave a diary entry between 1741 and 1746 to every twinge and ache, together with the effects of the remedies given by his doctor, and the health advice Wyndham himself gave to friends. Unfortunately, we have no means of knowing just how representative recorded experiences such as these were. In some cases the historical experience might have been reasonably common to many patients, but in others diverse and individual peculiarities warn us against generalizing from a small sample. We need also to bear in mind that we are looking at accounts of experience and not at the subjective experience itself, and, inevitably, the patient's experiential view has been subtly influenced by the medium—whether the written word or the varied forms of illustration—that recorded it.

In addition to the records of the affluent, literate, sufferer there are the records concerning poor patients in public asylums and hospitals which have been written up in a standardized format as cases in institutional registers, journals, and day books. These offer the possibility of a different kind of patient's history in the form of large-scale statistical analyses of treatments, patient stays, and outcomes. This chapter will focus on the period since the

| beginning of the seventeenth century in an attempt to capture some of the potentialities, as well as the ambiguities and limitations, of looking at medical history 'from below'.

Domestic and Alternative Medicine

The domestic perspective of the sufferer and the centrality of the household in the care of the sick have tended to be obscured by the spotlight placed on non-domestic innovations and advances in medicine, so that the professionalizing doctor and the hospital, the 'magic bullets' of pharmacological improvement, have relegated the less dramatic continuities of home nursing and the household medical chest to the wings of the historical stage. Yet, despite modern triumphs in vanquishing infectious diseases, self-management by the sufferer and the adoption of a healthy regimen retained their significance. At the end of the eighteenth century Mr Hyde declared, for instance, that despite being 104 he walked 12 miles a day and had 'never taken doctors stuff'. In many households a well-stocked medical chest, and its adjunct the household book of medical recipes, were staples. Through their miscellany of medicinal and culinary recipes the latter suggest the everyday centrality of the nurturing and healing housewife, and of other women, both in the household and frequently beyond it, in the care of ailing relatives and neighbours.

For some, selective self-medication by the sufferer might also be a reaction to the indiscriminate, heroic prescriptions of the medical faculty, which, until the mid-nineteenth century, was remunerated, not on the basis of skill and knowledge, but instead on the mountainous quantities of pills and potions prescribed. Pills for ills was not, of course, the prerogative of the practitioner, and the self-medications of the sufferer—with an eclectic recourse to boluses, mixtures, elixirs, and juleps—were publicized to relatives and friends. The letters of the past are wonderfully revealing on the frequency with which the discriminating exchange of favourite prescriptions and remedies made up the currency of discourse. Lay manuals reinforced this with their advice, as did the many editions of Buchan's *Domestic Medicine*, with the recommendation that 'It is always, however, in the power of the patient, or those about him, to do as much towards his own recovery as can be effected by the physician.' The doctor was very much an optional or late extra for many sufferers in a predominantly domestic—and thus lay—management of sickness.

Alternative medicine also flourished in this environment, so that only a minority of sufferers became patients of the regular medical faculty. There was a plurality of choices available to the sufferer, and more particularly the chronic invalid whose condition was outside the orthodox practitioner's skill to cure rather than palliate. Charles Darwin's adoption of the water cure followed on dissatisfaction with the advice of his consultant physicians. 'I feel certain that the water-cure is no quackery,' he stated firmly. Particularly for the poorer sufferer, recourse to apothecary, druggist, or chemist provided cheaper remedies for minor ailments.

The personal eloquence of the itinerant seller of 'secret remedies' in the early modern era was only gradually replaced by the printed puffs of patent

medicine advertisements, whose dubious catch-all claims to relieve sufferers' problems were trumpeted loudly in newspapers. Here there were bold asser- tions of the ability of a patent medicine to: cure sexual impotence; vanquish cancer; provide relief for 'all female complaints' (a well-known coding for abor- tifacients); offset 'brain fag', nervous debility, or lassitude; or relieve chronic skin conditions. These promises of immediate relief for intractable, serious, or chronic conditions were remarkably successful in extracting money from credulous sufferers, not least because they offered health as an accessible and cheap consumer commodity.

Rural and 'Frontier' Medicine

Calling out the doctor was an expensive matter in remote rural or frontier regions particularly, when a day or a half-day on horseback was needed for the doctor to reach the patient, so that only the more dire emergencies merited professional attention, the rest being succoured from the household medical chest. The versatility and enterprise of the frontier doctor, to whom economic survival was a greater imperative than professional preconceptions as to what was orthodox or quack medicine, meant that a heterodox range of treatments might be made available to the rural patient.

Sufferers in the American West, for example, could buy from drug stores owned by doctors the very quack medicines that were denounced by pro- fessional journals in the metropolis. For patients out in 'the sticks', the horse- back-doctor brought in his saddlebags only a restricted collection of surgical instruments and a range of well-tried medicaments. Depending on the skill and knowledge of the practitioner (many qualified only by a self-styled prefix as 'Doctor'), treatment was applied to human—and animal—patients with vary- ing degrees of audaciousness or discrimination. Some deficiencies in skill were perhaps counterbalanced in the patient's mind by more personal qualifications earned by the doctor's heroic encounters with floods, sand- storms, or blizzards in attempts to reach the isolated household. 'I sent for the doctor. He didn't git my word until three days later. . . . It took him two days more to git to us,' recollected an American parent who lived in snow-bound mountains, and whose twin babies died before the doctor reached the house- hold.

Indeed, the different personal and geographical terrain of frontier medicine frequently baffled practitioners whose urban or suburban past had habituated them to more frequent encounters between patient and 'family doctor'. One young immigrant doctor to South Africa was nostalgic for the intimacy of such past encounters, and contrasted it with the frontier colonial situation where 'a doctor looks on the patients as so many aids to making a fortune, and the patients on their doctors as necessary evils'. During the early twentieth cen- tury, distance shrank with modern technological innovation. 'We have expected to see you pass, which we have, but in a flying machine,' commented some Yorkshire patients disapprovingly, after their doctor had bought a car. In country practice especially, the car and telephone transformed the patient– doctor relationship, and American physicians reckoned that buying a car halved the journey time needed to reach the patient.

Views on Childbirth

Relationships between patient and practitioner were also remade in child-birth, although here the radical changes effected in roles and expectations took the form of more gradual historical transitions. Chagall's *The Birth* (1887) vividly depicts a Russian version of the customarily separate worlds of feminine childbirth and excluded masculinity. Until comparatively recently childbirth was quite a public event, like so many other encounters between patients and those dealing with their conditions in shops or surgeries. Traditionally, mothers were participants rather than patients in an egalitarian, lay, and all-female world of the lying-in chamber, where neighbours or gossips, presided over by an experienced 'old wife' or a licensed midwife, put into effect their customary rituals. The skills of an experienced midwife, such as the Dutch seventeenth-century Catharina Schrader, were welcomed by mothers, while in turn they received sympathetic care during their 'martyr's torment', as Catharina termed it. Mothers' belief that childbirth was not a 'medical' event was a resilient one. 'I'm afraid of a hospital and I am also afraid of a doctor. I don't just let people touch me, also not strip me naked. Our old wise women don't do that, no, they treat one properly,' commented an Afrikaner woman in the Cape during the 1930s.

Undermining this situation was a process beginning in the eighteenth century when the male surgeon, equipped with specialist instruments at first only for difficult births, gradually extended his practice to include normal births. This colonization of female territory went more slowly in the Netherlands than in the USA or Britain. Genteel Englishwomen were amongst the first to adopt the new custom and came to see this male management of their labour—in the words of Anne Norma Norris in 1812—as being 'in the newest and most approved style'. Her medical attendant doubtless trod delicately in the bedchamber in order to prevent any hint of impropriety or accusation of malpractice arising from social or physiological ignorance, for, if the mother's confidence was retained, attendance on the infant or child patient might ensue.

Children as Patients

Small children arrived relatively late on the medical scene as patients. The primary care resorted to by mothers was most likely to be in the form of home cures. Amongst black households in the southern plantations of the USA, for example, 'Whooping cough is treated by tying a leather string round the child's neck. A necklace of cork and mole's feet is used to make teething easy.' In the context of child illness, the medical profession was long both distrusted and distrustful. Like female patients, the young may have appeared as the Other—alien and mysterious as were their specialist diseases and pathology. And, like many poor patients in hospital, their inability to supply adequate accounts of symptoms meant that their conditions stood a relatively high chance of being misdiagnosed, more particularly before the advent of scientific measurement of such vital indicators as temperature, heartbeat, or pulse. Prudence by the doctor in any case meant a careful selectivity of accept-

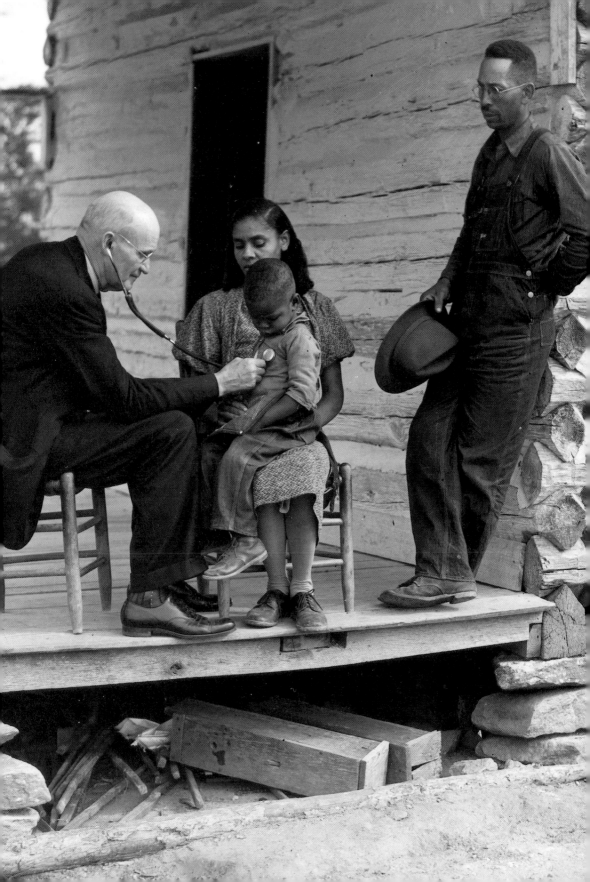

able cases, since, in a situation of obstinately high infant and child mortality, there were justifiable fears that a shadow might be cast over the professional reputation of any physician whose skill was found wanting.

The child patient was, therefore, likely to be visited frequently, spoken to gently, perhaps given the doctor's fob chain or even a small present as a distraction, while careful questions were put to the mother or nurse. To give added reassurance to a child who might be frightened by the unfamiliar entrance of a formally dressed stranger, apparently licensed to perform intrusive but intimate procedures, the sick child was often held by the mother or seated on her lap. Thus the doctor was mediated to the young patient through the mother in a tripartite encounter. In this situation, as in the many other circumstances where the secular power of Western medicine seemed deficient, an additional powerful but unseen presence could be felt in the sickroom. Thus, in 1798 Mary Taylor, aged 12, 'died in the utmost composure, as if she had a full assurance of now passing from this life to a better state'.

Medical Care and Religious Faith

Providential belief in a 'Great Physician in Gilead', who practised a divine art of healing, was widespread and long-lasting. Traditionally, patients in many cultures offered less a clinical than a religious opportunity to those who cared for them: hence the notable presence of nursing sisterhoods, as in France. In England, the continuing popularity of John Wesley's *Primitive Physic* (1747), with its advice to 'apply to a physician that fears God' and to 'add to the rest ... that old unfashionable medicine, prayer', indicated a belief in a symbiotic relationship of health and prayer within a providential view of healing. Until the scientific (and more particularly the surgical) achievements of the nineteenth and twentieth centuries endowed Western medicine with an enhanced authority based on greater therapeutic effectiveness, a providential worldview—where disease could be seen as the punishment for sin, and good health be seen as God's work—remained resilient.

In the early seventeenth century Lady Margaret Hoby believed that it was God's power that was manifest in her own lay healing, and wrote that 'I may truly conclude it is the Lord, and not the physician, who both ordains the medicine for our health and ordereth the ministering of it ... therefore let everyone—physician and patient—call upon the Lord for a blessing.' Providentialism was particularly likely to be invoked where medicine had been found wanting. The chaplain to an aristocratic English family wrote in 1794, for example, that since a patient's 'distemper has baffled all medical skill and assistance all we can do is by family prayer to recommend her to the Great Physician of Souls who alone can heal all our infirmities'. Picasso's painting of *Science and Charity* (1897) is a particularly late allegorical version of this tradition in Spain; the doctor (representing science) is depicted taking the pulse on one side of the patient's bedside whilst a nun is placed on the other. Increasing secularism during the nineteenth century, however, meant that in many other cultures the doctor gradually inherited the clerical mantle, so that, instead of psychological support for the patient being obtained by sacerdotalism, it was the doctor's professional rituals, his improved social presentation, and the mystique

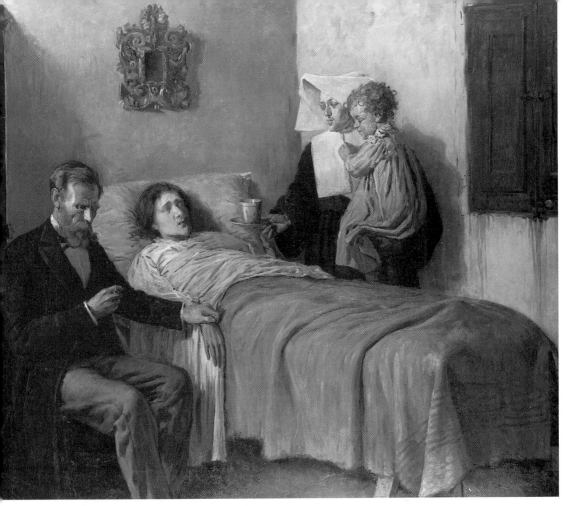

of his technical language that were designed to give patients reassurance that their recovery was safeguarded. In this context it is revealing that professional handbooks admonished the Victorian doctor on the importance of creating faith, since 'the faculty of keeping hope and confidence alive in the breast of the patient . . . carries him with you on the road to recovery'.

The Effects of Professionalization and Medical Institutions

Did the professionalizing process and its adjunct, the medical institution, 'carry' the patient with the doctor? Collectively the testimony of patients forms a kaleidoscope which needs considerable interpretative intervention by the historian to produce a synthesis. Nowhere is the evidence left by patients more elusive and fragmentary than in the record of the asylum inmate. John Perceval stated retrospectively that he had felt as if he 'were a piece of furniture, an image of wood, incapable of desire or will as well as of judgement' when he was a patient in English asylums during the 1830s. This comment encapsulates the helplessly abject reduction of the patient to the status of object. Verbal comments such as these can make up an anthology of patient experience, yet these may be so differentiated as to make it difficult to determine which (if any) is typical.

Science and charity. Originally entitled 'Visit to a Sick Woman', this allegorical painting by Picasso was inspired by the death of the painter's sister, Conchita; the doctor takes the pulse and represents science, while the nun offers soup to the patient and represents charity.

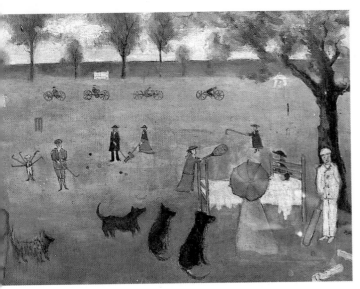

The insane patient. This painting by a psychiatric patient depicts the black dogs which are the threatening symbols of his mental illness together with the enjoyable therapeutic pursuits offered by the asylum in the 1890s, but his interpretation of their relationship, and thus of how effective he thought his treatment, remains ambiguous.

For example, amongst nineteenth-century patients at the York Retreat one recorded that 'the past year [in the asylum] has been the happiest of his life', whilst another stated that she looked upon 'her detention as a humiliation and a disgrace'. Even a pictorial record of his treatment by a third Retreat patient may impart not clarity but ambiguity. In his painting he depicted himself in a bed placed in the asylum's grounds, with his enjoyable therapeutic pursuits (such as croquet, golf, or bicycling) behind him, while the menacing symbols of his illness (in the shape of the large dogs mentioned as delusions in his admission certificate) occupy the foreground. Do these delusions obscure, and thus more than offset, his therapy or is the patient's interpretation one in which illness and therapy are evenly counterpoised?

The apparently transparent nature of the historical patient's narrative poses an obvious difficulty in the case of mad patients, since all too frequently the only record of the subject's experiences are the transcriptions within the doctor's clinical case notes—a professional prism through which the original viewpoint is refracted in shadowy form. More generally, however, the poor patient's narrative may also be problematic, since, with the birth of the clinic or modern hospital, it has been alleged that the patient was effectively silenced. This was because objective technological measurements of temperature or pulse and the medical narrative of the case history were interpreted as having replaced subjective patient testimony.

In my view, this overstates the case. Although a new epistemology reconceptualized specific disease entities so that the 'medical gaze' focused to a greater extent on their physical signs, the resilience of history-taking in medical encounters indicates that the patient's own story continued to be heard. For example, students were lectured in medical school on the need to be sensitive to the patient's account of pain—from the uneasy sensation to the violent spasm—and admonished about the relationship of these morbid symptoms to the likelihood of particular diseases. Since the nineteenth century, the patient's subjective account of his or her symptoms has become just the first stage in the diagnostic sequence. The patient's story and the doctor's interpretation of that story have become distinct but separate narratives. Not only the patient's body, but also the patient's story, have, as it were, become subjected to medical treatment. As a result, patients have often found that they can no longer understand the ways in which the disorders of their body are interpreted by doctors and feel profoundly alienated from medicine, and, more particularly perhaps, from surgery.

This has been a feature not only of twentieth-century medicine. Revealingly in this context, the Royal College of Surgeons in London was viewed during the early nineteenth century as 'that cutting shop in Lincoln's Inn Fields', whilst surgeons were termed slasher, sawbones, or fillgrave. That patients were reluctant to submit to surgery, except for minor conditions or as a last resort in more serious ones, was rational behaviour given the painfulness and uncertain outcome of many operations before mid-nineteenth-century anaesthetics and antiseptics reduced mortality from shock or sepsis. Hospital case notes might detail a sequence like that for William Doughty of Leeds, who was suffering from the stone. 'Refused operation . . . therefore on the 18th [September] he went out. October 28, he returned—the symptoms having become so severe, as to lead him to be willing for operation.' After an apparently successful operation he was discharged but returned six months later considering himself 'unrelieved and declaring that he would submit to *no* operation'. He later died, having refused his assent to any further surgical intervention.

Yet demand for admission into hospitals in Britain continually outstripped the supply of beds. The perceived utility to the poorer patients for whom they had been designed apparently outweighed their most obvious disadvantages, such as supplying clinical material for observation or teaching, being trial subjects of new procedures, or chance objects of cross-infection. And, whilst the hospital case notes of most poor patients leave us to infer subjective feelings, for the literate patient an experiential account may supplement or replace the official record. Thus, for the actor Joseph Wilde, in the Devon and Exeter Hospital at the beginning of the early nineteenth century, nurses were less caring than doctors: 'Her tongue kills more than ablest doctors cure.' It was middle-class patients, however, with operations in their own homes who left the most detailed accounts of their treatment. Fanny Burney, for instance, recorded in

Patient patients. There was a very rapid increase in the number of people who sought free treatment from London hospitals in the late nineteenth century. This shows the new outpatients' room of University Hospital, London, in 1872.

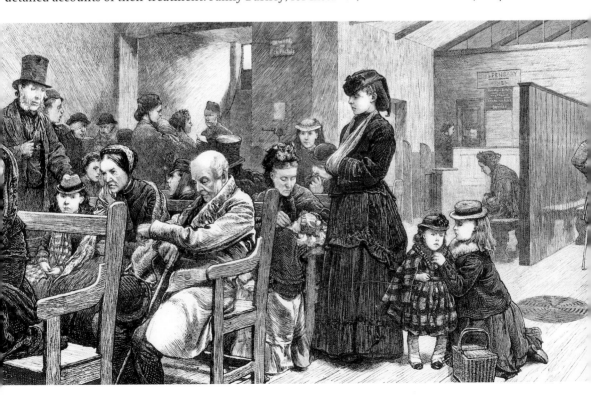

ghastly detail a major operation without anaesthesia. She wrote of being 'condemned' to a mastectomy, of the 'dreadful steel' being plunged into her breast, and of her discovery that so 'excruciating was the agony' that she could not prevent herself from screaming throughout the entire operation.

Medical and surgical advances contributed to a gradual change in emphasis from mortality to morbidity in the patient's perspective; the sixteenth- and seventeenth-century anxiety on how to die a good death became transmuted into an Enlightenment concern with how to stay well. The possibility of positive health and how to attain it became the staple of sufferers' letters and diaries at this time. 'I have applied myself very diligently to my health' or am 'laying in an additional stock of health' were veritable hallmarks of Georgian or Victorian sufferers' accounts. From bleeding to brimstone and treacle the long-term wisdom of lay medical culture enjoined purging as a regular servicing designed to keep the body ticking over efficiently. But for the chronic sufferer such periodic ministrations needed to be supplemented by a more continuous regimen with a prudent lifestyle of early rising, moderate application to business, restricted diet, cold bathing, and regular exercise.

Interestingly, the focus of twentieth-century patient concern differs cross-culturally, with the French typically worried about their liver, and the Germans focused on the condition of their hearts. Degenerative afflictions both present and past make health elusive, so that a pragmatic eclecticism might be practised in treatment, and, since the quality of care rather than a cure was a prime consideration, the social qualities of the doctor might assume greater importance. A patient-centred bedside medicine thus continued in private practice alongside the more illness-centred, or object-oriented, 'cases for treatment' of hospital medicine. Chronic patients looked to their practitioner for advice and reassurance, and became discriminating experts on their condition, at least in their own self-estimation. 'I had been bloodied several times but, I believe, not as often as I should . . . I remembered too what Sydenham says as to the cure of this distemper . . . And I believed that if I had been let blood once more I should have been perfectly cured,' critically reflected a Bedfordshire rector on the doctor's treatment of his rheumatism in 1739. The affluent thus frequently ended up patronizing several doctors. 'Restless from quack to quack they range | When 'tis themselves they ought to change,' aptly commented a versifying correspondent of the *Gentleman's Magazine* in 1751.

The Doctor's Bill

The dual business and clinical relationship of patient and practitioner has not yet received the academic attention it deserves, although the extent to which the patient's underlying financial anxieties on the cost of treatment impinged upon more overt clinical and social encounters was explored in contemporary cartoon representations, from Gillray, Cruickshank, and Rowlandson to *Punch*. Earlier medical bills usually itemized both visits and medicine, but interestingly they sustained a tradition of cartoons that outlived the practice by half a century and in which patients stated that they would pay for the medicines but return the visits. Patients themselves were very aware of the business side of the relationship, as with the old lady who was depicted as telling the doctor (in this case a specialist) what her income was before anything else was said. Predictably, it tended to be practices in poorer areas that made clear the fees that the practitioner would charge the patient, and poor British patients called their doctor the 'sixpenny' or the 'shilling' doctor.

Patients complained about the doctor's bill in their own homes, but occasionally might express their dissatisfaction to the doctor's face, as allegedly did an elderly, but stereotypically Scottish, patient who considered that his illness was 'varra expensive. I was wunnering if it was worthwhile at ma time of life.' Dissatisfaction by patients could lead to failure to pay bills and, more rarely, if the doctor attempted to reclaim his fees by legal action, to a counterclaim of malpractice. Inadvertently, non-payment was encouraged by the medical profession's habit of billing at infrequent intervals, often on a yearly basis, so that the patient's original gratitude had long since been forgotten. Unremunerative patients' attitudes were said to be:

> God and the doctor we alike adore
> When on the brink of danger, not before.
> The danger past, both are alike requited,
> God is forgotten and the doctor slighted.

In hard times patients found that doctors gave as little credit as possible, whilst patients themselves might avoid paying the doctor's bill by moving around from one unsuspecting practitioner to another. Sometimes a *rapprochement* or brokered deal was effected through payment in kind—stock from artisans, produce from farmers, or perhaps a (poached) rabbit or pheasant left anonymously at the back door by those too poor to pay even in kind. In England

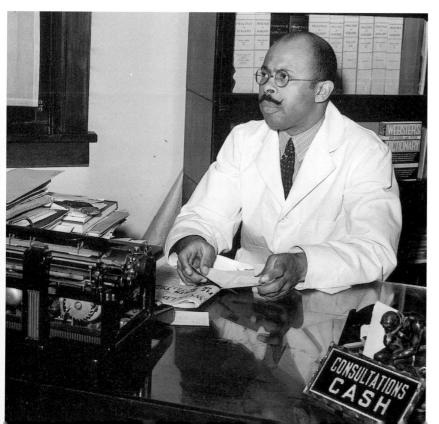

Consultations cash. In genteel practice the clinical preceded the business relationship but, in poorer areas, the patient was made aware that the economics of medicine took priority, as in the case of this Chicago practitioner in 1941.

301

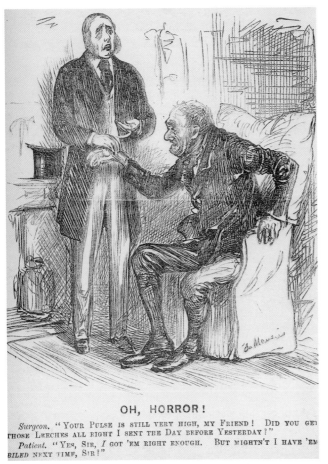

OH, HORROR!

Surgeon. "Your Pulse is still very high, my Friend! Did you get those Leeches all right I sent the Day before Yesterday?"

Patient. "Yes, Sir, I got 'em right enough. But mightn't I have 'em biled next time, Sir?"

A misunderstanding between a doctor and his working-class patient.
Surgeon, 'Your pulse is still very high, my friend! Did you get the leeches all right I sent the day before yesterday?'

Patient, 'Yes, sir, I got 'em right enough. But mightn't I have 'em biled [boiled] next time, sir?'

patients and doctors might operate an informal medical welfare state, since affluent patients paid inflated bills in the knowledge that this would help the doctor extend medical altruism to the poorer patient by way of low fees or free treatment. In the USA during times of depression doctors admitted that 'there wasn't a whole lot of money and there wasn't a whole lot of care' in poorer areas. When medical care that was free at the point of access was made available for a larger section of the population—whether by insurance or taxation—this was characterized by the standardized procedures and rapid throughput that had been features of earlier provision for the poor.

Patients set the financial cost of doctors against their utility in effecting a cure. Before professionalization, lay patient power had sometimes been sufficient to insist on payment by results, perhaps half the fee as down payment and the rest once a 'cure' had been effected. But this was subsequently denounced by the profession as the conduct of the quack, and thus fell into disuse (at any rate before the reintroduction in the 1990s of performance-related pay). That the medical profession could later be found wanting in a more indefinite exchange of pain for gain is suggested by a middle-class patient who received a bill and exclaimed, 'Good Lord. Have I been as near death as that?' One widespread problem that impeded patient satisfaction with the doctor was that patients found the professionalized doctor's technical language difficult if not impossible to understand. *Punch* satirized the process by suggesting that working-class patients asked for their leeches to be boiled next time, or found the boxes (containing medicines) unpalatable, whilst their middle-class counterparts also misunderstood the tenor of their doctor's advice, replying 'No, no, doctor! Anything but an operation' to a kindly suggestion that 'What you need is to be taken out of yourself.'

Patients in the more distant past felt a need to believe in their doctors, not least since hope was a resilient commodity and desperation an even more powerful one. However, patients might harbour a shrewd suspicion that practitioners' therapeutic competence was not always equal to the task in hand. The Honourable John Byng reflected one of the most sceptical of patient's perspectives when he wrote in 1794:

Mr G. was call'd in last night for his advice, and assistance to Mrs B; he is as full of advice and as assistant as any of the faculty: but what can they do? In youth we want them not, in middle age we must rid ourselves and in age who can aid us? Their profits arise from folly and idle imbecility; prevention will assist us for a time, and when prevention fails our end is nigh.

It is salutary to discover that the enduring literary ironies of the early modern period were that medicine was worse than the malady, and that physicians cured the disease but killed their patients. These were replaced by satiric views of the doctor in disagreement with colleagues or of the practitioner who can now name, but still not cure, a disease. Rowlandson's *A Physician by his Patient's Deathbed* lampooned the fashionable eighteenth-century Quaker physician John Lettsom through using a popular epigram as its subtitle—'I purge, I bleed and sweat 'em, then if they die I lets 'em'. And as late as 1926 a cartoon showed a distinguished physician saying, 'If this doesn't put you right, come to me again', to which the patient's riposte is 'How many guesses do you want?' In recent years popular scepticism over the positive healing power of the doctor has been intensified as a result of journalistic publicity of iatrogenic mishaps. But for some of the clearest examples of historical scepticism we must turn to role reversal—to the doctor who fell sick and became the patient of his erstwhile colleagues. 'You must excuse me for I will take no more medicines', prudently declared the eminent nineteenth-century surgeon Astley Cooper to the two physicians and three surgeons who had been treating him during his terminal illness. That doctors made bad patients is a truism that the historical record confirms: doctors knew only too well the extent of their colleagues' uncertainties and hence showed reluctance to submit to painful and often ineffectual treatments.

Traditionally, a practitioner's authority might be enhanced in the patient's eyes by psychological shrewdness, as through the use of bitter drugs which, because they tasted nasty must—the patient inferred—be doing good. In more recent times the addition of effective pharmaceuticals (notably antibiotics) and of potent medical technology has undoubtedly helped elevate the status of medicine, while doctors' 'gatekeeping' responsibilities in providing certification for insurance companies, benefit societies, or insurance schemes have enhanced the profession's power in society. The *Lancet*'s view in 1878 that 'The doctor with the advance of civilisation and of medical science, becomes more and more indispensable' is one to which many patients in the late twentieth century would probably still subscribe.

Conclusion: The Patient's View

Much medical history, like the coverage of this volume, has been mainly from the vantage-point gained from standing in the doctor's shoes, while this chapter has attempted instead to stand in those of the patient. How then should we conceptualize the patient and the patient's viewpoint? Models of the patient–doctor encounter are of only limited utility since so far they have been poorly defined historically, and have been beguiled by a desire for symmetry in roles. For example, one hypothesis suggested that historically the earliest stage was one of activity by the doctor and passivity by the patient; this was then succeeded by guidance and leadership by the doctor and obedience and admiration by the patient; and the third stage—allegedly reached by the twen-

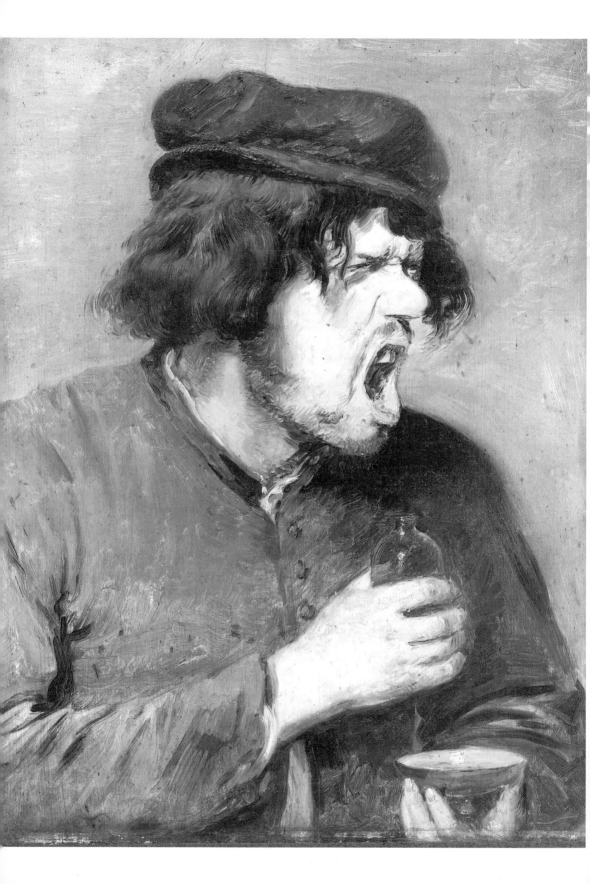

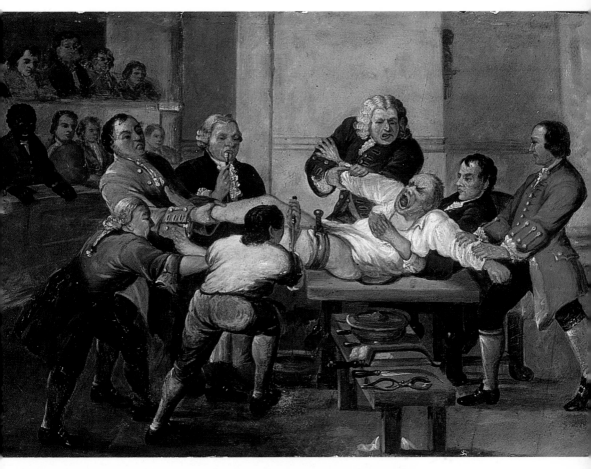

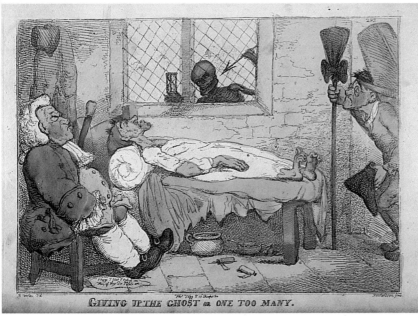

GIVING UP THE GHOST or ONE TOO MANY.

A scene in the men's operating theatre of the old St Thomas's Hospital in Southwark, London, which suggests very vividly the terror of the individual facing surgery in the period before anaesthesia offered a blissful non-awareness of the surgeon's operative techniques.

A Physician by his *Patient's Death-Bed*. Entitled 'Giving up the Ghost or One too Many' and subtitled 'I purge, I bleed and sweat 'em, then if they die I lets 'em.' This was a popular epigram, dating from the 1790s, on the highly successful Quaker practitioner, Dr John Coakley Lettsom (1744–1815).

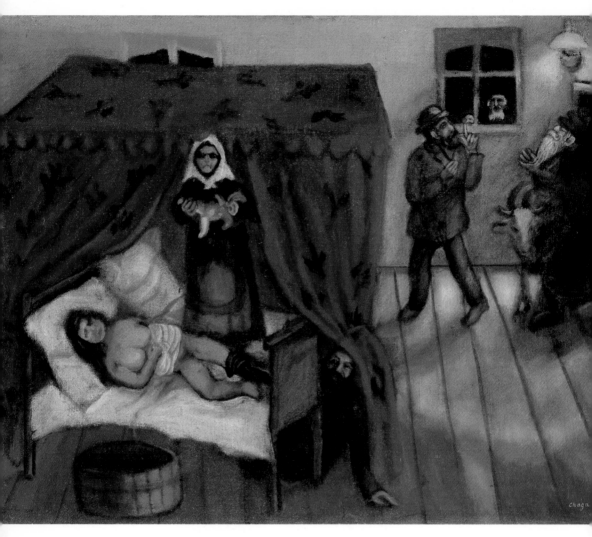

Marc Chagall, *The Birth*. This painting highlights
theatrically the separation between the female
terrain of traditional childbed, where a midwife
or oldwife attended the mother, and the
excluded world of masculinity. The hidden male
figure should be interpreted in a non-literal way
since, characteristically, Chagall's paintings
suggest the hidden meaning of life.

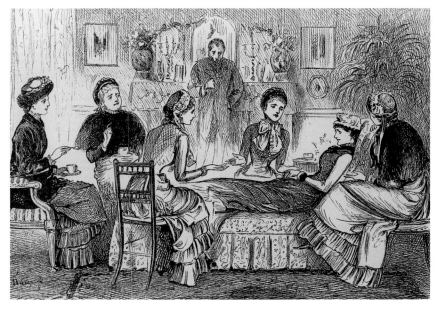

Female patients' perceptions of a good doctor. 'My dear Eliza, Sir Arthur Pillington is the man for your complaint. So clever, and a perfect gentleman.'. . .

'Why he nearly killed an aunt of mine! Send for Wilfrid Jones, Eliza. Trust me, there's nobody like him. He listens to every symptom!'

'No, no, Eliza, listen to me. . .'

tieth century—was one of mutual participation and interdependence between practitioner and patient.

Unfortunately, what we have seen in this chapter does not lend itself to such neat complementarity, but suggests instead both that patients had highly differentiated experiences, perspectives, and roles, and also that we need to focus not just on the patient but also on the sufferer. Since historical health care was centred in the household, the medical practitioner saw only a small sub-sample of those who were sick, and who designated themselves (or who were designated) as being sufficiently ill to merit the attention of a professional. The economics of medical care, it has also been argued, were vital constituents in this process, so that the business as well as the clinical relationship might be of central importance to the sufferer/patient viewpoint. Patients' class, race, gender, age, income, and status were balanced against medical expertise in the distribution of social, economic, and clinical power, and thus influenced whether patients were patrons, participants, or merely objects of medical attention. This suggests that patients were sometimes subjects but at other times objects: as patrons or participants they might control or influence their destiny, or alternatively—as with many hospital inmates or surgical patients— they might be subordinate to it.

Bitter medicine. Typically, patients thought that medicine did not do good unless it tasted bad. Doctors might employ shrewd psychology in achieving a high ratio of pain to gain in the mixtures their patients were prescribed.

FURTHER READING

1. Medicine in View: Art and Visual Representation

Ars Medica: Art, Medicine and the Human Condition (exhibition catalogue by D. Karp, Philadelphia Museum of Art, 1985).

I. B. Cohen, *Album of Science from Leonardo to Lavoisier* (New York, 1980).

B. Ford, *Images of Science* (The British Library, London, 1990).

D. Fox and C. Lawrence, *Photographing Medicine: Images and Power in Britain and America since 1840* (New York, 1988).

S. Gilman, *Seeing the Insane: A Cultural History of Psychiatric Illustration* (New York, 1982).

—— *Health and Illness: Images of Difference* (London, 1995).

L. Jordanova, *Sexual Visions: Images of Gender in Science and Medicine between the Eighteenth and Twentieth Centuries* (Madison, Wisc., 1989).

M. Lynch and S. Woolgar, *Representation in Scientific Practice* (Cambridge, Mass., 1990).

F. Marti-Ibañez (ed.), *The Epic of Medicine* (New York, 1962).

M. Masson, *A Pictorial History of Nursing* (London, 1985).

R. Mazzolini (ed.), *Non-Verbal Communication in Science prior to 1900* (Florence, 1993).

A. Newman, *The Illustrated History of Medical Curiosa* (New York, 1988).

K. Roberts and J. Tomlinson, *The Fabric of the Body: European Traditions of Anatomical Illustration* (Oxford, 1992).

B. Stafford, *Body Criticism: Imaging the Unseen in Enlightenment Art and Medicine* (Cambridge, Mass., 1992).

J. Thornton and C. Reeves, *Medical Book Illustration: A Short History* (Cambridge, 1983).

2. Medicine in the Classical World

W. A. Heidel, *Hippocratic Medicine: Its Spirit and Method* (New York, 1941).

R. Jackson, *Doctors and Diseases in the Roman Empire* (London, 1988).

W. W. Jaeger, 'Diocles of Carystus: A New Pupil of Aristotle', *Philosophical Review*, 49 (1940), 393–414, repr. in *Scripta Minora II* (Rome, 1960), 243–65.

G. E. R. Lloyd, 'Alcmaeon and the Early History of Dissection', *Sudhoffs Archiv*, 59 (1975), 113–47, and 'The Hippocratic Question', *Classical Quarterly*, NS 25 (1975) 171–92, repr. in G. E. R. Lloyd, *Methods and Problems in Greek Science* (Cambridge, 1991).

—— *Magic, Reason and Experience* (Cambridge, 1979).

J. Longrigg, *Greek Rational Medicine: Philosophy and Medicine from Alcmaeon to the Alexandrians* (London, 1993).

G. Majno, *The Healing Hand: Man and Wound in the Ancient World* (Cambridge, Mass., 1975).

V. Nutton, *From Democedes to Harvey* (London, 1988).

—— 'Healers in the Medical Market Place: Towards a Social History of Graeco-Roman Medicine', in A. Wear (ed.), *Medicine in Society: Historical Essays* (Cambridge, 1992), 15–58.

W. D. Smith, *The Hippocratic Tradition* (Ithaca, NY, 1979).

H. von Staden, *Herophilus: The Art of Medicine in Early Alexandria* (Cambridge, 1989).

J. T. Vallance, *The Lost Theory of Asclepiades of Bithynia* (Oxford, 1990).

3. Europe and Islam

G. C. Anawati, 'Science' in P. M. Holt, A. K. S. Lambton, and B. Lewis, *The Cambridge History of Islam*, ii: *The Further Islamic Lands, Islamic Society and Civilization* (Cambridge, 1970).

L. I. Conrad, 'The Arab–Islamic Medical Tradition' in L. I. Conrad, M. Neve, V. Nutton, R. Porter, and A. Wear, *The Western Medical Tradition, 800 BC to AD 1800* (Cambridge, 1995).

Norman Daniel, *The Arabs and Medieval Europe* (2nd edn., New York, 1979).

C. L. Elgood, *A Medical History of Persia and the Eastern Caliphate* (Cambridge, 1951; repr. Amsterdam, n.d.).

—— *Safavid Medical Practice, or The Practice of Medicine, Surgery and Gynaecology in Persia between 1500 AD and 1750 AD* (London, 1970).

D. R. Hill, *Islamic Science and Engineering* (Edinburgh, 1993).

T. E. Huff, *The Rise of Early Modern Science: Islam, China, and the West* (Cambridge, 1993).

D. Jacquart and F. Micheau, *La Médecine arabe et l'occident médiéval* (Paris, 1990).

Danielle Jacquart, 'The Influence of Arabic Medicine in the Medieval West', in R. Rashed (ed.), *Encyclopaedia of the History of Arabic Medicine*, iii, 963–84 (London,1996)

S. K. Jayyusi, *The Legacy of Muslim Spain* (Leiden, 1992).

Bernard Lewis, *The Muslim Discovery of Europe* (New York, 1982).

De Lacy O'Leary, *How Greek Science Passed to the Arabs* (London, 1949; repr. 1964).

E. Savage-Smith, *Islamic Culture and the Medical Arts* (Bethesda, Md., 1994).

M. Plessner, 'The Natural Sciences and Medicine' in J. Schacht and C. E. Bosworth (eds.), *The Legacy of Islam* (2nd edn., Oxford, 1974).

Nancy G. Siraisi, *Avicenna in Renaissance Italy: The* Canon *and Medical Teaching in Italian Universities after 1500* (Princeton, 1987).

Manfred Ullmann, *Islamic Medicine* (Islamic Survey, vol. 11; Edinburgh, 1978).

M. J. L. Young, J. D. Latham, and R. B. Serjeant (eds.), *Religion, Learning and Science in the Abbasid Period* (Cambridge, 1990).

4. Medicine in the Latin Middle Ages

Saul Nathaniel Brody, *The Disease of the Soul* (Ithaca, NY, 1974).

M. L. Cameron, *Anglo-Saxon Medicine* (Cambridge, 1993).

Ronald C. Finucane, *Miracles and Pilgrims: Popular Beliefs in Medieval England* (London, 1977).

Luis García-Ballester, Roger French, Jon Arrizabalaga, and Andrew Cunningham (eds.), *Practical Medicine from Salerno to the Black Death* (Cambridge, 1994).

Peter M. Jones, *Medieval Medical Miniatures* (Austin, Tex., 1985).

Edward J. Kealey, *Medieval Medicus: A Social History of Anglo-Norman Medicine* (Baltimore, 1981).

Loren C. MacKinney, *Medical Illustrations in Medieval Manuscripts* (Berkeley and Los Angeles, 1965).

Michael R. McVaugh, *Medicine before the Plague* (Cambridge, 1993).

Stanley Rubin, *Medieval English Medicine* (Newton Abbot, 1974).

Nancy G. Siraisi, *Medieval and Early Renaissance Medicine* (Chicago, 1990).

—— *Taddeo Alderotti and his Pupils* (Princeton, 1981).

Charles H. Talbot, *Medicine in Medieval England* (London, 1967).

5. Medicine and the Renaissance

Agnes Robertson Arber, *Herbals, their Origin and Evolution: A Chapter in the History of Botany, 1470–1670* (3rd edn.; Cambridge, 1986).

Giulia Calvi, *Histories of a Plague Year: The Social and the Imaginary in Baroque Florence*, trans. Dario Biocca and Bryant T. Ragan, Jr. (Berkeley and Los Angeles, 1989).

Piero Camporesi, *The Incorruptible Flesh: Bodily Mutation and Mortification in Religion and Folklore*, trans. Tania Croft-Murray and Helen Elsom (Cambridge, 1988).

Carol Maria Cipolla, *Miasmas and Disease: Public Health and the Environment in the Pre-Industrial Age* (New Haven, 1992).

—— *Public Health and the Medical Profession in the Renaissance* (Cambridge, 1976).

William Eamon, *Science and the Secrets of Nature: Books of Secrets in Medieval and Early Modern Culture* (Princeton, 1994).

Paula Findlen, *Possessing Nature: Museums, Collecting, and Scientific Culture in Early Modern Italy* (Berkeley and Los Angeles, 1994).

Robert S. Gottfried, *The Black Death: Natural and Human Disaster in Medieval Europe* (London, 1983).

—— *Doctors and Medicine in Medieval England, 1340–1530* (Princeton, 1986).

Anthony Grafton, April Shelford, and Nancy G. Siraisi (eds.), *New Worlds, Ancient Texts: The Power of Tradition and the Shock of Discovery* (Cambridge, Mass., 1992).

Monica Green, 'Documenting Medieval Women's Medical Practice', in Luis García-Ballester, Roger French, Jon Arrizabalaga, and Andrew Cunningham (eds.), *Practical Medicine from Salerno to the Black Death* (Cambridge, 1994), 322–52.

—— 'Women's Medical Practice and Health Care in Medieval Europe', in Judith M. Bennett, Elizabeth A. Clark, Jean F. O'Barr, B. Anne Vilen, and Sarah Westphal-Wihl (eds.), *Sisters and Workers in the Middle Ages* (Chicago, 1989), 39–78.

Peter Murray Jones, *Medieval Medical Miniatures* (Austin, Tex., 1985).

Charles D. O'Malley, *Andreas Vesalius of Brussels, 1514–1564* (Berkeley and Los Angeles, 1964).

Walter Pagel, *Paracelsus: An Introduction to Philosophical Medicine in the Era of the Renaissance* (Basel, 1958).

Katharine Park, *Doctors and Medicine in Early Renaissance Florence* (Princeton, 1985).

—— 'Healing the Poor: Hospitals and Medical Assistance in Renaissance Florence', in Jonathan Barry and Colin Jones (eds.), *Medicine and Charity before the Welfare State* (London, 1991), 26–45.

Linda Pollock, *With Faith and Physic: The Life of a Tudor Gentlewoman, Lady Grace Mildmay, 1552–1620* (London, 1993).

Claude Quetel, *History of Syphilis*, trans. Judith Braddock and Brian Pike (London, 1990).

Karen Meier Reeds, *Botany in Medieval and Renaissance Universities* (New York, 1991).

Guenter B. Risse, 'Medicine in New Spain', in Ronald L. Numbers (ed.), *Medicine in the New World: New Spain, New France, and New England* (Knoxville, Ten., 1987), 12–63.

K. B. Roberts and J. D. W. Tomlinson, *The Fabric of the Body: European Traditions of Anatomical Illustrations* (Oxford, 1992).

J. B. de C. M. Saunders and Charles D. O'Malley, *The Illustrations from the Works of Andreas Vesalius of Brussels* (New York, 1973).

Bernard Schultz, *Art and Anatomy in Renaissance Italy* (Ann Arbor, 1985).

Joseph Shatzmiller, *Jews, Medicine, and Medieval Society* (Berkeley and Los Angeles, 1994).

Nancy G. Siraisi, *Medieval and Early Renaissance Medicine: An Introduction to Knowledge and Practice* (Chicago, 1990). A fine survey with excellent bibliography.

Paul Slack, *The Impact of Plague in Tudor and Stuart England* (London, 1985).

Charles Webster (ed.), *Health, Medicine and Mortality in the Sixteenth Century* (Cambridge, 1979).

Philip Ziegler, *The Black Death* (London, 1969).

6. From the Scientific Revolution to the Germ Theory

Harold J. Cook, *The Decline of the Old Medical Regime in Stuart London* (Ithaca, NY, 1986).

Alain Corbin, *The Foul and the Fragrant: Odor and the French Social Imagination*, trans. Miriam Kochan (Cambridge, Mass., 1986).

Further Reading | Robert Darnton, *Mesmerism and the End of the Enlightenment in France* (Cambridge, Mass., 1968).

Anne Digby, *Making a Medical Living: Doctors and Patients in the English Market for Medicine, 1720–1911* (Cambridge, 1994).

Barbara Duden, *The Woman beneath the Skin: A Doctor's Patients in Eighteenth-Century Germany*, trans. Thomas Dunlap (Cambridge, Mass., 1991).

Michael W. Flinn, *The European Demographic System, 1500–1820* (Baltimore, 1981).

Michel Foucault, *The Birth of the Clinic: An Archaeology of Medical Perception*, trans. A. M. Sheridan Smith (New York, 1973).

Jean-Pierre Goubert, *The Conquest of Water: The Advent of Health in the Industrial Age*, trans. Andrew Wilson (Princeton, 1989).

Colin Jones, *The Charitable Imperative: Hospitals and Nursing in Ancien Régime and Revolutionary France* (London, 1989).

Lester S. King, *The Road to Medical Enlightenment, 1650–1695* (New York and London, 1970).

Coral Lansbury, *The Old Brown Dog: Women, Workers, and Vivisection in Edwardian England* (Madison, 1985).

Mary Lindemann, *Patriots and Paupers: Hamburg, 1712–1830* (New York, 1990).

Irvine Loudon, *Medical Care and the General Practitioner, 1750–1850* (Oxford, 1986).

Hilary Marland, *Medicine and Society in Wakefield and Huddersfield 1780–1870* (Cambridge, 1987).

——(ed.), *The Art of Midwifery: Early Modern Midwives in Europe* (London, 1993).

Dorothy Porter and Roy Porter, *Patient's Progress: Doctors and Doctoring in Eighteenth-Century England* (Stanford, 1989).

Roy Porter, *Health for Sale: Quackery in England 1650–1850* (Manchester, 1989).

Matthew Ramsey, *Professional and Popular Medicine in France, 1770–1830: The Social World of Medical Practice* (Cambridge, 1988).

Charles Webster, *The Great Instauration: Science, Medicine and Reform 1626–1660* (London, 1975).

Dora B. Weiner, *The Citizen-Patient in Revolutionary and Imperial Paris* (Baltimore, 1993).

7. From the Germ Theory to 1945

J. Austoker and L. Bryder (eds.), *Historical Perspectives on the Role of the MRC* (Oxford, 1989).

Claude Bernard, *An Introduction to the Study of Experimental Medicine* (1865; first English translation, New York, 1927; 1957).

C. C. Booth, 'Clinical Research', in W. F. Bynum and R. S. Porter (eds.), *Companion Encyclopaedia of the History of Medicine*, i (London, 1993), 205–29.

W. F. Bynum, *Science and the Practice of Medicine in the Nineteenth Century* (Cambridge, 1994).

W. Coleman and F. L. Holmes (eds.), *The Investigative Enterprise: Experimental Physiology in Nineteenth-Century Medicine* (Berkeley and Los Angeles, 1988).

G. W. Corner, *A History of the Rockefeller Institute, 1901–1953: Origins and Growth* (New York, 1964).

Anne Hardy, *The Epidemic Streets: Infectious Disease and the Rise of Preventive Medicine, 1856–1900* (Oxford, 1993).

Robert E. Kohler, *From Medical Chemistry to Biochemistry: The Making of a Biomedical Discipline* (Cambridge, 1982).

J. Parascandola, *The Development of American Pharmacology: John J. Abel and the Shaping of a Discipline* (Baltimore, 1992).

Arthur M. Silverstein, *A History of Immunology* (San Diego, Calif., 1989).

A. Landsborough Thomson, *Half a Century of Medical Research*, i. *Origins and Policy of the Medical Research Council (UK)* (London, 1973); ii. *The Programme of the Medical Research Council (UK)* (London, 1975).

M. Weatherall, *In Search of a Cure* (Oxford, 1990).

8. Medicine in the Second Half of the Twentieth Century

I. Illich, *Medical Nemesis* (London, 1975).

I. Kennedy, *The Unmasking of Medicine* (London, 1981).

T. McKeown, *The Role of Medicine: Dream, Mirage, or Nemesis?* (Oxford, 1979).

—— *The Origins of Human Disease* (Oxford, 1988).

J. Walton, J. Barondess, and S. Lock (eds.), *The Oxford Medical Companion* (Oxford, 1994).

J. D. Watson, *The Double Helix* (London, 1968).

9. The Growth of Medical Education and the Medical Profession

Howard S. Becker, Blanche Geer, Everett C. Hughes, and Anselm L. Strauss, *Boys in White: Student Culture in Medical School* (New Brunswick, NJ, 1977).

Thomas Neville Bonner, *To the Ends of the Earth: Women's Search for Education in Medicine* (Cambridge, 1992).

—— *Becoming a Physician: Medical Education in Great Britain, France, Germany and the United States 1750–1945* (New York, 1995).

Toby Gelfand, *Professionalizing Modern Medicine: Paris Surgeons and Medical Science and Institutions in the 18th Century* (Westport, Conn., 1980).

Charles E. McClelland, *The German Experience of Professionalization: Modern Learned Professions and their Organizations from the Early Nineteenth Century to the Hitler Era* (Cambridge, 1991).

Herbert M. Morais, *The History of the Negro in Medicine* (New York, 1968).

C. D. O'Malley (ed.), *The History of Medical Education* (Berkeley and Los Angeles, 1970).

Felix Platter, *Beloved Son Felix: The Journal of Felix Platter, a Medical Student in Montpelier in the Sixteenth Century* (London, 1961).

Lisa Rosner, *Medical Education in the Age of Improvement: Edinburgh Students and Apprentices, 1760–1826* (Edinburgh, 1991).

10. The Rise of the Modern Hospital

H. Beukerand and J. Moll (eds.), *Clinical Teaching, Past and Present* (Amsterdam, 1989).

N. Bosanquet, 'Health Economics: Finance, Budgeting, and Insurance', in W. F. Bynum and R. Porter (eds.), *Companion Encyclopedia of the History of Medicine*, ii (London, 1993), 1373–90.

W. F. Bynum, *Science and the Practice of Medicine in the Nineteenth Century* (Cambridge, 1994).

N. Finzsch and R. Jütte (eds.), *Institutions of Confinement: Hospitals, Asylums and Prisons in Western Europe and North America, 1500–1900* (Cambridge, 1996).

L. Granshaw and R. Porter (eds.), *The Hospital in History* (London, 1989).

C. Jones, *The Charitable Imperative: Hospitals and Nursing in Ancien Régime and Revolutionary France* (London, 1989).

Y. Kawakita, S. Sakai, and Y. Otsuka (eds.), *History of Hospitals* (Tokyo, 1989).

G. B. Risse, *Hospital Life in Enlightenment Scotland: Care and Teaching at the Royal Infirmary of Edinburgh* (Cambridge, 1986).

M. Tew, *Safer Childbirth? A Critical History of Maternity Care* (London, 1990).

J. D. Thompson and G. Goldin, *The Hospital: A Social and Architectural History* (New Haven, 1975).

U. Tröhler, 'Quantification in British Medicine and Surgery 1750–1830, with Special Reference to its Introduction into Therapeutics' (Ph.D. thesis, London, 1978).

J. Woodward, *To Do the Sick No Harm: A Study of the British Voluntary Hospital System to 1875* (London, 1974).

11. Epidemics and the Geography of Disease

Roy M. Anderson and Robert M. May, *Infectious Diseases of Humans: Dynamics and Control* (Oxford, 1991).

Virginia Berridge and Philip Strong (eds.), *AIDS and Contemporary History* (Cambridge, 1993).

Andrew D. Cliff, Peter Haggett, and Matthew Smallman-Raynor, *Measles: An Historical Geography of a Major Human Viral Disease from Global Expansion to Local Retreat, 1840–1990* (Oxford, 1993).

Charles Creighton, *A History of Epidemics in Britain* (2 vols., 2nd edn., London 1965; originally published Cambridge, 1891–4).

Alfred W. Crosby, *The Columbian Exchange: Biological Consequences of 1492* (Westport, Conn., 1972).

Philip D. Curtin, *Death by Migration: Europe's Encounter with the Tropical World in the Nineteenth Century* (Cambridge, 1989).

Daniel Defoe, *A Journal of the Plague Year*, ed. Kenneth Hopkins (Oxford, 1990; first published 1772).

Mary J. Dobson, *Contours of Death and Disease in Early Modern England* (Cambridge, 1996).

Anne Hardy, *The Epidemic Streets: Infectious Disease and the Rise of Preventive Medicine 1856–1900* (Oxford, 1994).

Arno Karlen, *Plague's Progress: A Social History of Man and Disease* (London, 1995)

Kenneth F. Kiple (ed.), *The Cambridge World History of Human Disease* (Cambridge, 1993).

Vincent J. Knapp, *Disease and its Impact on Modern European History* (New York, 1989).

Thomas McKeown, *The Modern Rise of Population* (New York, 1976).

William McNeill, *Plagues and Peoples* (New York, 1976).

Andrew Nikiforuk, *The Fourth Horseman: A Short History of Epidemics, Plagues and Other Scourges* (London, 1993).

Terence O. Ranger and Paul Slack, *Epidemics and Ideas: Essays on the Historical Perception of Pestilence* (Cambridge, 1992).

Charles E. Rosenberg, *Explaining Epidemics and other Studies in the History of Medicine* (Cambridge, 1992).

Paul Slack, *The Impact of Plague in Tudor and Stuart England* (Oxford, 1990).

Robert Wilkins, *The Fireside Book of Deadly Diseases* (London, 1994).

12. Nurses and Ancillaries in the Christian Era

B. Abel-Smith, *A History of the Nursing Profession* (London, 1960).

M. Baly, *Florence Nightingale and the Nursing Legacy* (London, 1986).

L. L. Dock and M. A. Nutting, *A History of Nursing* (2 vols.; New York, 1907).

C. Jones, *The Charitable Imperative: Hospitals and Nursing in Ancien Régime and Revolutionary France* (London, 1989).

C. Maggs, *The Origins of General Nursing* (London, 1983).

S. Reverby, *Ordered to Care: The Dilemma of American Nursing, 1850–1945* (Cambridge, 1987).

A. Summers, *Angels and Citizens: British Women as Military Nurses 1854–1914* (London, 1988).

13. Childbirth

Mary Breckinridge, *Wide Neighbourhoods: A Story of the Frontier Nursing Service* (New York, 1952, repr. Lexington, Ky., 1981).

R. Campbell and A. Macfarlane, *Where to Be Born?* (Oxford, 1987).

K. Codell Carter and Barbara Carter, *Childbed Fever: A Scientific Biography of Ignaz Semmelweis* (Westport, Conn., 1994).

J. Garcia, R. Kilpatrick, and M. Richards, *The Politics of Maternity Care: Services for Childbearing Women in Twentieth-Century Britain* (Oxford, 1990).

O. W. Holmes, *Puerperal Fever as a Private Pestilence* (Boston, 1855).

J. W. Leavitt, *Brought to Bed: Childbearing in America, 1750 to 1950* (Oxford, 1986).

J. Lewis, The Politics of Motherhood (London, 1980).

J. B. Litoff, *The American Midwife Debate: A Sourcebook on its Modern Origins* (New York, 1986).

I. Loudon, *Death in Childbirth: An International Study of Maternal Care and Maternal Mortality 1800–1950* (Oxford, 1992).

—— *Childbed Fever: A Documentary History* (New York, 1995).

H. Marland (ed.), *The Art of Midwifery: Early Modern Midwives in Europe* (London, 1993).

I. Porter, *Alexander Gordon, MD, of Aberdeen, 1752–1799* (Aberdeen University Studies, no. 139; Edinburgh, 1958).

Philip Rhodes, *A Short History of Clinical Midwifery* (Hale, Cheshire, England, 1995).

M. Sandelowski, *Pain and Pleasure in American Childbirth: From Twilight Sleep to the Read Method, 1914–1960* (Westport, Conn., 1984).

I. P. Semmelweis, *The Etiology, Concept and Prophylaxis of Childbed Fever*, slightly abridged version, trans. with an introduction by K. Codell Carter (Madison, Wis., 1983).

R. W. Wertz and D. C. Wertz, *Lying-in: A History of Childbirth in America* (New York, 1977).

Adrian Wilson, *The Making of Man-Midwifery: Childbirth in England, 1660–1770* (Cambridge, Mass., 1995).

14. Children in Hospital

A. Davis, 'British Paediatrics', in Buford L. Nichols, Angel Ballabriga, and Norman Kretchmer (eds.), *History of Pediatrics 1850–1950* (Nestlé Nutrition Workshop Series, 22; New York, 1991).

Jules Kosky, *Queen Elizabeth Hospital for Children: 125 Years of Achievement* (London, 1992).

—— and Raymond J. Lunnon, *Great Ormond Street and the Story of Medicine* (London, 1991).

Buford L. Nichols, Angel Ballabriga, and Norman Kretchmer (eds.), *History of Pediatrics 1850–1950* (Nestlé Nutrition Workshop Series, 22; New York, 1991).

E. Seidler, 'An Historical Survey of Children's Hospitals', in L. Granshaw and Roy Porter (eds.), *The Hospital in History* (London, 1989).

15. Medicine and the Mind

W. F. Bynum, 'Psychiatry in its Historical Context', in M. Shepherd and O. L. Zangwill (eds.), *Handbook of Psychiatry: General Psychopathology*, i (Cambridge, 1986), 11–38.

Sander Gilman, *Seeing the Insane* (New York, 1982).

Jan Goldstein, *Console and Classify: The French Psychiatric Profession in the Nineteenth Century* (Cambridge, 1990).

Stanley W. Jackson, *Melancholia and Depression: From Hippocratic Times to Present Times* (New Haven, 1989).

Michael MacDonald, *Mystical Bedlam: Madness, Anxiety, and Healing in Seventeenth-Century England* (Cambridge, 1981).

Mark S. Micale, *Approaching Hysteria: Disease and its Interpretation* (Princeton, 1995).

H. C. Eric Midelfort, *Mad Princes of Renaissance Germany* (Charlottesville, Va., 1994).

Roy Porter, *Mind-Forg'd Manacles: A History of Madness in England from the Restoration to the Regency* (London, 1987; pbk. edn. Harmondsworth, 1990).

Jack D. Pressman, 'Concepts of Mental Illness in the West', in Kenneth F. Kiple (ed.), *The Cambridge World History of Human Disease* (Cambridge, 1993), 59–83.

Andrew Scull, *The Most Solitary of Afflictions: Madness and Society in Britain, 1700–1900* (New Haven, 1993).

Elaine Showalter, *The Female Malady: Women, Madness, and English Culture, 1830–1980* (London, 1987).

Thomas Szasz, *The Myth of Mental Illness* (New York, 1974).

Owsei Temkin, *Hippocrates in a World of Pagans and Christians* (Baltimore, 1991).

Elliot S. Valenstein, *Great and Desperate Cures: The Rise and Decline of Psychosurgery and Other Radical Treatments for Mental Illness* (New York, 1986).

16. The Spread of Western Medicine

David Arnold (ed.), *Imperial Medicine and Indigenous Societies* (Manchester, 1988).

—— *Colonizing the Body: State Medicine and Epidemic Disease in Nineteenth-Century India* (Berkeley and Los Angeles, 1993).

John Z. Bowers, *Western Medicine in a Chinese Palace: Peking Union Medical College, 1917–1951* (New York, 1972).

—— *'When the Twain Meet': The Rise of Western Medicine in Japan* (Baltimore, 1980).

Marcus Cueto, *Missionaries of Science: The Rockefeller Foundation and Latin America* (Bloomington, Ind., 1994).

Philip Curtin, *Death by Migration: Europe's Encounter with the Tropical World in the Nineteenth Century* (Cambridge, 1989).

Donald Denoon, *Public Health in Papua New Guinea: Medical Possibility and Social Constraint, 1884–1984* (Cambridge, 1989).

Nancy E. Gallagher, *Medicine and Power in Tunisia, 1780–1900* (Cambridge, 1983).

Mark Harrison, *Public Health in British India: Anglo-Indian Preventive Medicine, 1859–1914* (Cambridge, 1994).

Arthur Kleinman, *Patients and Healers in the Context of Culture: An Exploration of the Borderland between Anthropology, Medicine and Psychiatry* (Berkeley and Los Angeles, 1980).

Charles Leslie (ed.), *Asian Medical Systems: A Comparative Study* (Berkeley and Los Angeles, 1976).

AmElissa Lucas, *Chinese Medical Modernization: Comparative Policy Continuities, 1930s–1980s* (New York, 1982).

Roy MacLeod and Milton Lewis (eds.), *Disease, Medicine and Empire: Perspectives on Western Medicine and the Experience of European Expansion* (London, 1988).

Ronald Numbers (ed.), *Medicine in the New World: New Spain, New France and New England* (Knoxville, Ten., 1987).

Paul U. Unschuld, *Medicine in China: A History of Ideas* (Berkeley and Los Angeles, 1985).

M. Vaughan, *Curing their Ills: Colonial Power and African Illness* (Cambridge, 1991).

17. Unofficial and Unorthodox Medicine

Michael Anderson, *Approaches to the History of the Western Family, 1500–1914* (Basingstoke, 1980).

Harriet Bradley, *Men's Work, Women's Work* (Cambridge, 1989).

William F. Bynum and Roy Porter (eds.), *Medical Fringe and Medical Orthodoxy, 1750–1850* (London, 1987).

Roger Cooter (ed.), *Studies in the History of Alternative Medicine* (Basingstoke, 1988).

Harris L. Coulter, *Divided Legacy: A History of the Schism in Medical Thought* (3 vols.; Washington, 1973–7).

Valerie I. J. Flint, *The Rise of Magic in Early Medieval Europe* (Oxford, 1993).

Stephen Fulder, *The Handbook of Complementary Medicine* (London, 1984).

David Gentilcore, *From Bishop to Witch: The System of the Sacred in Early Modern Terra d'Otranto* (Manchester, 1992).

Wayland D. Hand (ed.), *American Folk Medicine* (Berkeley and Los Angeles, 1976).

Brian Inglis, *Natural Medicine* (London, 1979).

Alison K. Lingo, 'Empirics and Charlatans in Early Modern France: The Genesis of the Classification of the "Other" in Medical Practice', *Journal of Social History*, 19 (1986), 583–603.

Michael MacDonald, *Mystical Bedlam: Madness, Anxiety and Healing in Seventeenth-Century England* (Cambridge, 1981).

Hilary Marland (ed.), *The Art of Midwifery: Early Modern Midwives in Europe* (London, 1993).

Vivian de Sola Pinto, *The Famous Pathologist or the Noble Mountebank* (Nottingham University Miscellany, 1; Nottingham, 1961).

Roy Porter, *Health for Sale: Quackery in England, 1660–1850* (Manchester, 1989).

Matthew Ramsey, *Professional and Popular Medicine in France, 1770–1830* (Cambridge, 1988).

Lyndal Roper, *Oedipus and the Devil: Witchcraft, Sexuality and Religion in Early Modern Europe* (London, 1994).

Pam Schweitzer (ed.), *Can We Afford the Doctor?* (London, 1985).

Sean Shesgreen (ed.), *The Criers and Hawkers of London: Engravings and Drawings by Marcellus Laroon* (Aldershot, Hants, 1990).

Reinhard Spree, *Health and Social Class in Imperial Germany*, trans. S. McKinnon-Evans (Oxford, 1988).

Keith Thomas, *Religion and the Decline of Magic* (London, 1971; pbk. edn. Harmondsworth, 1980).

—— *Man and the Natural World: Changing Attitudes in England, 1500–1800* (London, 1983).

Andrew Wear, Johanna Geyer-Kordesch, and Roger French (eds.), *Doctors and Ethics: The Earlier Historical Setting of Professional Ethics* (Amsterdam, 1993).

Charles Webster (ed.), *Caring for Health: History and Diversity* (Buckingham, 1993).

18. Medicine, Politics, and the State

Brian Abel-Smith and R. M. Titmuss, *The Cost of the NHS* (Cambridge, 1956).

Rashi Fein, *Medical Care, Medical Costs: The Search for Health Insurance Policy* (Cambridge, Mass., 1986).

Julian Le Grand and William Bartlett, *Quasi-Markets and Social Policy* (Basingstoke, 1993).

Frank Honigsbaum, *The Division in British Medicine* (London, 1979).

Ivan Illich, *Medical Nemesis: The Expropriation of Health* (London, 1975).

Rudolf Klein, *The Politics of the National Health Service* (London, 1983).

Thomas McKeown, *The Modern Rise of Population* (London, 1976).

Calum Paton, *Competition and Planning in the NHS: The Danger of Unplanned Markets* (London, 1992).

M. Jeanne Peterson, *The Medical Profession in Mid-Victorian London* (Berkeley and Los Angeles, 1978).

Paul Starr, *The Social Transformation of American Medicine* (New York, 1982).

R. M. Titmuss, *Essays on the Welfare State* (London, 1958).

Charles Webster, *The Health Services since the War*, i. *The Problems of Health Care: The National Health Service before 1957* (London, 1988).

19. The Patient's View

L. M. Beier, *Sufferers and Healers: The Experience of Illness in the Seventeenth Century* (London, 1987).

A. Digby, *Madness, Morality and Medicine: The York Retreat, 1790–1914* (Cambridge, 1985).

—— *Making a Medical Living: Doctors and Patients in the English Market for Medicine, 1720–1911* (Cambridge, 1994).

M. Fissell, *Patients, Power, and the Poor in Eighteenth-Century Bristol* (Cambridge, 1991).

D. Peterson (ed.), *A Mad People's History of Madness* (Pittsburgh, 1982).

D. Porter and R. Porter, *Patient's Progress: Doctors and Doctoring in Eighteenth-Century England* (London, 1989).

—— —— *In Sickness and in Health* (London, 1988).

R. Porter, 'The Patient in England, c.1660–1800', in A. Wear (ed.), *Medicine in Society: Historical Essays* (Cambridge, 1992).

—— (ed.), *Patients and Practitioners: Lay Perceptions of Medicine in Pre-Industrial Society* (Cambridge, 1985).

R. Richardson, *Death, Dissection and the Destitute* (London, 1988).

J. D. Stoeckle and G. A. White, *Plain Pictures of Plain Doctors* (Cambridge, Mass., 1985).

A. Wear, 'Interfaces: Perceptions of Health and Illness in Early Modern England', in A. Wear (ed.), *Problems and Methods in the History of Medicine* (Cambridge, 1987).

CHRONOLOGY

828–765 BC	Hesiod, *Works and Days*
6th cent. BC	Cult of Asclepius of Epidaurus
*c.*500 BC	Alcmaeon
492–432 BC	Empedocles
*c.*450–370 BC	Hippocrates
*c.*440 BC	Diogenes of Apollonia
430–426 BC	Plague of Athens
428–347 BC	Plato
384–322 BC	Aristotle
350 BC	Diocles of Carystos publishes the first Green Herbal
fl. *c.*320 BC	Praxagoras of Cos
fl. *c.*280 BC	Herophilus
fl. *c.*270 BC	Erasistratus
234–149 BC	Cato the Elder
219 BC	Archagathus, the first Greek doctor to settle in Rome and practise as a wound specialist
46 BC	Julius Caesar introduces decree conferring citizenship on all who practise medicine at Rome
1st cent. BC	Asclepiades of Bithynia d. before 91 BC
1st cent. AD	Rufus of Ephesus, Greek physician in Asia Minor
*c.*77	Dioscorides completes his Greek treatise on medicinal substances
129–216	Galen
395–1453	Byzantine Empire
6th cent.	Rise of monastic medicine
542	Plague of Rome
634	Expansion of Islam begins with the invasion of Syria and Iraq
651	Hôtel Dieu founded in Paris
*c.*786–809	Earliest documented Islamic hospital built in Baghdad
9th cent.	Ḥunayn ibn Isḥāq (809–73/7) translates Greek and other medical books into Arabic
872	First hospital founded in Egypt
873 or 877	Death of Ḥunayn ibn Isḥāq, physician and translator, in Baghdad
903	Abū Bakr Muḥammad ibn Zakarīyā' al-Rāzī, known as Rhazes, writes *Book of Medicine Dedicated to Manṣūr*
11th cent.	Constantine the African (d. *c.*1087), a monk at Monte Cassino who translated Arabic works into Latin
*c.*1000	*Canon of Medicine* written by Avicenna (980–1037)
*c.*1009	Albucasis, author of the medico-chirurgical treatise *Altasrif*, dies in Spain
12th cent.	Formation of the canon of medical writings known as the *Ars medica* or *Articella*
1137	Foundation of St Bartholomew's Hospital in London
*c.*1170	Rise of universities
1180	Roger Frugardi of Parma produces his *Practica chirurgiae* sig-

nalling the beginning of European study of anatomy and surgery

1187	Death of Gerard of Cremona, prolific translator of Arabic works into Latin
13th cent.	Beginning of a system of licensing medical practitioners in certain Mediterranean towns
1215	Magna Carta
1215	Foundation of St Thomas's Hospital in London
1215	Fourth Lateran Council places severe restrictions on churchmen practising surgery or studying medicine
1270–80	Introduction of spectacles, one of the great blessings to mankind, by the glass workers of Venice
1288	Death in Cairo of Ibn al-Nafis, who first described the pulmonary circulation
*c.*1300	Galen's writings more broadly incorporated into the medical curriculum at Montpellier and Bologna, and Henry de Mondeville teaches anatomy at Montpellier
1346–53	Outbreak of plague later known as the Black Death
*c.*1350	A few medieval hospitals begin to devote themselves exclusively to the treatment of the sick
1362–92	Lesser epidemics of plague (less, that is, than the Black Death) in Britain
*c.*1370	John of Arderne produces surgical treatises
1400	Death of Chaucer
1440–50	Invention of printing
1452–1519	Leonardo da Vinci
1454	Gutenberg bible printed
1490	Introduction of virulent syphilis into Europe
1490–1553	François Rabelais, priest, physician, and author of *Gargantua* and *Pantagruel*
1499	Ludovico dal Pozzo Toscanelli publishes the first European official pharmacopoeia
16th cent.	Paracelsus (1493–1541) substitutes an alchemical model for the humoral model of Galen, becoming one of the precursors of chemical pharmacology
*c.*1500	Thomas Linacre (1460–1524), an English physician and physician to Henry VIII, writes Latin versions of the works of Galen
1506–88	Jean Fernel, sometimes described as the greatest French physician of the Renaissance
1507	Copernicus (1473–1543) describes the rotation of the earth round the sun
1529–30	Mysterious illness known as the sweating sickness spreads throughout Europe
1540	Clinical teaching by Giovanni Battista della Monte in Padua, who made a critical exegesis of difficult passages of Latin and Greek
1543	Andreas Vesalius (1514–64), anatomist and author of *De humani corporis fabrica* (Fabric of the Human Body), establishes illustration at the heart of anatomical learning
1575	Leiden University established
1577–1644	Jan Baptiste van Helmont suggests that physiological activities are based on chemical processes
1590	Compound microscope invented

1596–1650	René Descartes claims to have established a separation of body and mind
17th cent.	Rapid growth in the number of university-trained physicians
1601	Establishment in England of the 'old' or 'Elizabethan' poor-law system based on parish relief
1624–89	Thomas Sydenham, an English physician who founded the theory of 'epidemic constitution' (that atmospheric conditions affected the nature of illness) and who named scarlet fever and differentiated it from measles
1628	Publication of *De motu cordis et sanguinis* by William Harvey (1578–1657), an anatomical disquisition on the motion of the heart and blood in animals
1632	Cinchona or Jesuit's bark (containing the active agent quinine) brought from Peru to Europe
1642–9	Civil War in England
mid-17th cent.	François de la Boë Sylvius (1614–72) extends van Helmont's ideas on the chemical basis of physiology
1660–1734	Georg Ernst Stahl, believer in the life force or vital principle in which the body is guided by an immortal soul
1661	Publication by Robert Boyle (1627–91) of *The Sceptical Chymist*
1664	Publication of *Cerebri Anatome* by the physician Thomas Willis (1621–75) of Oxford and London, a pioneer of the anatomy of the nervous system
1665	Great Plague of London, in which over 100,000 died
1667	End of plague in England
1668	Publication of *Traité des Maladies des Femmes Grosses* by François Mauriceau (1637–1709), one of the earliest writers of note on obstetrics
1668–1738	Hermann Boerhaave, professor of medicine, botany, and chemistry at Leiden at the height of the medical school's reputation
1685	Publication of *Novum Lumen*, an early treatise on obstetrics by Hendrik van Deventer of Holland (1651–1724)
18th cent.	Rise of the Edinburgh Medical School to a position of prominence
1682–1771	Giovanni Battista Morgagni, who introduced 'the idea of anatomy' to the study of pathology
1700–2	Gerhard van Swieten establishes what was to become the famous medical school of Vienna modelled on the school of Leiden
1708–77	Albrecht von Haller, eminent mostly as a physiologist but also as an anatomist, botanist, and bibliographer
1710–90	William Cullen, a Scottish physician and nosologist who wrote extensively on fevers, insanity, and nervous disorders
1720	Introduction of smallpox inoculation in England by Mary Wortley Montagu (1689–1762)
1728–93	John Hunter, anatomist and surgeon
1728	Foundation of Edinburgh Infirmary
*c.*1740	Beginning of obstetrics in England, in the sense that it becomes accepted as part of standard medical practice by a large majority of practitioners, accompanied by the establishment of lying-in hospitals
*c.*1740	Beginning of the voluntary hospital movement in England
1745	Foundation of the Company of Surgeons in England

1751	Discovery of the art of percussion of the chest by Leopold Auenbrugger of Vienna (1722–1809)
1751	First university hospital of obstetrics established at Göttingen
1752	Publication of *A Treatise on the Theory and Practice of Midwifery* by William Smellie (1697–1763), one of the earliest teachers of midwifery in London
1754	The cure for scurvy in the Royal Navy discovered by the work of James Lind (1716–94)
1768	Publication by François Boissier de Sauvages de la Croix (1706–67) of *Nosologica methodica*, which classified diseases into classes, genera, and species
1768	William Heberden describes angina pectoris
1774	Publication of *The Anatomy of the Gravid Uterus* by William Hunter (1718–83), anatomist and obstetrician
*c.*1780	Mesmerism introduced by Franz Anton Mesmer (1734–1815)
1785	Introduction of digitalis by William Withering of Birmingham (1741–99)
1788	Publication of *Elements of Medicine* by John Brown of Edinburgh (1735–88), who asserted that diseases were caused by too much or too little external stimulation, requiring treatment by depressants or stimulants respectively
1790s	Work of Philippe Pinel (1745–1826) in France, and later of William Tuke (1732–1822) in York, England, begins the era of treating mental illness with kindness and care instead of incarceration and chaining to the wall
1794	Foundation of the mental hospital known as the Retreat in York
1794	French hospitals absorbed by the state
1795	Reformed medical education established in France
1795	Alexander Gordon of Aberdeen (1752–99) publishes his *Treatise on the Epidemic Fever of Aberdeen*, which showed that puerperal fever was contagious
1795	Thomas Denman of London publishes *An Introduction to the Practice of Midwifery*, which became the standard text on midwifery for many years
1796	Introduction by Edward Jenner (1749–1823) of smallpox vaccination using material from cowpox; his treatise describing vaccination was published in 1798
1799	Marie François Xavier Bichat (1771–1802) publishes *Treatise on Membranes*, one of the major works in the foundation of modern pathology
1800	Foundation of the Royal College of Surgeons of London
1812	Foundation of the *New England Journal of Medicine*, the oldest medical periodical still published in the 1990s
*c.*1800	Introduction of homoeopathy by Samuel Hahnemann (1755–1843)
1815	Apothecaries Act, which introduced the LSA (Licence of the Society of Apothecaries) as the legally required qualification for general practitioners
1819	Introduction of 'mediate' auscultation by means of the stethoscope by René-Théophile-Hyacinthe Laënnec (1781–1826)
1823	Foundation of the *Lancet*
1829	J. J. Lister invents the achromatic microscope

1830	The use of hypnotism in surgical operations by John Eliotson (1791–1868)
1831–2	Cholera, spreading across Europe from the Indian subcontinent, reaches England, Canada, and the USA, to be followed by later epidemics in 1847, 1853, and the 1860s
1832	Foundation of the British Medical Association (initially with the title the Provincial Medical and Surgical Association)
1832	Anatomy Act, introduced because of the scandal of 'body-snatching' from graveyards
1834	Introduction of the new poor-law system in England
1835	Publication of *Recherches sur les effects de la saignée* by Pierre-Charles-Alexandre Louis (1787–1872), the founder of the statistical method in medicine
1836	Creation of the Registrar General's Office in England, which recorded births, deaths, and marriages
1839	Beginning of photography
1839	William Farr (1807–83) appointed Compiler of Abstracts at the Registrar General's Office and creates the system of vital statistics in Britain
1843	Royal College of Surgeons of London becomes Royal College of Surgeons of England
1843	McNaghten case defines the grounds on which a plea of insanity can be entered in criminal cases
1844	Horace Wells (1815–48), a dentist in Connecticut who used nitrous oxide as an anaesthetic, is probably the first to use an anaesthetic in surgery
1846	The anaesthetic ether is used for the first time in surgery by William Morton (1819–68) in Boston
1847	Elizabeth Blackwell enters the medical school in Geneva, New York State, and becomes the first British-born woman to qualify in medicine
1847	Ignaz Phillip Semmelweis shows that puerperal fever is contagious but does not publish his treatise, *Etiology, Concept and Prophylaxis of Childbed Fever*, until 1861
1847	Foundation of the American Medical Association
1847	Introduction of chloroform anaesthesia by James Young Simpson in Britain
1848	Demonstration of the function of the liver by the French physiologist Claude Bernard (1813–78), who was responsible for many important advances in the science of physiology in the mid-nineteenth century
1850	Introduction of the ophthalmoscope by Hermann von Helmholtz (1821–94)
1850	Opening of the Women's Medical College of Philadelphia
1850s	Rudolph Virchow (1821–1902) develops the concept of cellular pathology and publishes *Die Cellularpathologie* in 1858
1854–6	The Crimean War, in which Florence Nightingale (1820–1910) first became famous
1854	John Snow (1813–58) traces cholera to the pump in Broad Street in London
1855	Oliver Wendell Holmes (1809–94) publishes *Puerperal Fever as a Private Pestilence*, a work which demonstrated forcibly the contagiousness of puerperal fever
1858	Introduction of the Medical Act to regulate medical education

	and medical practice in the UK, and to publish a list of registered medical practitioners
1859	Charles Darwin's *Origin of Species*
1860	Florence Nightingale (1820–1910) opens a School of Nursing at St Thomas's Hospital in London
1860s	Louis Pasteur (1822–95) begins the work which, with the work of Robert Koch (1843–1910), laid the foundations of the germ theory
1863	Foundation of the International Red Cross on the initiative of five private Swiss citizens led by Henri Dunant (1828–1910)
1865	Antisepsis is introduced in surgery by Joseph (Lord) Lister (1827–1912), followed later by asepsis
1865	Opening of the Women's College of the New York Infirmary
1866	Sanitary Act in the UK introduced by Sir John Simon (1816–1904)
1874	Opening of the London School of Medicine for Women
1890s	Introduction of safe Caesarean section, an operation which formerly had been almost uniformly fatal
1891	Foundation of the British Institute for Preventive Medicine, later renamed as the Lister Institute
1895	Discovery of X-rays by Wilhelm Konrad Röntgen (1845–1923)
1896	Introduction of the sphygmomanometer by the Italian physician Scipione Rive-Rocci, preceded by the sphygmograph in the 1870s
1897	Ronald Ross (1857–1932) discovers that malaria is transmitted by mosquitoes of the genus Anopheles
1899	Publication by Sigmund Freud (1856–1939) of *The Interpretation of Dreams*, leading to the introduction of psychoanalysis
1899	Introduction of Aspirin as a drug
1900	Paul Ehrlich (1854–1915) makes early and important contributions to chemotherapy, including the discovery of Salvarsan (1909) for the treatment of syphilis
1901	Introduction of electrocardiography by Willem Einthoven (1860–1927)
1902	Introduction of the Midwives Act in the UK to regulate the training and to supervise the practice of midwives
1906	Food and Drug Act, USA, replaced by a new Act in 1938, which led shortly after the Second World War to the Food and Drug Administration (FDA) of the USA
1906–12	Work by Frederick Gowland Hopkins (1861–1947) on 'accessory food factors' and by Christiaan Eijkman of Denmark (1858–1930) leads to the discovery of vitamins
1911	Introduction of National Health Insurance in the UK
1913	Formation of the Medical Research Committee in England
1918–19	Pandemic of influenza which probably killed more people in the course of two years than any epidemic at any time before or since
1920	Medical Research Committee in England reconstituted as the Medical Research Council
1922–3	Discovery of insulin by Frederick Banting (1891–1941) and Charles Best (1899–1978)
1926	Discovery by George Minot (1885–1950) and William Murphy (1892–1987) that pernicious anaemia can be cured by eating large amounts of raw liver, which leads to treatment first by

	liver extract and in 1949 by the active agent, vitamin B_{12} or cobalamin
1928	Alexander Fleming (1881–1955) discovers that a mould of the genus Penicillium produces an antibacterial agent, penicillin
1929	Foundation of the Royal College of Obstetricians and Gynaecologists
1931	'Lübeck disaster', when live tuberculosis bacilli contaminated some batches of BCG (used for vaccination against tuberculosis) causing many deaths in children
1932	Gerhard Domagk (1895–1964) discovers that a dye called Prontosil Red destroys haemolytic streptococcal infection in mice, which leads to the development of the sulphonamides, the first of the antibacterial chemotherapeutic agents or antibiotics
1932	Vitamin C, lack of which causes scurvy, is isolated and its chemical structure identified
1933	First isolation of the causative virus of influenza
1936–7	First major and highly successful clinical trial of the sulphonamides by Leonard Colebrook (1883–1967) in cases of puerperal fever in Queen Charlotte's Hospital, London
1938	Howard Florey (1898–1968), Ernst B. Chain (1906–79), and Norman Heatley (b. 1911) begin work on penicillin which leads to its first successful trials on humans in 1940–1 and its subsequent large-scale use by the mid-1940s
1939–45	The Second World War. The urgencies of war lead to various medical advances, such as improvements in plastic surgery and the treatment of wounds, anaesthesia, and the widespread availability of blood transfusion to civilians as well as the armed services
1941	Roosevelt creates the Committee on Medical Research in the USA
1942	Beveridge Report
1944	Discovery of streptomycin by Selman Waksman (1888–1973) in the USA, the first antibiotic which was effective against tuberculosis
1945–85	'Therapeutic Revolution', which consisted of the introduction of a very wide range of effective drugs including numerous antibiotics, antihistamines, anticoagulants, antihypertensives, new anaesthetic agents, drugs for the treatment of depression, mania, and schizophrenia, sedatives, agents for the treatment of a wide range of malignant diseases, drug treatment for peptic ulcer, for Parkinsonism, and for certain viral infections, and the contraceptive pill
1946	Introduction of the National Institutes of Health in the USA
1946	First randomized trial carried out in the UK by Austin Bradford Hill to determine the effectiveness of streptomycin
1948	Establishment of the World Health Organization as a special agency of the United Nations
1950s	Introduction of hip replacement as a routine operation by Sir John Charnley
1952	Foundation of the Royal College of General Practitioners
1953	Development of the heart–lung machine, an essential prerequisite for cardiac surgery

| 1953 | J. D. Watson and F. Crick describe the structure of DNA | Chronology |

1953   J. D. Watson and F. Crick describe the structure of DNA

1960s   Beginnings of cardiac-bypass surgery for coronary artery disease

1961   Discovery that thalidomide taken in pregnancy can cause severe deformities in babies ushers in a new era of concern over the safety of medicines

1964   Declaration of Helsinki is a landmark in medical ethics

1967   Cicely Saunders opens a hospice in south London for the palliative care of the terminally ill, thereby initiating the hospice movement

1967   First successful heart transplant by Christiaan Barnard in South Africa

1974   First major reorganization of the National Health Service in the UK

1975   Ivan Illich publishes *Medical Nemesis*, an attack on the established views and values of orthodox medicine

1979   Smallpox eradicated from the world

1980   Introduction of endoscopic, 'minimally invasive', or 'keyhole' surgery

1980s–1990s Beginnings of the rapid growth of medical genetics and molecular medicine

1981   Recognition of AIDS as a new disease

early 1990s Establishment of a university chair in alternative medicine in London and an office of alternative medicine in the USA at the National Institutes of Health

GLOSSARY

accoucheurs a term of French origin introduced in the eighteenth century by British obstetricians to describe themselves in preference to 'men-midwives' (*q.v.*)

anal fistula *see* fistula-in-ano

antisepsis and **asepsis** antisepsis consists of using chemical antiseptics to kill bacteria that are already present on the skin of the patient or elsewhere during a surgical operation or an obstetric delivery. Asepsis consists of the use of heat, or chemicals, or radiation, to sterilize syringes and needles, surgical gloves and instruments, gowns, dressings and drapes, and so on. Surgical antisepsis was introduced in 1865 by Joseph (Lord) Lister and asepsis followed soon after

aphasia loss of, or defect in, the power of speech

apothecaries in England the apothecaries separated themselves from the Company of Grocers and established the Society of Apothecaries in 1615. The role of the apothecaries was to make up medicines from prescriptions written by physicians. From the seventeenth century, however, they tended more and more to treat patients directly, both by providing them with medicines in their shops and by visiting them in their homes, thereby acting in effect as general practitioners (*see* surgeon-apothecaries)

barber-surgeons barbers and surgeons can be identified as craftsmen from the classical period onwards. From at least the fourteenth century, they were organized in guilds in major European towns, but they were amongst the most widely dispersed of occupations, and barbers were found even in villages. Before the decline of the guild structure and the general transfer to university-based training in surgery in the eighteenth century, there was no strict distinction between barbers and surgeons in institutional terms. However, it was usual in cities to find small élite groups of surgeons at one end of the spectrum, and, at the other, humble practitioners who were clearly barbers rather than barber-surgeons

Black Death this term was first introduced into medical literature by Babington's translation of Hecker's *Der Schwarze Tod* in 1833, since when it has been the name given to the outbreak of plague which wiped out a huge proportion of the population in Europe in the mid-fourteenth century. It is occasionally used more broadly as the name for later epidemics of plague as well as the mid-fourteenth-century epidemic (*see* plague)

CAT scan CAT (Computerized Axial Tomography) is a radiological technique in which an X-ray image of a cross-section of the body or head at any particular depth is reconstructed electronically and displayed on a computer screen

cataract, couching for cataract, which is loss of vision due to opacities in the lens of the eye, was treated in the past by 'couching', which consisted of removal or displacement of the lens

childbed fever *see* puerperal fever

China root the root of China smilax, which came from America and was introduced as a drug in Europe in the early sixteenth century

chlorosis or **'Green Sickness'** known since the sixteenth century as a disease of young women (and more especially as a disease of virgins) characterized by amenorrhoea, nervous behaviour, and appetite disturbance, and 'cured' by sexual intercourse and marriage. According to a recent view, it was a disorder closely similar to anorexia nervosa and was known as Green Sickness because the word 'green' referred to the innocence of youth. But the traditional view, dating from the mid-nineteenth century, is that it was a form of anaemia, common in young women, especially servants and other members of the working class, which was accompanied by a green tinge of the skin; it disappeared in the 1920s

cholera a disease due to the micro-organism *Vibrio cholera*, which causes profuse watery diarrhoea and death by dehydration. There were famous epidemics in Britain of what was then known as 'Asiatic Cholera' in 1830, 1847, 1853, and the 1860s. It is still a common disease in the developing world

cinchona, Jesuit's bark, Peruvian bark the active ingredient of this substance, which was brought from Peru to England in the seventeenth century, probably by Jesuit missionaries, was quinine, which is active against malaria (*see* malaria)

consumption the word indicates loss of weight and wasting, but it was widely used for what later became known as pulmonary tuberculosis or TB

couching *see* cataract

dispensary the term had two meanings: (1) a room in which medicines were made up and 'dispensed'; (2) a type of medical institution, first established in the mid-eighteenth century, similar to the voluntary hospitals (*q.v.*) except for the absence of in-patient beds. Physicians and surgeons saw outpatients at the dispensary or, in response to requests for a home visit, they attended the sick poor in their homes

doxographer a writer who collected and recorded the opinions of the ancient Greek philosophers

ECT (electroconvulsive therapy) consists of passing an electric current through the brain to induce a generalized epileptiform convulsion. It is usually performed under light anaesthesia and a muscle relaxant. It was introduced as a therapy for various forms of psychiatric illness in the 1930s, but its main use in the second half of the twentieth century has been for the treatment of severe depression

empirics another name for irregular practitioners or quacks (*q.v.*)

fistula-in-ano an infection of the rectum leading to a channel or fistula from the inside of the rectum to an opening through the skin in the peri-anal region. It appears to have been common in the medieval period, but this may be an illusion due to the fact that, when surgical operations were few, the surgical treatment of fistula was one of the standard procedures

French pox see *morbus gallicus*

hospice historically, this usually applied to pre-eighteenth-century institutions established to care for the poor, the disabled, and the old, and only incidentally and occasionally for the sick. During the thirteenth and fourteenth centuries a few hospices in Europe began to become hospitals in the modern sense by devoting themselves largely or solely to treating the sick. The term has recently been revived in the UK to describe institutions which provide palliative care for dying patients—a form of care pioneered by Dame Cicely Saunders

hospitalism a term coined by Joseph (Lord) Lister in the mid-nineteenth century to describe diseases due to, or exacerbated by, admission to hospitals

hydrotherapy the use of water, mainly cold water, in the treatment of diseases, which became popular in the eighteenth century, and is still much used on the Continent

iatrogenic disease literally 'disease caused by doctors', it consists of diseases induced by the use or misuse of medical or surgical treatments, including, for instance, side effects of prescribed drugs

infant mortality the death of children in the first year of life expressed numerically as the number of deaths under the age of 1 per 1,000 live births. Death in the first month is called 'neonatal mortality' (and death in the first week as 'early neonatal mortality'); death between the end of the first month and the end of the first year is called post-neonatal mortality

infirmary a synonym for 'hospital'. There has never been a distinction between the two in terms of stucture, organization, or function

intermittent fever a term used in the past to cover several infectious diseases, including malaria. The success of 'the bark' (*see* cinchona) in treating malaria led to its wide use in the treatment of intermittent fevers in particular and fevers in general

itch, the scabies

Jesuit's bark *see* cinchona

lock hospitals lock hospitals were used for the treatment of venereal disease. The origin of the word 'lock' in this context is obscure, but it is possible that lock hospitals evolved from hospitals for leprosy, and that 'lock' is a corruption of 'leper'

lues venerea syphilis (see *morbus gallicus*)

malaria an illness that derives its name from the old belief that it was due to 'bad air' especially in damp marshy ground. It is due to infection with protozoa of the genus *Plasmodium*, transmitted by the bites of mosquitoes of the genus *Anopheles*. There are three main forms: tertian malaria due to *Plasmodium vivax*, quartan malaria due to *Plasmodium malariae*, and the dangerous malignant tertian form due to *Plasmodium falciparum*

materia medica the branch of medicine dealing with drugs, and especially with their source and preparation, and their uses. The term is obsolete, the modern equivalent being pharmacology

maternal mortality deaths of women during pregnancy, labour, or the postnatal period, which is commonly the first six weeks after delivery. The maternal mortality rate (or more strictly the maternal mortality *ratio*) was calculated as the number of maternal deaths per 1,000 or 10,000 births in the past, but today, when maternal deaths have become rare, as maternal deaths per 100,000 births

melancholia a term commonly used for what would now be called depression

men-midwives when medical men started to undertake the practice of midwifery or obstetrics (the terms are synonymous) in the eighteenth century, they were often referred to, with more than a touch of scorn, as 'men-midwives'. Most British obstetricians, however, preferred the more elegant French usage of *accoucheurs*. Although the terms 'obstetrics' and 'obstetricians' can be found in the eighteenth century, they came into general use only in the nineteenth century

miasmas vapours arising from the air, the soil, drains, sewers, or diseased bodies which, it was believed, could cause disease. Miasmas were described as being invisible, inodorous, and capable of clinging to the body or to clothes

morbus gallicus the French pox. An early name for syphilis, probably due to the fact that some of the earliest descriptions of the disease came from France. Understandably it was not a term favoured in France, where it was usually called the *lues venerea* or even the *lues hispanica*, blaming the Spanish

mountebank an irregular practitioner or quack (*q.v.*), so named because he advertised his wares while mounted on a high place or platform

National Health Insurance introduced in 1911, and sometimes known as the Lloyd George Act, this was a health insurance scheme in the UK which paid workers below a certain wage level, both sickness benefit and the cost of treatment by general practitioners. A list or 'panel' of general practitioners who were willing to accept National Health Insurance patients was published: hence the terms 'panel doctor', 'panel patients', and 'being on the panel' for being off work through sickness. National Health Insurance did not cover the dependants of workers

neonatal mortality *see* infant mortality

nosology the study of the nomenclature and classification of diseases

phthisis like consumption (*q.v.*), this means a wasting-away of the body, and was used as a synonym for pulmonary tuberculosis or TB

physicians the hallmark of the physician was the possession of a university degree in medicine, usually an MD. Physicians undertook the diagnosis and treatment of medical disorders by listening to the patient's story, and by inspection of the patient and the patient's urine and faeces. The routine of physical examination was not introduced until the nineteenth century. Physicians undertook no manual activities (which distinguished them from surgeons), and they prescribed but never dispensed medicines (dispensing medicines was the role of the apothecaries). The Royal College of Physicians of London, founded in 1518, claimed a monopoly of treating the sick in London and a seven-mile radius around

plague a disease of rodents caused by the bacillus *Yersinia pestis* which can spread to human populations, chiefly by means of the oriental flea from an infected black rat, *Rattus rattus*. It usually occurred in the bubonic form (a 'bubo' is a swollen lymph gland, especially in the groin or armpit) but could also occur in the pneumonic form (which was contagious and could be transmitted directly from human to human) and the septicaemic form (*see* Black Death)

post-neonatal mortality *see* infant mortality

puerperal fever (also known as 'childbed fever') is an infection of the genital tract in women who have just had a baby. Most of the severe and fatal cases in the past were due to infection with *Streptococcus pyogenes*, which was usually introduced by the hands or instruments of the birth attendant. Until the introduction of the sulphonamides in the mid-1930s, it was by far the most common cause of maternal mortality

quack an irregular practitioner, an empiric, or an impostor. The origin of the term is obscure. It has been suggested that it may be derived from 'quacksalver' as a corruption of 'quicksilver' or mercury (used in the treatment of syphilis); or because the irregulars 'quacked' their salves (a 'salve' was an ointment) like noisy ducks. Neither suggestion is wholly convincing

quicksilver mercury, which was used for the treatment of syphilis, either by mouth or by inunction, when mercury was incorporated in an ointment and rubbed into the skin

quinine *see* cinchona

schistosomiasis a tropical disease due to the penetration of human skin by larval forms of worms of the genus *Schistosoma*. The disease is carried by certain freshwater snails which produce the larval forms which infect man, and the larvae and their eggs can cause long-term damage to the liver and the urinary system. Deaths from the disease are not common, but it was estimated in the 1980s that about 200 million people in Asia, Africa, the Caribbean, and South America are infected with this disease

smallpox or **variola** a deadly and disfiguring virus disease now eliminated from the world. It acquired the name smallpox in the early sixteenth century to distinguish it from the 'Great Pox', which was yet another synonym for syphilis (*q.v.*)

smallpox inoculation in the eighteenth century smallpox inoculation (as opposed to smallpox vaccination) consisted of taking fluid from the vesicles (blisters) in a case of smallpox and injecting the fluid into the arm of a healthy individual. The aim of this process, which was known as variolation, was to produce a mild attack of the disease which conferred immunity. It was first introduced into England from the Middle East *c.*1720 by Lady Mary Wortley Montagu (1689–1762). It is debatable whether the risk of smallpox inoculation was less than the risk of exposure to the disease, but most historians believe it was, at least to a limited extent, beneficial. It must not be confused with smallpox vaccination (*q.v.*), which superseded inoculation at the end of the eighteenth and beginning of the nineteenth century

sphygmomanometer an instrument for measuring blood pressure. The modern form of the instrument, preceded in the 1870s by the sphygmograph, was introduced in 1896 by an Italian physician, Scipione Rive-Rocci

syphilis or **the great pox** see *morbus gallicus*

surgeon-apothecaries in the early eighteenth century rank-and-file medical practitioners, who had previously been known as 'apothecaries' or 'barber-surgeons', began to call themselves 'surgeon-apothecaries' to emphasize that they were willing and able to practise all of the three main branches of medicine: physic, surgery, and pharmacy. The surgeon-apothecaries were the direct precursors of the general practitioners, the latter term first coming into use in the second decade of the nineteenth century

surgery and **surgeons** surgery was described in the eighteenth century as the branch of medicine which dealt with external diseases and disorders requiring manual activities such as manipulation or operation. In England the surgeons formally separated themselves from the barber-surgeons (*q.v.*) by forming the Company of Surgeons in 1745. The Royal College of Surgeons of London was founded in 1800 and by royal charter became the Royal College of Surgeons of England in 1843. The rise in the status of surgeons was closely associated with the foundation of the voluntary hospitals (*q.v.*)

uroscopy in the past, physicians believed they could tell a great deal about diseases by inspecting a patient's urine in a flask held up to the light

vaccination the therapeutic prevention of certain infectious diseases by the process of injecting micro-organisms, either killed, or living but modified to reduce pathogenicity, to stimulate the production of antibodies and provide protection against a disease. In smallpox vaccination, introduced by Edward Jenner (1749–1823) in 1796, fluid from the vesicles of cowpox, closely related to smallpox, was scratched into the surface of the skin, a process described as scarification (*see* smallpox inoculation)

variolation *see* smallpox inoculation

venesection the opening of a vein, usually in the arm, for the purpose of bloodletting

voluntary hospitals in contrast to continental Europe, where most hospitals were funded by the state or local government, most of the hospitals, including all the teaching hospitals founded in the UK and North America in the eighteenth and nineteenth centuries, were charitable institutions funded by the voluntary contributions from the public. The medical staff at these hospitals, the 'honorary' physicians and surgeons, gave their services free or were paid only a nominal sum

ILLUSTRATION SOURCES

The editor and publishers wish to thank the following who have kindly given permission to reproduce the illustrations on the following pages:

INDEX

Note: Page numbers in *italic* indicate references to black and white illustrations and page numbers in **bold** refer to the colour illustrations.

Abel-Smith, Brian 287
abortion 128
abuse 175
academic/popular medicine 61–4
accidents 123
accoucheurs 209–11
acetylcholine 117
action portraits 19–21
acupuncture 124, 139, *261*, 263
administrators, hospital 167–9
adrenaline 113, 117
advertisements 84, 86, 292–3
Africa:
   epidemics in 176, 180–2
   spread of Western medicine 251, 253–6,
     258, 261–2
age of hospital patients 165, 170
ageing population 132, 184, 205, 287
AIDS (acquired immune deficiency syndrome)
     10, 124, *136*, 139–40, *141*, 142, 175–6, 184,
     187, 191
Aiguillon, Duchesse d' 196
al-Antaki, Da'ud 51
al-Ghafiqi, Ahmad *48*
al-Husayni, Muzaffar ibn Muhammad 53
al-Qayrawan Hospital, Tunisia 50
al-Rashid, Harun 50
albarello 18, *49*
Alberti, Leon Battista 78
Albinus *6, 12*
Albucasis **33**, 46, 58, *60*, 63
alchemy 77
Alcmaeon of Croton 29–30
alcohol dependency 135, 175
Alderotti, Taddeo 58
Alexandria, medical science in 33, 36–7
allergies 111
Allgemeines Krankenhaus, Vienna 161
Alonso de Sedano **96**
Alpago, Andrea 45, 47
alternative medicine 80, 138–9, 255, 263, 272,
     275–6, 292
American Federation of Labor 285
American Indians 81, 177, 180–1, 251
American Medical Association 156, 284, 286
amino acids 118
amputation 88
anaemia 118, 120, 126
anaesthetics *96*, 111–12, 126–7, 129–30, *175*,
     213–15, 217, 219, 299–300
anaphylaxis 111

anatomy:
   childbirth 209, 211
   classical medicine 35–9
   Islamic medicine 44, 47, 52
   medical education and 153
   Middle Ages 63, *64*
   Renaissance 75–6, *78*
   scientific revolution 84–6, 93–4, *97*
   teaching of 147–9
   visual representation 1, 3–4, 12, *13*, 15, 17
   Western medicine 254, *261*
Anatomy Act (UK) 94
Anaximander 30–1
Anaximenes 32
Anderson, Elizabeth Garrett 213
antenatal clinics 216
Anthony, St 1
anthrax 103
anti-cancer drugs 131–2, 144
anti-coagulants 121, 127
anti-depressants 247
anti-hypertensives 127
anti-Semitism 74
anti-vivisection 90, 96, 100, 113
antibiotics 118, 121, 123–4, 126–8, 133, 144,
     183–4, 303
antihistamines 126–7
antisepsis 111–12, 120, 213, 215–17, 219, 299
antitoxins 103–5, 109–12, 113–14, 117
aphasia 245
apothecaries 18, 62–3, 68–9, 73, 81–2, 86, 90–1,
     149, 209, 266, 268, 272, 292
Apothecaries Act (UK) 91
appendectomy 112
apprentice:
   midwives 73, 208–10, 274
   physician 73, 270
   as servants *149*, 150
   student 152
   surgeon 153
Arabic texts **33**, 40–1, 43–9, 51–3, 56, 58–9, **65**,
     71, 74
Archagathus 38
architecture:
   of body *6, 12*
   of hospitals *161, 167, 175*
Aristotle *14,* 34–5, 39, 43, 58–9, 79
Armstrong, George 221, 222
Army Medical Service 200
Arnau de Vilanova 58
aromatherapy 139

331

women:
  healers 62, 68
  health care and 271–4
  itinerant 84
  liberation movement 128
  physicians 73, 80, 92, 150, 154–7, *172*, 256
  portraiture 20
  protest groups 284
  in research 107
  rights 90
Women's College, New York Infirmary 155
Women's Hospital Medical College, Chicago
  155
Women's Medical College of Philadelphia 155
woodcuts *8*, 78, 84
workhouses 163, 165, 212, *213*, 241
World Health Organization 115, 142–3, 183,
  187, *189*, 259
Wortley Montagu, Lady Mary 53, 89

wounds 33, 114, 121
'wound man' 3
Würzburg University 170
Wyndham, John 291

X-rays 9, *10*, 11, 17, 102, 109, 112, 161, *230*

yaws 180
yellow fever 115, 142, 177–8, 180, 182, 251,
  258, 259, 261–2
York Retreat 93, 236, *237*, 248, 298
Youville, Marguerite d' 196
Yunani medical colleges 53

Zhdanov, Victor 143
zodiacman *63*
Zurich University 155

Index compiled by Judi Barstow